Clinical Obstetrics
A Case-based Approach

Editors

Pushpa Mishra
Senior Medical Officer
Department of Obstetrics and Gynecology
Maulana Azad Medical College and
Lok Nayak Hospital
New Delhi, India

Niharika Dhiman
Assistant Professor
Department of Obstetrics and Gynecology
Maulana Azad Medical College and
Lok Nayak Hospital
New Delhi, India

Anjali Tempe
Director Professor and Head
Department of Obstetrics and Gynecology & IVF Center
Maulana Azad Medical College and
Lok Nayak Hospital
New Delhi, India

Foreword
Siddarth Ramji

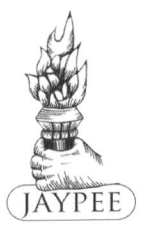

JAYPEE The Health Sciences Publisher
New Delhi | London | Panama

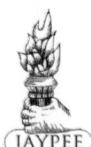 **Jaypee Brothers Medical Publishers (P) Ltd**

Headquarters

Jaypee Brothers Medical Publishers (P) Ltd
4838/24, Ansari Road, Daryaganj
New Delhi 110 002, India
Phone: +91-11-43574357
Fax: +91-11-43574314
Email: jaypee@jaypeebrothers.com

Overseas Offices

J.P. Medical Ltd
83 Victoria Street, London
SW1H 0HW (UK)
Phone: +44 20 3170 8910
Fax: +44 (0)20 3008 6180
Email: info@jpmedpub.com

Jaypee Brothers Medical Publishers (P) Ltd
17/1-B Babar Road, Block-B, Shaymali
Mohammadpur, Dhaka-1207
Bangladesh
Mobile: +08801912003485
Email: jaypeedhaka@gmail.com

Jaypee-Highlights Medical Publishers Inc
City of Knowledge, Bld. 235, 2nd Floor, Clayton
Panama City, Panama
Phone: +1 507-301-0496
Fax: +1 507-301-0499
Email: cservice@jphmedical.com

Jaypee Brothers Medical Publishers (P) Ltd
Bhotahity, Kathmandu
Nepal
Phone: +977-9741283608
Email: kathmandu@jaypeebrothers.com

Website: www.jaypeebrothers.com
Website: www.jaypeedigital.com

© 2018, Jaypee Brothers Medical Publishers

The views and opinions expressed in this book are solely those of the original contributor(s)/author(s) and do not necessarily represent those of editor(s) of the book.

All rights reserved. No part of this publication and DVD-ROM may be reproduced, stored or transmitted in any form or by any means, electronic, mechanical, photocopying, recording or otherwise, without the prior permission in writing of the publishers.

All brand names and product names used in this book are trade names, service marks, trademarks or registered trademarks of their respective owners. The publisher is not associated with any product or vendor mentioned in this book.

Medical knowledge and practice change constantly. This book is designed to provide accurate, authoritative information about the subject matter in question. However, readers are advised to check the most current information available on procedures included and check information from the manufacturer of each product to be administered, to verify the recommended dose, formula, method and duration of administration, adverse effects and contraindications. It is the responsibility of the practitioner to take all appropriate safety precautions. Neither the publisher nor the author(s)/editor(s) assume any liability for any injury and/or damage to persons or property arising from or related to use of material in this book.

This book is sold on the understanding that the publisher is not engaged in providing professional medical services. If such advice or services are required, the services of a competent medical professional should be sought.

Every effort has been made where necessary to contact holders of copyright to obtain permission to reproduce copyright material. If any have been inadvertently overlooked, the publisher will be pleased to make the necessary arrangements at the first opportunity. The **CD/DVD-ROM** (if any) provided in the sealed envelope with this book is complimentary and free of cost. **Not meant for sale**.

Inquiries for bulk sales may be solicited at: jaypee@jaypeebrothers.com

Clinical Obstetrics: A Case-based Approach

First Edition: **2018**

ISBN: 978-93-5270-274-9

Printed at: Paras Offset Pvt. Ltd., New Delhi

Dedicated to

*All our students
past, present and future*

Contributors

Aastha Raheja
Resident
Department of Obstetrics and Gynecology
Maulana Azad Medical College and
Lok Nayak Hospital
New Delhi, India

Anjali Tempe
Director Professor and Head
Department of Obstetrics and
Gynecology & IVF Center
Maulana Azad Medical College and
Lok Nayak Hospital
New Delhi, India

Anubhuti Rana
Senior Resident
Department of Obstetrics and Gynecology
Maulana Azad Medical College and
Lok Nayak Hospital
New Delhi, India

Aparna Setia
Resident
Department of Obstetrics and Gynecology
Maulana Azad Medical College and
Lok Nayak Hospital
New Delhi, India

Ashish Jain
Assistant Professor
Department of Neonatology
Maulana Azad Medical College and
Lok Nayak Hospital
New Delhi, India

Ashok Kumar
Director Professor
Department of Obstetrics and Gynecology
Maulana Azad Medical College and
Lok Nayak Hospital
New Delhi, India

Asmita Muthal Rathore
Director Professor
Department of Obstetrics and Gynecology
Maulana Azad Medical College and
Lok Nayak Hospital
New Delhi, India

Bidisha Singha
Specialist
Department of Obstetrics and Gynecology
Maulana Azad Medical College and
Lok Nayak Hospital
New Delhi, India

Chetna Arvind Sethi
Specialist
Department of Obstetrics and Gynecology
Maulana Azad Medical College and
Lok Nayak Hospital
New Delhi, India

Chinmoyee Sonowal
Resident
Department of Obstetrics and Gynecology
Maulana Azad Medical College and
Lok Nayak Hospital
New Delhi, India

Deepali Dhingra
Fellow of National Board of Examinations
(Reproductive Medicine)
Department of Obstetrics and Gynecology
Maulana Azad Medical College and
Lok Nayak Hospital
New Delhi, India

Deepti Goswami
Director Professor
Department of Obstetrics and Gynecology
Maulana Azad Medical College and
Lok Nayak Hospital
New Delhi, India

Devender Verma
Professor
Department of Obstetrics and Gynecology
Maulana Azad Medical College and Lok Nayak Hospital
New Delhi, India

Divya Arora
Resident
Department of Obstetrics and Gynecology
Maulana Azad Medical College and Lok Nayak Hospital
New Delhi, India

Divya Singh
Resident
Department of Obstetrics and Gynecology
Maulana Azad Medical College and
Lok Nayak Hospital
New Delhi, India

Gazala Shahnaz
Fellow of National Board of Examinations
(High-Risk Pregnancy)
Department of Obstetrics and Gynecology
Maulana Azad Medical College and
Lok Nayak Hospital
New Delhi, India

Gauri Gandhi
Director Professor
Department of Obstetrics and Gynecology
Maulana Azad Medical College and
Lok Nayak Hospital
New Delhi, India

Kashika Kathuria
Fellow of National Board of Examinations
(Reproductive Medicine)
Department of Obstetrics and Gynecology
Maulana Azad Medical College and
Lok Nayak Hospital
New Delhi, India

Komal Rastogi
Senior Resident
Department of Obstetrics and Gynecology
Maulana Azad Medical College and
Lok Nayak Hospital
New Delhi, India

Krishna Agarwal
Professor
Department of Obstetrics and Gynecology
Maulana Azad Medical College and
Lok Nayak Hospital
New Delhi, India

Latika Sahu
Professor
Department of Obstetrics and Gynecology
Maulana Azad Medical College and
Lok Nayak Hospital
New Delhi, India

Madhavi M Gupta
Professor
Department of Obstetrics and Gynecology
Maulana Azad Medical College and
Lok Nayak Hospital
New Delhi, India

Meenakshi Goel
Senior Resident
Department of Obstetrics and Gynecology
Maulana Azad Medical College and
Lok Nayak Hospital
New Delhi, India

Neelam Yadav
Senior Resident
Department of Obstetrics and Gynecology
Maulana Azad Medical College and
Lok Nayak Hospital
New Delhi, India

Niharika Dhiman
Assistant Professor
Department of Obstetrics and Gynecology
Maulana Azad Medical College and
Lok Nayak Hospital
New Delhi, India

Nilanchali Singh
Assistant Professor
Department of Obstetrics and Gynecology
Maulana Azad Medical College and
Lok Nayak Hospital
New Delhi, India

Nupur Ahuja
Senior Resident
Department of Obstetrics and Gynecology
Maulana Azad Medical College and
Lok Nayak Hospital
New Delhi, India

Nuzhat Zaman
Resident
Department of Obstetrics and Gynecology
Maulana Azad Medical College and
Lok Nayak Hospital
New Delhi, India

Pallavi Sharma
Senior Resident
Department of Obstetrics and Gynecology
Maulana Azad Medical College and
Lok Nayak Hospital
New Delhi, India

Poonam Kashyap
Specialist
Department of Obstetrics and Gynecology
Maulana Azad Medical College and
Lok Nayak Hospital
New Delhi, India

Poonam Sachdeva
Senior Specialist
Department of Obstetrics and Gynecology
Maulana Azad Medical College and
Lok Nayak Hospital
New Delhi, India

Preeti Singh
Associate Professor
Department of Obstetrics and Gynecology
Maulana Azad Medical College and
Lok Nayak Hospital
New Delhi, India

Priyanka Chaudhary
Senior Resident
Department of Obstetrics and Gynecology
Maulana Azad Medical College and
Lok Nayak Hospital
New Delhi, India

Priyanka Khandey
Senior Resident
Department of Obstetrics and Gynecology
Maulana Azad Medical College and Lok Nayak Hospital
New Delhi, India

Pushpa Mishra
Senior Medical Officer
Department of Obstetrics and Gynecology
Maulana Azad Medical College and
Lok Nayak Hospital
New Delhi, India

Rachna Sharma
Senior Specialist
Department of Obstetrics and Gynecology
Maulana Azad Medical College and
Lok Nayak Hospital
New Delhi, India

Renu Tanwar
Professor
Department of Obstetrics and Gynecology
Maulana Azad Medical College and
Lok Nayak Hospital
New Delhi, India

Ruchi Gupta
Fellow of National Board of Examinations
(High-Risk Pregnancy)
Department of Obstetrics and Gynecology
Maulana Azad Medical College and
Lok Nayak Hospital
New Delhi, India

Sangeeta Bhasin
Chief Medical Officer (NFSG)
Department of Obstetrics and Gynecology
Maulana Azad Medical College and
Lok Nayak Hospital
New Delhi, India

Sangeeta Gupta
Director Professor
Department of Obstetrics and Gynecology
Maulana Azad Medical College and
Lok Nayak Hospital
New Delhi, India

Shakun Tyagi
Associate Professor
Department of Obstetrics and Gynecology
Maulana Azad Medical College and
Lok Nayak Hospital
New Delhi, India

Shristi
Resident
Department of Obstetrics and Gynecology
Maulana Azad Medical College and
Lok Nayak Hospital
New Delhi, India

Simar Kaur
Fellow of National Board of Examinations
(High-Risk Pregnancy)
Department of Obstetrics and Gynecology
Maulana Azad Medical College and
Lok Nayak Hospital
New Delhi, India

Sneha Sharma
Senior Resident
Department of Obstetrics and Gynecology
Maulana Azad Medical College and
Lok Nayak Hospital
New Delhi, India

Snigdha Pathak
Senior Resident
Department of Obstetrics and Gynecology
Maulana Azad Medical College and
Lok Nayak Hospital
New Delhi, India

Sparsha
Resident
Department of Obstetrics and Gynecology
Maulana Azad Medical College and
Lok Nayak Hospital
New Delhi, India

Sudha Prasad
Director Professor and IVF Coordinator
Department of Obstetrics and Gynecology
Maulana Azad Medical College and
Lok Nayak Hospital
New Delhi, India

Tarang Preet Kaur
Resident
Department of Obstetrics and Gynecology
Maulana Azad Medical College and
Lok Nayak Hospital
New Delhi, India

Vandana Sehrawat
Senior Resident
Department of Obstetrics and Gynecology
Maulana Azad Medical College and
Lok Nayak Hospital
New Delhi, India

Foreword

The idea of a book which captures the essentials of the postgraduate course in obstetrics and gynecology is a welcome one. The case presentation format will facilitate problem-based learning among the students. This will not only be useful for their examinations, but also subsequently in their clinical practice. This will complement their learning from direct observations of patients in the clinical setting.

Siddarth Ramji
Director Professor and Dean
Maulana Azad Medical College
New Delhi, India

Preface

The Department of Obstetrics and Gynecology and faculty of Maulana Azad Medical College has been instrumental in writing various books on different aspects of obstetrics and gynecology in last 20 years. Our books have been received by the students with great excitement and enthusiasm. It has been our practice to choose relevant topics for discussion which are useful to undergraduates and postgraduates of obstetrics and gynecology.

In this book, it is our endeavor to deal with clinical aspects of obstetrics, mainly the case discussion in high-risk pregnancy and medical disorders associated with pregnancy. There are many books on obstetrics in the market but this book is written with the view of making all obstetric cases simple in diagnosis and management for the young obstetricians. This book also covers other practical aspects which deal with specimens, instruments, drugs and viva voce.

The DVD-ROM which has been enclosed includes the obstetric examination of the pregnant patient and basic obstetric procedures. We hope that this will be useful to all postgraduates and undergraduates for their examinations as well as to the young practicing obstetricians.

Pushpa Mishra
Niharika Dhiman
Anjali Tempe

Preface

Contents

Chapter 1. **Anemia in Pregnancy** — 1
Ashok Kumar, Ruchi Gupta, Divya Arora

Chapter 2. **Hypertension in Pregnancy** — 15
Anjali Tempe, Komal Rastogi

Chapter 3. **Diabetes in Pregnancy** — 25
Krishna Agarwal, Aastha Raheja

Chapter 4. **Fetal Growth Restriction** — 33
Simar Kaur, Sangeeta Gupta

Chapter 5. **Multifetal Pregnancy** — 47
Renu Tanwar, Shristi

Chapter 6. **Pregnancy with Intrauterine Demise** — 58
Madhavi M Gupta, Sparsha

Chapter 7. **Rh Negative Pregnancy** — 62
Sudha Prasad, Meenakshi Goel

Chapter 8. **Pregnancy with Previous Cesarean Section** — 72
Bidisha Singha

Chapter 9. **Morbidly Adherent Placenta** — 78
Devender Verma

Chapter 10. **Preterm Labor** — 83
Poonam Sachdeva, Niharika Dhiman, Sneha Sharma

Chapter 11. **Preterm Premature Rupture of Membranes** — 90
Shakun Tyagi, Vandana Sehrawat

Chapter 12. **Pregnancy with Fetal Congenital Anomaly** — 96
Gazala Shahnaz, Asmita Muthal Rathore

Chapter 13. **Recurrent Pregnancy Loss** — 106
Deepali Dhingra, Anjali Tempe, Komal Rastogi

Chapter 14. **Pregnancy in Extremes of Ages** — 111
Komal Rastogi, Niharika Dhiman, Nupur Ahuja, Pushpa Mishra

Chapter 15. **Postdated Pregnancy** — 116
Neelam Yadav, Preeti Singh

Chapter 16.	**Antepartum Hemorrhage**	**121**
	Gauri Gandhi, Snigdha Pathak, Divya Singh	
Chapter 17.	**HIV with Pregnancy**	**132**
	Pushpa Mishra, Priyanka Chaudhary	
Chapter 18.	**Pregnancy with Heart Disease**	**140**
	Chetna Arvind Sethi	
Chapter 19.	**Thyroid Diseases in Pregnancy**	**152**
	Deepti Goswami, Chinmoyee Sonowal	
Chapter 20.	**Neurological Disorder in Pregnancy**	**162**
	Latika Sahu, Tarang Preet Kaur	
Chapter 21.	**Renal Diseases in Pregnancy**	**174**
	Sangeeta Bhasin, Neelam Yadav	
Chapter 22.	**Liver Disorders in Pregnancy**	**182**
	Kashika Kathuria, Anjali Tempe	
Chapter 23.	**Critically Ill Patients**	**194**
	Nilanchali Singh, Priyanka Khandey	
Chapter 24.	**Postnatal and Postoperative Ward Round**	**205**
	Pallavi Sharma, Pushpa Mishra	
Chapter 25.	**Neonatal Resuscitation for an Obstetrician**	**213**
	Ashish Jain	
Chapter 26.	**Postpartum Contraception**	**220**
	Rachna Sharma, Anubhuti Rana	
Chapter 27.	**Surgeries in Obstetrics**	**226**
	Pushpa Mishra, Aparna Setia	
Chapter 28.	**Gynecological Disorders in Pregnancy**	**243**
	Niharika Dhiman	
Chapter 29.	**Miscellaneous**	**253**
	Poonam Kashyap, Nuzhat Zaman	
Chapter 30.	**Common Mistakes in Case Presentation**	**260**
	Nilanchali Singh, Pushpa Mishra	

Appendices *265*

Plate 1

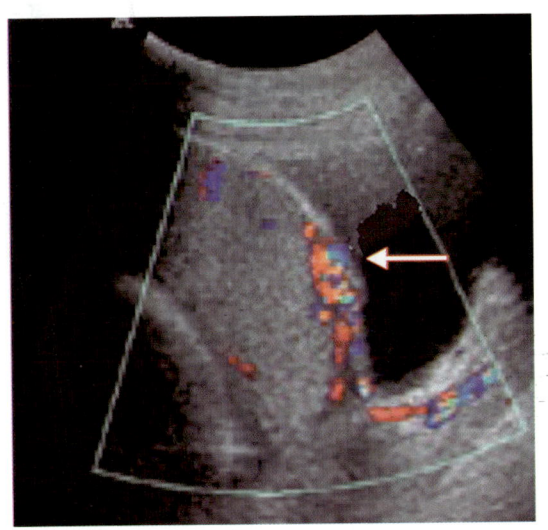

Fig. 9.1: Hypervascularity at bladder and lower segment junction with loss of intervening myometrium (marked with arrow)

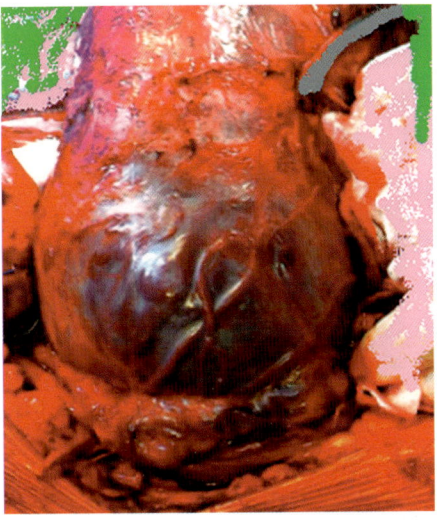

Fig. 9.2: Bulging lower segment of uterus with high vascularity

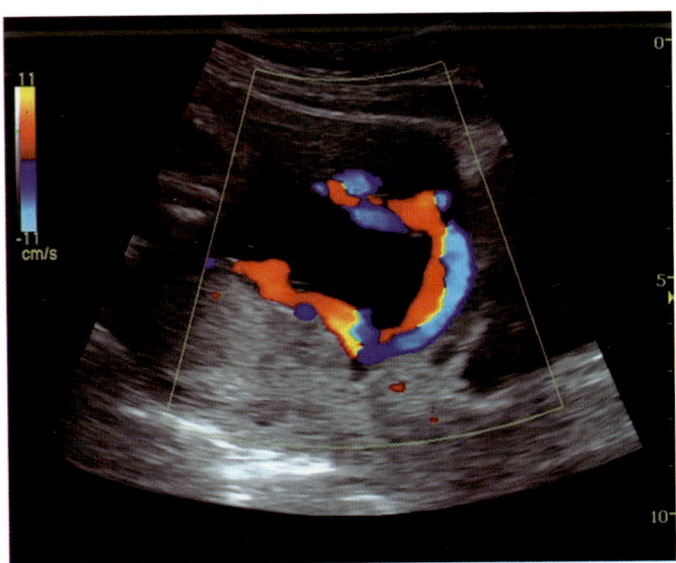

Fig. 29.2: Vasa previa

Plate 2

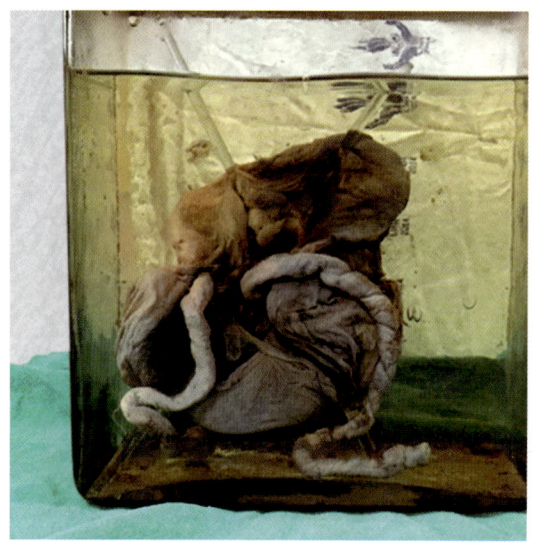

Fig. 29.16: Monochorionic, diamniotic placenta

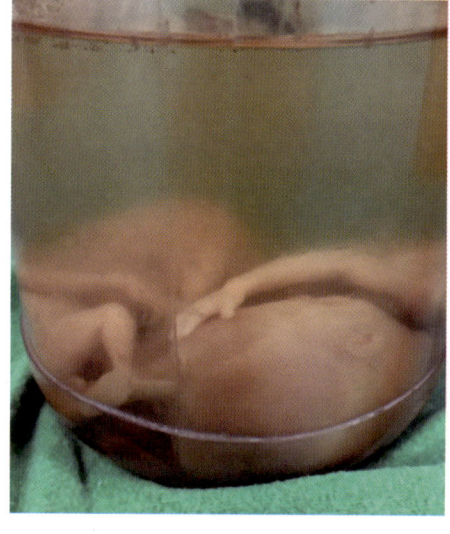

Fig. 29.17: Conjoined twins

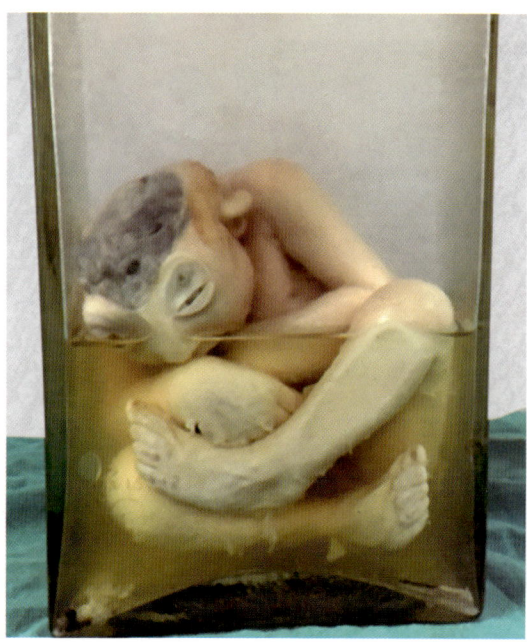

Fig. 29.18: Anencephaly

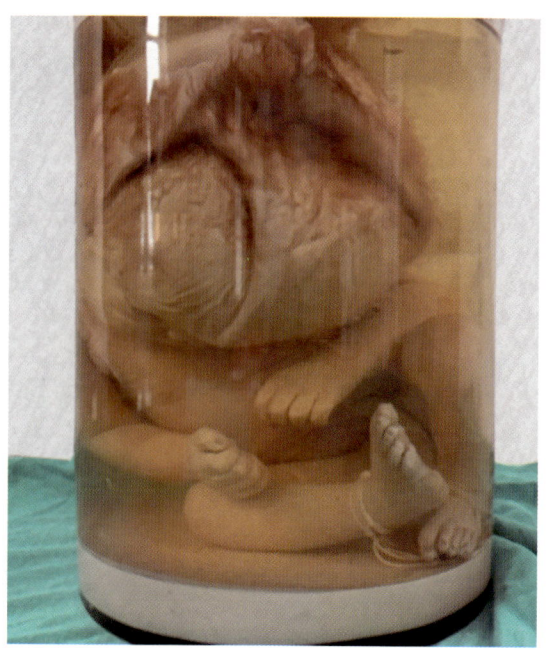

Fig. 29.19: Hydrocephalus

CHAPTER 1

Anemia in Pregnancy

Ashok Kumar, Ruchi Gupta, Divya Arora

CASE SCENARIO

G3P2L1A0 with 8 months amenorrhea with previous two lower segment cesarian section (LSCS) with severe hemoglobin.

A 30 years old, Mrs X, wife of Mr Y resident of Sonipat, Haryana, a housewife, came to gyne casualty on 12/05/2017 with complaints of:
- Amenorrhea 8 months
- Weakness and fatigue since one month
- Breathlessness since 3 days.

Her last menstrual period (LMP) was 13/10/2016 so making her period of gestation 30 weeks and 1 day on 12/05/2017.

History of Present Complaints

- Patient was a booked antenatal case in some private hospital in Sonipat since 4 months amenorrhea.
- She got all her routine antenatal investigations done at 5 months amenorrhea and diagnosed with moderate hemoglobin.
- She was non compliant with oral iron tablets and was transfused 6 doses of iron sucrose and with that her hemoglobin improved.
- Again at 8 month of pregnancy she, became symptomatic and was referred to Lok Nayak Hospital (LNH) in view of severe anemia.

Course in the Hospital

- She was admitted to labor room after her general, physical and abdominal examination.
- Her blood sample [full blood count (FBC), blood group cross match, liver function test, kidney function test, serum electrolytes] was taken and patient was evaluated. She was diagnosed with moderate anemia with microcytic hypochromic picture in peripheral smear.
- She was shifted to clean maternity ward, to be investigated and evaluated for the cause of anemia.

History of Present Pregnancy

Spontaneous conception, planned pregnancy.

First Trimester

- Pregnancy was confirmed, at home by urine pregnancy test when she was overdue by 10 days.
- She had no history of any bleeding or discharge per vaginum, pain lower abdomen, fever with rashes, bladder and bowel symptoms, self-medication or radiation exposure.
- Folic acid (FA) was started once her pregnancy test came positive after she consulted in local dispensary. Her FA intake was occasional.
- She reported mild symptoms of morning sickness and managed with dietary modification.
- Ultrasonography was done in first trimester that showed positive cardiac activity.

Second Trimester

Amenorrhea Continued

- Quickening felt at around 5 months. Iron and calcium started. FA not taken. Two doses of tetanus toxoid were received.
- Blood and urine test were done and patient was diagnosed with moderate anemia. As she was noncompliant due to nausea and vomiting, i.e. intolerance after oral iron, injectable iron (six doses) was transfused. Her anemia got corrected. There is no history of any blood transfusion.

- Level II ultrasound was done in fifth month of pregnancy and was normal.
- No history of breathlessness, easy fatigability, burning micturition, blood from any orifices, passage of worms in stools, swelling over feet, bleeding or leaking per vaginum or increased blood sugar was there.
- She visited antenatal clinic thrice and her blood pressure was normal on all visits.

Third Trimester
Amenorrhea Continued
- She was intolerant to oral iron. FA not taken. Calcium intake was normal.
- She had breathlessness and fatigability at eighth month of amenorrhea. She was investigated and diagnosed with severe anemia.
- She was referred to LNH in view of severe anemia and nonavailability of blood bank in dispensary.

Obstetric History
Married since 12 years, consanguineous marriage.

G3P2L1A0
- G1—booked at Ambedkar hospital at 2 months amenorrhea, had preterm intrauterine demise (IUD) at 8 months, delivered by induction of labor 10 years back. Baby was female, 1.8 kg birth weight, history of diabetes mellitus or hypertension was there, no morphological abnormality was detected in baby. Breast suppression was given, postnatal period was uneventful. Discharged in satisfactory condition on postpartum day 3.
- G2—booked at LNH at four months amenorrhea. She had preterm lower segment cesarean section (LSCS) in view of severe preeclampsia with moderate hemoglobin with poor bishops score eight years back, baby was female 2 kg birth weight, admitted in nursery for 6 days. No history of PPH or any blood loss (surgical). Two units of packed cell transfused post-LSCS in view of severe anemia. SRC out on day 2, complete stitch removal on day 10. Uneventful postpartum period. Baby six months breastfed, is alive and healthy with normal milestones, immunized till date.
- G4—present pregnancy.

Menstrual History
- Menarche—14 years of age
- LMP—13/10/2016
- Estimated date of delivery (EDD)—20/07/2017
- No history of dysmenorrhea, menorrhagia.

Medical History
No history of chronic hypertension, diabetes mellitus (DM), tuberculosis, asthma or any seizure disorder in past, or any chronic gastrointestinal complaints.

Surgical History
Not significant.

Family History
Not significant.

Personal History
- She is a housewife with normal bowel and bladder pattern with normal sleep pattern.
- Nonvegetarian, nonalcoholic and no other addictions.

Socioeconomic History
She lives in a nuclear family of four, pukka house, Municipal Corporation of Delhi (MCD) water supply with modern sanitation and electricity facilities. As per modified Kuppuswamy scale she belongs to lower middle class.

Dietery History
- Patient takes approximately 2200 kcal.
- Her protein intake is approximately 60 g.

Diagnosis on History
G3P2L1A0 with POG 30 week 2 days with moderate anemia with previous lower segment cesarean section (LSCS).

Examination
Patient is conscious, oriented, sitting comfortably in bed, average built with normal gait, normal hair line, average orodental hygiene.
- Gestational carrier (GC)—good
- Weight—65 kg.
- Height—150 cm.
- Body mass index (BMI)—28.8 kg/m^2 [according to prepregnancy weight]
- Pallor—present, clinically 7-8 g%.
- Icterus—absent.
- Cyanosis—absent.
- Clubbing—absent.

- Pedal edema—absent.
- Pulse rate—90/min, regular, rhythmic, no radioradial or radiofemoral delay.
- Blood pressure (BP)—110/80 mm Hg in right arm in sitting.
- Respiratory rate—16/min.
- Thyroid—normal
- Lymph nodes—not palpable.

Respiratory System

Trachea centrally placed, no added sounds.

Cardiovascular System

S1, S2 normal with no abnormal sound.

Abdominal Examination

Inspection

- Abdomen is uniformly distended with all quadrants moving with respiration.
- Linea nigra and stria gravidarum present, transverse scar of previous LSCS present.
- Umbilicus is central and everted, no herniation observed.

Palpation

- Fundal height—30 weeks
- Symphysio fundal height—28 cm
- Abdominal girth—31.5 inches
- Fundal grip—a soft broad ballotable structure felt at fundus, suggestive of breech
- Lateral grip—smooth and curved structure felt on right lateral side of abdomen, suggestive of back
- Multiple nobby parts felt on left side, suggestive of limbs
- Pelvic grips—a hard, globular and smooth structure is felt on palpation, suggestive of head, was freely mobile and not engaged.

Auscultation

Fetal heart sounds were heard at right spinoumbilical line, 130 beats/min, regular.

Perineal Examination

- External genitalia—normal
- No bleeding and no leaking observed.

Per Speculum Examination

- Os closed
- Cervix long
- No abnormal discharge or bleeding observed.

Diagnosis After Examination

G3P2L1A0 with POG 30 week 2 days with cephalic presentation with moderate anemia with previous LSCS, not in failure.

Her blood investigations are as follows:
- Hemoglobin (Hb)—8 g%
- Hematocrit (Hct)—30%
- Mean corpuscular volume (MCV)—74 fL
- Mean corpuscular hemoglobin (MCH)—24 pg
- Mean corpuscular hemoglobin concentration (MCHC)—29%
- Peripheral smear shows microcytic hypochromic red blood cells (RBCs) rest unremarkable
- Nestroft—negative
- High performance liquid chromatography (HPLC)—normal
- Stool ova and cyst—not observed, no occult blood seen
- Serum protein—6 g%
- Lactate dehydrogenase (LDH)—320 IU/L

Treatment

As patient was intolerant to oral iron, injectable iron was given to her on alternate days for 8 doses calculated according to her prepregnancy weight. Patient was discharged on day 19 with Hb 10.1 g/dL.

Calculation of dose of iron (mg) = (2.4 ×[target Hb - actual Hb] × prepregnancy weight (kg)) + 10 mg /kg for stores replenishment.[1]

Q1. Define anemia and its epidemiology.

Anemia in pregnancy is defined by hemoglobin levels, trimester wise as:
- First trimester <11.0 g/L
- Second and third trimesters <10.5 g/L
- Postpartum period <10.0 g/L.[2]

According to World Health Organization (**WHO**): Hemoglobin of <11 g/dL, or hematocrit <33%, irrespective of trimesters.[3]

Center of disease control and prevention (CDC)—according to Hb and Hct:

- First and third trimesters—Hb <11 g/dL, Hct <33%
- Second trimester—Hb <10.5 g/dL, hematocrit <32%.[4]

The **WHO** defines hemoglobin for all:
- Severe hemoglobin Hb <7 g/dL
- Very severe hemoglobin Hb <4 g/dL.[5]

National Family Health Survey IV
- Non-pregnant female (15–49 years of age)—Hb <12 g%.[6]
- Pregnant women (15–49 years of age)—Hb <11 g%.[6]

In India, prevalence of hemoglobin by WHO estimates was 65–75%. 50% of maternal deaths, worldwide due to anemia, occur in South Asian countries, 80% being contributed by India.[7]

Q2. How will you classify anemia according to severity?

The severity of anemia is based on the patient's Hb/hematocrit:[5]

Pregnancy state	Normal (g/dL)	Mild (g/dL)	Moderate (g/dL)	Severe (g/dL)
First trimester	11 or higher	10–10.9	7–7.9	Lower than 7
Second trimester	10.5 or higher			
Third trimester	11 or higher	10–10.9	7–7.9	Lower than 7

Q3. What are the causes of anemia?

Causes of Anemia[8]

Acquired Causes
- Iron deficiency anemia—dietary/chronic blood loss/worm infestation
- Megaloblastic anemia—vitamin B_{12} and folic acid deficiency
- Anemia of inflammation or malignancies, e.g. chronic renal disease, tuberculosis, etc.
- Aplastic or hypoplastic anemia
- Drug induced, e.g. alkylating agents like vincristine, chloramphenicol, anticonvulsants especially primidone, quinine, alpha methyldopa, etc.
- Anemia caused by acute blood loss—postpartum hemorrhage (PPH)/ectopic/abortions, etc.

Hereditary Causes
- Thalassemia
- Sickle cell hemoglobinopathy and hemoglobinopathies
- Hereditary hemolytic anemia.

Q4. How will you diagnose iron deficiency clinically?

Symptoms and signs are usually nonspecific.
- *Symptoms*—fatigue, weakness, headache, dizziness, palpitations, irritability, poor concentration, hair loss.
- *Signs*—pallor, tachycardia, dyspnea, glossitis, stomatitis, restless leg syndrome, pica.[9-11]

Q5. Laboratory tests for diagnosis of iron deficiency anemia.

Full Blood Count (FBC)[2]
- ↓Hb and Hct
- ↓MCV
- ↓MCH
- ↓MCHC.

Blood Film
Microcytic hypochromic RBCs.

Serum Ferritin[2,7]
- Earliest laboratory marker to become abnormal
- Best test for iron deficiency anemia (IDA) with cut off of 30 µg/L.[12] The values <15 µg/L indicates severe deficiency.
- Sensitivity was 92% and specificity 98%.[13]
- Serum ferritin initially rises followed by gradual fall till 32 weeks, slight increase is observed in third trimester.

Serum Iron (Fe) and Total Iron Binding Capacity (TIBC)
Unreliable indicators of tissue iron levels as fluctuation in levels observed with recent ingestion of Fe, diurnal rhythm and other.

Zinc Protoporphyrin (ZPP)
Unaffected by hemodilution. It increases with decrease in serum iron ZPP as zinc, is incorporated into the protoporphyrin ring in place of iron.

Reticulocyte Hemoglobin Content and Reticulocytes
It decreases in iron deficiency.

Soluble Transferrin Receptor (sTfR)
Sensitive marker[13]

A meta-analysis of ten studies of sTfR showed that it had a sensitivity of 86% and a specificity of 75%.[14]

Bone Marrow Iron[2]
Gold standard but clearly too invasive and not practical for any but can be done for most complicated cases in pregnancy.

Q6. What do you understand by trial of iron therapy?
- In trial of iron therapy first we measure serum ferritin and rule out hemolysis with Nestroft.
- If negative a trial of iron preparation either oral or injectable depending on period of gestation was given.

- Response to therapy was assessed by demonstrating a rise in Hb after 2 weeks. It is both diagnostic and therapeutic.
- If no improvement is observed in Hb by 2 weeks, one should rule out other causes.[3]

Q7. Enumerate the factors influencing iron absorption.

Factors Inhibiting Iron Absorption
- Foods rich in calcium
- Tannins in tea
- Phytates in cereals.

Factors Enhancing Iron Absorption
- Heme iron
- Ferrous iron
- Ascorbic acid
- Low iron stores.

Q8. What are the maternal and fetal effects of iron deficiency?

Effects of iron deficiency anemia have been described on:

Maternal Effects
- Decrease immunity with increased susceptibility to infections[15]
- Decrease work capacity and performance[16]
- Postpartum emotional and cognition disturbances.[17]

Fetal Effects
- Relatively unaffected.[18]
- Impaired psychomotor and/or mental development.
- Social emotional behaviour of infant is negatively affected.[19]

Effects on Pregnancy Outcome
Increase risk of preterm delivery,[20] low birth weight,[21] possibly placental abruption and increased peri-partum blood loss.[22]

Q9. Describe in brief the management of iron deficiency anemia.

Dietary Advice
- Mothers should be advised to take food rich in iron
- Due to very high requirement of iron, iron and folic acid should be given to all pregnant patients as prophylaxis to prevent anemia
- To optimize absorption of iron, its intake should be spaced properly with meals rich in phytats, tannins, calcium
- Maternal iron requirements are approximately 1000 mg in singleton pregnancies (500 mg for maternal hemoglobin, 300 mg for placenta and fetus, and 200 mg that is shed normally through gut, urine and skin)
- Approximately 10 mg iron is absorbed from food, i.e. 15% of dietary iron
- Pregnant women iron requirements are thrice as high as menstruating women[23]
- Iron absorption increases by three-fold with progressive gestation, with iron requirements increasing from 1–2 mg to 6 mg per day in third trimester[24]
- The main sources of dietary heme iron are from nonvegetarian foods like red meats, fish and poultry
- Heme iron is 2- to 3-fold readily absorbed than nonheme iron sources which contributes approximately 95% of dietary iron[25]
- Vitamin C markedly enhances iron absorption from non-heme foods[26]
- Germinated and fermented food decreases phytate thereby improving bioavailability of nonheme iron
- Tea and coffee (tannins) if taken with a meal or shortly after it decreases iron absorption
- Deworming should be done in all patients
  - Tablet albendazole 400 mg single dose
  - Tablet mebendazole 500 mg single dose or 100 mg twice daily for 3 days.

Oral Iron Supplements
- In pregnancy increased iron demands cannot be fulfilled by dietary changes alone and hence iron supplements are required
- Ferrous iron salts cheap, effective, and safer way to replace iron and are the preparation of choice. The effective oral dose should be 100–200 mg of elemental iron daily.

Dose and elemental iron content per tablet of oral iron preparations:

Iron salt	Dose per tablet	Elemental iron
Ferrous ascorbate	500 mg	100 mg
Carbonyl iron		45 mg
Ferrous fumarate	200 mg	65 mg
Ferrous gluconate	300 mg	35 mg
Ferrous sulfate (dried)	200 mg	65 mg
Ferrous sulfate	300 mg	60 mg
Ferrous feredetate (Sytron)	190 mg/5 mL elixir	27.5 mg/5 mL elixir

Counseling should be done on how to take oral iron.
- Preferably empty stomach
- At least 1 hour prior meals
- Along with vitamin C
- Avoid other drugs like antacids.

Q10. What are the Indications for oral iron supplementation?

- All antenatal women should have a FBC taken at the booking and at 28 weeks [National Institute of Health and Clinical excellence (NICE), 2008][27]
- Trial of therapeutic iron replacement should be offered to women with a Hb <11 g% until 12 weeks or <10.5 g% beyond 12 weeks
- In a women with hemoglobinopathy trial of iron therapy can be offered if the ferritin is <30 µg/L
- *The patient who are **intolerant** to oral iron,* i.e. having excessive nausea and vomiting, lot of upper gastrointestinal (GI) discomfort to the extent patient avoid taking oral iron. Such patients are advised to take iron tablets after meals
- To be given for 6 months in countries with prevalence <40% and additional 3 month postpartum where the prevalence >40%.

Q11. Enumerate non-anemic women with increased predisposition for anemia.

- Inter-conceptional anemia
- Frequent pregnancies ≤1 year interval in between
- Vegetarians
- Teenagers
- Women with bleeding disorders
- Known hemoglobinopathy.

Q12. How will you assess response to oral iron supplementation?

Clinical improvement is assessed as:
- Increased sense of well being
- Increase in work capacity
- Improvement of other symptoms.

Laboratory parameters:
- Reticulocyte count—increase up to 5% in 5–7 days.
- Hb—increase @ 0.8–1 g/dL/ week after 2–3 weeks.
- RBCs indices—improvement in MCV/MCH/MCHC after 2–3 weeks.
- Peripheral smear—normocytic normochromic picture in 6–8 weeks.

Q13. Describe in brief regarding indications and contraindications of parenteral iron therapy.

Indications
- Poor compliance to oral iron
- Intolerance to oral iron therapy
- Lack of response
- Postpartum hemoglobin
- Women with GI disorders that hampers oral iron absorption
- Proven malnutrition.

Contraindications
- Hypersensitivity to parenteral iron therapy
- First trimester of pregnancy
- Noniron deficiency hemoglobin
- Active acute or chronic infection
- Chronic liver disease.

Q14. Describe in brief various injectable iron preparations.

Injectable iron preparations available

	Iron hydroxide dextran complex	*Iron hydroxide sucrose complex*	*Iron carboxymaltose*	*Iron isomaltoside*
Dose of elemental iron	50 mg/mL	20 mg/mL	50 mg/mL	100 mg/mL
Test dose	Yes	Yes	No	No
Routes of administration	Slow intravenous injection/ Intravenous infusion/ Intramuscular injection	Slow intravenous injection/ Intravenous infusion	Slow intravenous injection/ Intravenous infusion	Slow intravenous injection/ Intravenous infusion
Able to administer total Dose	Yes (up to 20 mg/kg bodyweight over 4–6 h)	No	Yes [up to 20 mg/kg bodyweight (maximum of 1000 mg/week) over 15 min]	Yes (up to 20 mg/kg bodyweight over 1 h)
Dosage	100–200 mg per IV injection up to 3 times a week	Total IV single dose no more than 200 mg, can be repeated up to 3 times in 1 week	1000 mg by IV injection up to 15 mg/kg per week	100–200 mg per IV injection up to 3 times a week Total dose infusion up to 20 mg/kg body weight per week
	Total dose infusion up to 20 mg/kg bodyweight over 4–6 h) (100 mg IM into alternate buttocks daily in active patients in bed ridden up to 3 times a week)		Total dose infusion up to 20 mg/kg bodyweight. Maximum weekly dose of 1000 mg, which can be administered over 15 min	Doses up to 10 mg/kg bodyweight can be administered over 30 min, doses >10 mg/kg body weight should be administered over 60 min
Adverse effects	5%	0.5–1.5%	3%	1%

Q15. Describe fast-acting intravenous iron preparations.

Iron III Carboxymaltose
- It facilitates controlled delivery of iron within the cells of the reticuloendothelial system
- Followed by delivery to the iron binding proteins ferritin and transferrin.

Iron III Isomaltoside
This compound has strongly bound iron in spheroid iron-carbohydrate particles, allowing slow release of bioavailable iron to iron binding proteins thereby increasing reticulocyte count with in few days.

Q16. What are the recommendations for parenteral iron administrations and how to calculate the dose?[2]

Consider parenteral iron administration from second trimester onwards and postpartum period in case of failure or intolerance to oral iron.
- The dose to be calculated on the basis of prepregnancy weight, with a target Hb of 11 g/mL.
- Written informed consent should be there regarding potential side-effects.

Calculation of dose of iron (mg) =
- [2.4 × (target Hb-actual Hb) × prepregnancy weight (kg)] + 10 mg/kg for stores replenishment.[1]
- Iron (mg)–{weight (kg) × (14 – Hb) × (2.145)}

C—concentration of elemental iron (mg/mL) in the product being used, e.g. iron sucrose 20 mg /mL.

Q17. Indications of blood transfusion in a women with anemia.

Royal College of Obstetrics and Gynecologists (RCOG) blood transfusion guideline recommends blood transfusion in labor or immediate postpartum period if Hb <7 g/dL.[28]

Indications of Blood Transfusion In Pregnancy[29,30]

Antepartum Period
- Pregnancy <34 weeks
  - Hb <5 g/dL with/without signs of cardiac failure or hypoxia
  - 5–7 g/dL—in presence of impending heart failure.
- Pregnancy >34 weeks
  - Hb <7 g/dL even without signs of cardiac failure or hypoxia
  - Severe anemia with decompensation.
- Anemia not due to hematinic deficiency
  - Hemoglobinopathy or bone marrow failure syndromes
  - Hematologist should always be consulted.
- Acute hemorrhage
  - Always indicated if Hb <6 g/dL
  - If the patient become hemodynamically unstable due to ongoing hemorrhage.

Intrapartum Period
- Hb <7 g/dL (in labor)
- Decision of blood transfusion depends on medical history or symptoms.

Postpartum Period
- Anemia with signs of shock/acute hemorrhage with signs of hemodynamic instability
- Hb <7 g/dL (postpartum): Decision of blood transfusion depends on medical history or symptoms.

Q18. Strategies for prevention of iron deficiency anemia.

A summary of recommendations by WHO and MoHFW:[31-33]

During Pregnancy

	Prophylaxis	Treatment
WHO	Daily 60 mg iron + 400 µg folic acid till term	Daily 120 mg iron + 400 µg folic acid—3 months
MoHFW	Daily 100 mg iron + 500 µg folic acid—6 months	Mild anemia—2 IFA tablets/day—100 days Moderate anemia—IM iron therapy + oral folic acid Severe anemia—IV sucrose

During Postpartum

WHO	Daily 60 mg iron and 400 µg folic acid—3 months
MoHFW	Daily 100 mg iron and 500 µg folic acid—6 months

Q19. What are the differential diagnosis of microcytic hemoglobin and how will differentiate them?

Differential diagnosis of various microcytic RBCs etiologies:[34,35]

Indicator	Iron deficiency hemoglobin (IDA)	Beta thalassemia (BT)	Dimorphic hemoglobin	Acute/chronic infections (ACI)
Hb	Decreased	Normal or decreased	Decreased	Decreased
Ferritin	Decreased	Normal	Decreased or normal	Normal or increased
Serum iron	Decreased	Normal or increased	Normal or decreased	Normal or decreased
TIBC	Increased	Normal	Increased	Slightly decreased

Contd...

Contd...

Indicator	Iron deficiency hemoglobin (IDA)	Beta thalassemia (BT)	Dimorphic hemoglobin	Acute/chronic infections (ACI)
TS	Decreased	Normal to increased	Normal or decreased	Normal to slightly decreased
sTfR	Increased in severe IDA	>100 mg/L	normal	Normal
FEP	Increased	Normal	Normal/increased	Increased
MCV	Decreased	Decreased	Normal/increased/decreased	Normal or decreased
RDW	Increased	Normal to increased	Increased	Normal
Reticulocytes	Decreased	-	Decreased	Normal or decreased

Abbreviations: TIBC, total iron binding capacity; sTfR, soluble transferrin receptor; FEP, free erythrocyte protoporphyrin; MCV, mean corpuscular volume; RDW, red cell distribution width

CASE SCENARIO

G4P2L1A1 with eight month amenorrhea with moderate anemia.

A 28 years old, Mrs X, wife of Mr Y, resident of Turkman Gate, Delhi, a housewife, came to gyne casualty on 3/5/17 with complaints of:
- Amenorrhea 8 months
- Easy fatigability and difficulty in breathing on exertion since 1 month.

Her LMP was 17/9/16, so making her period of gestation 32 weeks 4 days on 3/5/17.

History of Presenting Complaints

- Patient was a booked antenatal case of same hospital
- She complained of easy fatigability and breathlessness on exertion since 1 month
- No history of any blood loss from any site
- No history of any cardiac illness in present or past
- No history of any respiratory disorders
- No complains of any bleeding or leaking per vaginum.

Course in the Hospital

- She was admitted to the labor room after her general and abdominal examinations.
- Her blood samples [full blood count (FBC), blood group cross match, liver function test, kidney function test, serum electrolytes] was taken and patient was evaluated. She was diagnosed with moderate anemia with macrocytic normochromic picture in peripheral smear.
- She was shifted to clean maternity ward, investigated and evaluated for the cause of anemia.

History of Present Pregnancy

Spontaneous conception, planned pregnancy.

First Trimester

- Pregnancy was confirmed, at home by urine pregnancy test when she was overdue by 20 days
- No intake of folic acid in first trimester. Rest unremarkable.

Second Trimester

Unremarkable.

Third Trimester

- Amenorrhea continued and patient develops gradual onset weakness, fatigability, and breathlessness over a period of 1 month
- Her iron intake was occasional, folic acid not taken.

Obstetric History

- Married since 11 years
- Non-consanguinous marriage.

G4P2L1A1

- G1—was a supervised pregnancy at LNH, had full-term emergency LSCS in view of fetal distress, 9 years back
- G2—was a supervised pregnancy at LNH, had full-term vaginal delivery, 4 year back
- Baby was male, 2.6 kg birth weight, cried after birth
- Died at 6 month of age due to drowning
- G3—spontaneous abortion
- G4—present pregnancy.

Menstrual History

- Menarche—14 years of age
- LMP—17/09/2016
- Estimate date of death delivery (EDD)—24/06/2017.
- No history of dysmenorrhea, menorrhagia.

Medical History/Surgical History/Family History/Personal History

Unremarkable.

Socioeconomic History

Unremarkable.

Dietery History

- Patient takes approximately 1,700 kcal as per 24 hour recall method.
- Her protein intake is approximately 40 g. Her calorie deficit was 500 kcal and her protein deficit was 20 g. Diet modification to include increase protein and calories explained.

Diagnosis on History

G4P2L1A1 with POG 32 weeks 4 days with moderate anemia with previous one LSCS not in failure.

Examination

Patient is conscious, oriented, sitting comfortably in bed, average built with normal gait, normal hair line, average orodental hygiene.

- GC—good
- Weight—50 kg
- Height—150 cm
- BMI—22.2 kg/m
- Pallor—present, clinically 7–8 g%
- Rest unremarkable
- Systemic examination—unremarkable.

Abdominal Examination

Inspection

Unremarkable.

Palpation

- Fundal height—32 weeks
- Symphysio fundal height—30 cm
- Abdominal girth—32.3 inches
- Grips—unremarkable.

Auscultation

Fetal heart sounds were heard at right spino umbilical line, 140 beats/min, regular.

Perineal Examination

Unremarkable.

Per Speculum Examination

Unremarkable

Diagnosis after Examination

G4P2L2A0 with period of gestation (POG) 32 week 4 days with cephalic presentation with moderate anemia with previous LSCS not in failure.

Her blood investigations are as follows:
- Hb—7.2 g%
- Hct—24%
- Mean corpuscular volume (MCV)—106 fl
- Mean corpuscular hemoglobin (MCH)—21 pg
- Mean corpuscular hemoglobin concentration (MCHC)—27%.

Peripheral smear shows macrocytic normochromic RBCs with anisopoikilocytosis, macro-ovalocytes, with hypersegmented neutrophils.
- Nestroft—negative
- HPLC—normal.

Treatment

Diagnosis of megaloblastic anemia is made based on examination and laboratory investigations. Injectable iron is also given along as there is increased requirement during erythropoisis.

7 doses of injection elderwit (B_{12}—2500 µg, 0.7 mg folic acid, 150 mg vitamin C/1.5 mL) given alternately with injection iron sucrose. Patient was discharged on 17th day with Hb 9.5 g/dL.

Q1. How will you confirm the diagnosis of megaloblastic hemoglobin?

Peripheral smear and FBC will suggest type of anemia followed by serum B_{12} and folate levels measurement for confirmation.
- Serum B_{12} level <100 pg/mL suggest B_{12} deficiency.
- Serum folate level <2 ng/mL suggests folate deficiency anemia.
- Fasting serum folate level <6 µg/L and RBC folate <165 µg/L are diagnostic of folate deficiency.

Q2. Causes of megaloblastic hemoglobin?

Megaloblastic hemoglobin is usually caused by a deficiency of folic acid or vitamin B_{12}.

Other less common causes are:[36]
- Alcohol abuse
- HIV infection
- Certain inherited disorders
- Atrophic gastritis and achlorhydria
- Pernicious hemoglobin
- Pancreatic insufficiency
- Zollinger-Ellison syndrome
- Inflammatory bowel syndrome
- Tropical sprue
- Blind loop syndrome
- Drugs that affect DNA, such as chemotherapy drugs
- Leukemia
- Myelodysplastic syndrome
- Myelofibrosis
- The anticonvulsant drug dilantin.

Q3. Describe the pathophysiology of megaloblastosis?

Due to deficiency of B_{12} and folic acid, a defect in DNA synthesis in rapidly dividing cells with RNA and protein causes megaloblastosis.

Arrest in nuclear maturation causes unbalanced cell growth and impaired cell division.

It causes intramedullary hemolysis.[37,38]

Q4. What are the symptoms and signs of megaloblastic hemoglobin?

Symptoms[39]
- Weakness, fatigue
- Gastrointestinal—loss of appetite, weight loss, nausea, constipation
- Neurological—numbness, pain, tingling, and burning in a patient's hands and feet stocking or glove neuropathy.

Signs[41]
- Lemon color complexion
- Palpitations, glossitis
- Hyperpigmentation of skin and abnormal hair pigmentation
- Peripheral neuropathy, psychosis, abnormal gait, speech impairment, loss of propioceptive and vibratory senses
- Weight loss, abdominal distension, diarrhea, and steatorrhea.

Q5. Enumerate the dietary sources of vitamin B_{12} and folic acid.

The primary sources of cobalamin (Clb), a cobalt-containing vitamin, are meat, fish, and dairy products and not vegetables and fruit.

The folate is found in fresh vegetables, fruits, and animal protein. Dietary folic is usually conjugated, polyglutamate folates, and are converted to dihydrofolic acid, so they can be absorbed.

Q6. What are the daily requirement of folic acid and vitamin B_{12} during pregnancy?

- Daily 400 µg of folic acid.[40]
- Daily vitamin B_{12} 2.6 µg.

Q7. Enumerate the differential diagnosis of macrocytic picture in peripheral smear.

Serum and vitamin B_{12} deficiency
- Hypothyroidism
- Liver disease
- Myelodysplasia
- Hydroxyurea
- Alcoholism
- Lesch-Nyhan syndrome
- Homocystinuria.

Q8. What are the maternal and fetal effects of folate and cobalamin deficiency.

Folic acid deficiency increases risk of neural tube defects (NTDs), low birth weight, and small for gestational age (SGA).
- Maternal vitamin B_{12} status affects fetal growth and development.
- Low cobalamin increases risk of fetal low lean mass and excess adiposity, increased insulin resistance and impaired neurodevelopment.
- Maternal risks include fatigue, pallor, tachycardia, poor exercise tolerance and suboptimal work performance.
- Depleted blood reserves during delivery may increase the need for blood transfusion, preeclampsia, placental abruption, cardiac failure and related death.

Q9. How will you treat B_{12} deficiency in pregnant women?

- *Oral:* 1000 µg of vitamin B_{12}, daily should be given to patient with serum levels to be monitored to ensure adequate repletion.
- *Sublingual:* For patients with absorption disorder, i.e. bariatric surgery, steatorrhea, malabsorption syndromes.
- *Parenteral:* Non-responders and patients with neurological features.

Treatment of clinical vitamin B_{12} deficiency has traditionally been accomplished by intramuscular injection of crystalline vitamin B_{12} at a dosage of 1 mg weekly for eight weeks, followed by 1 mg monthly for life.[41]

Q10. What is the difference in response to oral and intramuscular treatment with B_{12}?

In a 2005 Cochrane review, patients who received high dosages of oral vitamin B_{12} (1–2 mg daily) for 90–120 days had an improvement in serum vitamin B_{12} similar to patients who received intramuscular injections of vitamin B_{12}.[42]

Q11. How will you treat a folate deficiency?

As little as 1 mg of folic acid administered once daily, produces a striking hematological response by 4–7 days after beginning of treatment. The reticulocyte count increases with leukopenia and thrombocytopenia correction.

Q12. How will you monitor response of the treatment?

Clinically improvement assessed as:
- Increased sense of well being
- Improved working capacity
- Improvement of glossitis
- Improvement of depigmentation
- Improvement of neurological symptoms.

Laboratory parameters to assess improvement are:
- Decrease in LDH levels by 3–4 days
- Increase in reticulocyte count by 5–7 days
- Increase in hemoglobin 0.8–1 g/dL/week
- Peripheral smear shows normocytic normochromic RBCs.

Q13. Any counseling do you want to give to folate deficiency patients for prevention of NTDs in next pregnancy?

Preconceptional folic acid 4 mg daily is advised for 3 months and should be continued in first trimester.

CASE SCENARIO

G3P1L1E1 with 9 months amenorrhea with severe anemia.

A 28 years old, Mrs X, wife of Mr Y, resident of Najafgarh, New Delhi, a housewife, came to gyne casualty on 6/5/17 with complaints of:
- Amenorrhea 9 months
- Breathlessness since 2 months
- Palpitations since one month
- Marked weakness since 10 days.

Her LMP was 16/08/16 so making her period of gestation 37 weeks and 4 days on 6/5/17.

History of Presenting Complaints

- She was a booked antenatal case in government hospital, Najafgarh, New Delhi
- She had breathlessness since 2 months. It was gradual in onset and increased progressively
- She had palpitations since 1 month
- She had weakness which was gradual in onset and markedly increased since 10 days
- She had no history of any cardiac disorder in present or past
- She had no history of any respiratory illness in present or past
- She had no history of bleeding per vaginum or blood loss from any other orifices.

Course in the Hospital

- She was admitted to labor room after her general physical and abdominal examination which showed severe pallor, PR 100/min, RR 18/min, hemic murmur on cardiovascular system (CVS) examination with bilateral chest clear and presence of abdominal wall edema with pedal edema, rest unremarkable.
- She was evaluated again in labor room, propped up, oxygen saturation done (100%), continued oral intake with monitoring of vitals, input, output, chest auscultation to detect earliest symptoms and signs of cardiorespiratory failure.
- Intermittent oxygen by mask continued.
- Fetal monitoring continued as routine (NST at admission, DFMC, intermittent auscultation)
- Her blood samples [full blood count (FBC), blood group cross match, liver function test, kidney function test, serum electrolytes] was taken and patient was evaluated. She was diagnosed with severe anemia with microcytic hypochromic picture in peripheral smear.
- All other reports normal except serum proteins 5 g/dL.
- Patient was evaluated and investigated and diagnosed with severe hemoglobin not in failure.

Her blood investigations on 7/5/17 are as follows:
- ABO Rh—B+
- Hb—5.1 g/dL
- Hct—14.9%
- MCV—57 Fl
- MCH—14.8 pg
- MCHC—26.1%
- RDW—16.7
- TLC—14900/cumm
- Platelet—1.69/cumm

- Serum total bilirubin—1.6
- Aspartate transaminase (AST)—10
- Alanine transaminase (ALT)—22
- Serum proteins—5 g/dL
- Blood urea—22 mg/dL
- Serum creatinine—1.2 mg/dL
- Prothrombin time (PT)—14.4
- International normalized ratio (INR)—1.12
- Hepatitis B surface antibody (HBsAg)—Nonreactive
- Venereal disease research laboratory (VDRL)—nonreactive
- Human immunodeficiency virus (HIV)—nonreactive.

Decision of packed cell transfusion is made. Patient was transfused 3 units of packed RBCs under lasix cover. Her post-BT Hb was 8 g/dL. She went into labor two days after that and was delivered vaginally uneventfully. Her postnatal Hb was 7.6 g/dL. She was given 5 doses of iron sucrose in view of postnatal hemoglobin.

She was discharged on 24/5/17.

History of Present Pregnancy

Spontaneous conception, unplanned pregnancy.

First Trimester

Unremarkable.

Second Trimester

Blood and urine test were done and patient was diagnosed with moderate anemia. As she was intolerant to oral iron. Rest unremarkable.

Third Trimester

- Amenorrhea continued.
- She was intolerant to oral iron. FA not taken. Calcium intake was normal.
- She had breathlessness and fatigability at eighth month of amenorrhea. She was investigated and diagnosed with severe anemia.
- She was referred to LNH in view of severe anemia and nonavailability of blood bank in Najafgarh hospital.

Obstetric History

G3P1L1E1

- G1—was a supervised pregnancy at LNH, had full-term emergency LSCS in view of Naval Physical and Oceanographic Laboratory (NPOL) distress, 10 years back. Baby was female, 2.8 kg birth weight 6 months breastfed. SRC out on day 2rd, stitch removal on day 7. Discharged satisfactory on day 7th.
- G2—diagnosed with unruptured left tubal ectopic pregnancy. Treated medically at LNH, 7 year back.
- G3—present pregnancy.

Menstrual History

History of menorrhagia present. 7–8 days of bleeding, every 24–25 days with 6–7 pads soaked daily for 5–6 days.

Dietery History

Patient takes approximately 1500 kcal as per 24 hour recall method.

Her protein intake is approximately 35 g. Her calorie deficit was 700 kcal and protein deficit was 25 g. Dietary advice given.

Diagnosis on History

G3P1L1E1 with POG 37 week 4 days with severe anemia with hypoproteinemia with previous one LSCS, not in failure.

Examination

Patient is conscious, oriented, average built with normal gait, normal hair line, average orodental hygiene.

General Condition

- GC—good
- Weight—50 kg
- Height—150 cm
- BMI—22.2
- Pallor—present, clinically 3–4 g%
- Icterus—absent
- Cyanosis—absent
- Clubbing—absent
- Pedal edema—present
- Pulse rate—104/min, regular, rhythmic, no radioradial or radiofemoral delay
- BP—110/80 mm Hg in right arm in sitting
- Respiratory rate—22/min
- Cardiovascular examination—S1, S2 normal, hemic murmur heard.

Abdominal Examination

Inspection

Unremarkable.

Palpation

- Fundal height—40 weeks
- Symphysiofundal height—34 cm
- Abdominal girth—35.46 inches
- Presentation—cephalic.

Auscultation

Fetal heart sounds were heard at right spinoumbilical line, 150 beats/min, regular.

Perineal Examination

Unremarkable.

Per Speculum Examination

Unremarkable.

Diagnosis after Examination

G3P1L1E1 with POG 37 weeks 4 days with cephalic presentation with severe anemia with previous LSCS not in failure.

Q1. How will you manage the patient of severe anemia in labor?

1st Stage

- Patient should be propped up
- Intermittent oxygen should be given
- High-risk consent
- The patient should be in bed preferably in position comfortable to her
- Send urgent hemogram with BGCM
- Arrange and transfuse adequate packed cell
- Intermittent chest auscultation
- Strict asepsis should be followed
- Fluid restriction (IV fluid)
- Watch for symptoms and sign of cardiac failure.

2nd Stage

- Partogram to be maintained
- Concentrated oxytytocin should be given if required.

3nd Stage

- Active management of third stage of labor (AMSTL)
- Avoid postpartum hemorrhage (PPH).
- Avoid any genital trauma. Prophylactic episiotomy to be given, if required.

4nd Stage

- Patient should be kept in observation for at least 6 hours postpartum
- Prophylactic antibiotics can be considered to prevent sepsis
- Iron and folic acid should be continued 6 month postpartum
- Contraception advice
- Barrier methods
- POPs
- Sterilization if family completed.

Q2. How will you manage hypoproteinemia?

Hypoproteinemia is characterized by low protein level. It causes fluid loss from intravascular to interstitial space resulting in edema.

Causes

- Malnutrition as part of nutritional anemia
- Hypertensive disorders
- Deranged blood sugars/hyperglycemias
- Infections
- Liver diseases
- Renal diseases
- Nutritional deficiency
- Malabsorption
- Septicemia

Diagnosis

Serum protein-albumin and globulin.

Treatment

- *Nonspecific:* Dietary protein supplementation irrespective of cause is the most common way of treatment.
- *Specific:* Treating underlying cause.

REFERENCES

1. Adamson JW. Iron deficiency and other hypoproliferative anemias. In: Braunwald E, Fauci AS, Kasper DL (Eds). Harrison's textbook of internal medicine. 17th edn. New York:McGraw Hill; 2008; pp. 628-33.
2. Pavard S, Myers B, Robinson S, et al. Oppenheimer C British Journal of Haematology. 2012;156(5):588-600.
3. WHO. Iron Deficiency Anaemia Assessment, Prevention and Control. A guide for programme managers; 2001.
4. Recommendations to prevent and control iron deficiency in the United States. Centres for disease control and prevention. MMWR Recomm Rep. 1998;47(RR -3):1-29.
5. WHO. Haemoglobin concentrations for the diagnosis of anaemia and assessment of severity. Vitamin and Mineral Nutrition Information System, Vol 1. Geneva: World Health organisation;2011
6. National Family Health Survey 4; 2015-16.
7. WHO. The Global Prevalence of Anaemia in 2011. Geneva: World Health Organization; 2015.
8. Williams Textbook of Obstetrics, 23rd edition.
9. Bermejo F, García-López S. A guide to diagnosis of iron deficiency and iron deficiency anemia in digestive diseases. World J Gastroenterol. 2009;15:4638-43.

10. Gupta R, Dhyani M, Kendzerska T, et al. Restless legs syndrome and pregnancy: prevalence, possible pathophysiological mechanisms and treatment. Acta Neurol Scand. 2016;133: 320-9.
11. Upadhyaya SK, Sharma A. Onset of obsessive compulsive disorder in pregnancy with pica as the sole manifestation. Indian J Psychol Med. 2012;34:276-8.
12. Pavord S, Myers B, Robinson S, et al. UK guidelines on management of iron deficiency in pregnancy. Br J Haematol. 2012;156:588-600.
13. Choi J, Im M, Pai S. Serum transferrin receptor concentrations during normal pregnancy. Clinical Chemistry. 2000;46:725-7.
14. Infusino I, Braga F, Dolci A, Panteghini M. Soluble transferrin receptor (sTfR) and sTfR/log ferritin index for the diagnosis of iron-deficiency anemia. A meta-analysis. Am J Clin Pathol. 2012;138(5):642-9.
15. Ekiz E, Agaoglu L, Karakas Z, et al. The effect of iron deficiency anemia on the function of the immune system. The Hematology Journal. 2005;5:579-83.
16. Haas JD, Brownlie T. Iron deficiency and reduced work capacity: a critical review of the research to determine a causal relationship. Journal of Nutrition. 2001;131,676S-90S.
17. Beard JL, Hendricks MK, Perez EM, et al. Maternal iron deficiency anemia affects postpartum emotions and cognition. Journal of Nutrition. 2005;135:267-72.
18. Gambling L, Danzeisen R, Gair S, et al. Effect of iron deficiency on placental transfer of iron and expression of iron transport proteins in vivo and in vitro. Biochemical Journal. 2001;356:883-9.
19. Perez EM, Hendricks MK, Beard JL, et al. Mother-infant Interactions and infant development are altered by maternal iron deficiency anemia. Journal of Nutrition. 2005;135:850-55.
20. Scholl TO, Hediger ML. Anemia and iron-deficiency anemia: compilation of data on pregnancy outcome. American Journal of Clinical Nutrition.1994;59:S492-S501.
21. Cogswell ME, Parvanta I, Ickes L, et al. Iron supplementation during pregnancy, anemia, and birthweight: a randomised controlled trial. American Journal of Clinical Nutrition. 2003;78:773-81.
22. Arnold DL, Williams MA, Miller RS, et al. Maternal iron deficiency anaemia is associated with an increased risk of abruption placentae – a retrospective case control study. Journal of Obstetrics and Gynaecology Research. 2009;35: 446-52.
23. Tapiero H, Gaté L, Tew KD. Iron: deficiencies and requirements. Biomedicine and Pharmacotherapy. 2001;55:324-32.
24. Bothwell TH. Iron requirements in pregnancy and strategies to meet them. American Journal Clinical Nutrition. 2000;72:257S-64S.
25. Pasricha S, Flecknoe-Brown S, Allen K. Diagnosis and management of iron deficiency anaemia: a clinical update. Medical Journal of Australia. 2010;193:525-32.
26. Lynch SR. Interaction of iron with other nutrients. Nutritional Review. 1997;55:102-10.
27. NICE. Antenatal Care. Clinical Guideline CG62. National Institute for Health and Clinical Excellence, London; 2008.
28. Stolzfus RJ, Dreyfuss M. Guidelines for the Use of Iron Supplementation to Prevent and Treat Iron Deficiency Anemia. International Nutritional Anemia Consultative Group (INACG). ILSI Press, Washington, DC; 1998.
29. no.47 RCoOaGBtioG-tg. 2015.
30. Candio F, Hofmeyr GJ. Treatments for iron-deficiency anaemia in pregnancy: RHL commentary. The WHO Reproductive Health Library; Geneva: World Health Organization; 2007.
31. WHO. Guideline: Daily iron and folic acid supplementation in pregnant women. Geneva, Switzerland; 2012.
32. Ministry of Health and Family Welfare GoI, Office memorandum. Revised Operational strategy for oral iron for pregnant women-reg; November 2014.
33. Kapil U, Bhadoria AS. National Iron-plus initiative guidelines for control of iron deficiency anaemia in India, 2013. Natl Med J India. 2014;27:27-9.
34. Thomas C, Thomas L. Biochemical markers and hematologic indices in the diagnosis of functional iron deficiency. Clin Chem. 2002;48:1066-76.
35. AC Anemia: When Is it Iron Deficiency? Pediatr Nurs. 2003;29(2).
36. Dali-Youcef N, Andres E. An update on cobalamin deficiency in adults. QJM. 2009;102(1):17-28.
37. Antony AC. Megaloblastic Anemias. In: Hoffman R, Benz EJ Jr, Silberstein LE, Heslop HE, Weitz JI, Anastasi J (Eds). Hematology: Basic Principles and Practice. 6th edn. Philadelphia, PA:Elsevier.2013; 473-504.
38. Wang YH, Yan F, Zhang WB, et al. An investigation of vitamin B12 deficiency in elderly inpatients in neurology department. Neurosci Bull. 2009;25(4):209-15.
39. Hoffbrand AV. Megaloblastic Anemias. In: Kasper DL, Fauci AS, Hauser SL, Longo DL, Jameson JL, Loscalzo J (Eds) Harrison's Principles of Internal Medicine. 19th ed. New York, NY: McGraw-Hill Education; 2015.
40. Sharbi A, Cohen E, Sulkes J, et al. Replacement therapy for vitamin B12 deficiency: comparison between the sublingual and oral route. Br J Clin Pharmacol.2003;56(6):635-8.
41. Evatt ML, Mersereau PW, Bobo JK, et al. Centers for Disease Control and Prevention. Why vitamin B_{12} deficiency should be on your radar screen. http://www.cdc.gov/ncbddd/b12/index.html. Accessed August 20, 2010.
42. Toh BH, van Driel IR, Gleeson PA. Pernicious anemia. N Engl J Med. 1997;337(20):1441-8.

2

Hypertension in Pregnancy

Anjali Tempe, Komal Rastogi

Hypertensive disorders complicate 5–10% of all pregnancies and contribute significantly to perinatal and maternal morbidity and mortality. According to a systematic review by the World Health Organization (WHO), hypertensive disorders account for 16% of the maternal deaths in developed countries.[1] Of these disorders, the preeclampsia syndrome, either alone or superimposed on chronic hypertension, is the most dangerous.

CASE SCENARIO

Mrs A, 28 years old lady, Primigravida at 33 weeks of gestation comes to antenatal OPD and on routine checkup, she is found to be having blood pressure of 150/100 mm Hg. On repeating the blood pressure measurement after four hours, it is 156/100 mm Hg.

Q1. What important points should be asked in the history for this patient.

- Age: Young and nulliparous women are at increased risk of developing preeclampsia whereas older women >35 years are at increased risk of developing chronic hypertension with superimposed preeclampsia
- Any complaint of headache, epigastric pain, blurring of vision, decreased urine output
- Any complaint of easy fatiguability, dyspnea, orthopnea (signs of congestive heart failure)
- Any complaint of pain abdomen, leaking per vaginum, bleeding per vaginum and decreased fetal movements.

Obstetric History

- *Parity:* Nulliparous women are at a greater risk of developing preeclampsia
- *Present pregnancy related risk factors:* The incidence of gestational hypertension and preeclampsia is higher in women with twin gestation as compared to those with singletons. The incidence of gestational hypertension is 13% in twin gestation versus 6% in singletons, and the incidence of preeclampsia is 13% in twin gestation versus 5% in singletons.[2] Hydatidiform mole and hydrops fetalis are also associated with increased risk of hypertension in pregnancy.
- *History of hypertension in previous pregnancy:* Women with history of gestational hypertension in previous pregnancy have 16–47% risk of developing gestational hypertension in subsequent pregnancy.
- Longer interval between pregnancies (more than 10 years) is also one of the risk factors for preeclampsia.

Past History

Presence of underlying medical disorders: Diabetes, autoimmune diseases such as systemic lupus erythematosus (SLE) or antiphospholipid antibody syndrome, chronic kidney disease, maternal hyperhomocysteinemia and metabolic syndrome[4] are also the risk factors associated with preeclampsia.

Family History

Family history of hypertension: There is two-to four-fold increase in the risk of preeclampsia in patients having first-degree relative with medical history of the disorder.

Personal History

Smoking reduces the risk of hypertension during pregnancy because it upregulates placental adrenomedullin expression, which regulates volume homeostasis.[5]

Q2. Elaborate the important points in examination.

General Physical Examination

- Vital parameters like pulse, blood pressure, temperature, respiratory rate
- Pallor, icterus, pedal edema

- *Body mass index (BMI) of the patient:* The relationship between the risk of developing preeclampsia and maternal weight is progressive. It increases from 4.3% for women with a BMI <20 kg/m^2 to 13.3% in those with a BMI >35 kg/m^2.[6,7]
- Any thyroid enlargement should be noted and investigated.

Respiratory System, Cardiovascular System and Central Nervous System Examination
- Look for signs of congestive heart failure like dyspnea, basal crepitations, tachypnea, raised jugular venous pressure (JVP)
- Fundus examination
- Check deep tendon reflexes.

Abdominal Examination
Symphysiofundal height and abdominal girth to monitor fetal growth. Fetal growth restriction is commonly associated with hypertensive disorders in pregnancy. Fundal height more than period of gestation is suggestive of molar pregnancy, twins and hydraminos, these conditions may also be associated with hypertension in pregnancy.

Q3. What is the classification of hypertensive disorders in pregnancy?

Hypertension is defined as either systolic BP of ≥140 mm Hg or a diastolic BP of ≥90 mm Hg, or both, at least two readings four hours apart. Hypertension is considered mild until blood pressure levels reach or exceed 160/110 mm Hg. Hypertension during pregnancy is classified into four categories as per recommendations of National High Blood Pressure Education Program (NHBPEP, 2000), which are as follows:

1. *Gestational hypertension:* New-onset hypertension developing after 20 weeks of gestation, without proteinuria in a previously normotensive nonproteinuric woman and hypertension resolves by 12 weeks postpartum.
2. Preeclampsia and eclampsia syndrome.

Table 1: Diagnostic criteria for preeclampsia (ACOG, 2013)

Blood pressure	≥140/90 mm Hg on two occasions at least 4 hours apart after 20 weeks of gestation in a previously normotensive woman
	≥160/110 mm Hg, hypertension can be confirmed within a short interval (minutes) to facilitate antihypertensive therapy, and
Proteinuria	300 mg or more in 24-hour urine collection
	or
	Dipstick reading of 1+
	Protein/creatinine ratio ≥ 0.3

Contd...

Contd...

Or, in the absence of proteinuria, new-onset hypertension with any of the following:	
Thrombocytopenia	Platelet count < 100,000/mm^3
Impaired liver function	Elevated liver transaminases to twice the normal concentration
Renal insufficiency	Serum creatinine > 1.1 mg/dL
Cerebral or visual symptoms	
Pulmonary edema	

According to the task force recommendation, the term "mild preeclampsia" has now been replaced by the term "preeclampsia without severe features" as it is never mild and causes increased morbidity and mortality and rapid progression is possible.

Eclampsia is defined as the development of grand mal seizures in a woman with preeclampsia, in absence of other causes of convulsions.

3. Hypertension in a female prior to pregnancy or appearing before 20 weeks of gestation or persisting more than 12 weeks postpartum.
4. *Chronic hypertension with superimposed preeclampsia:*
   - Onset of proteinuria in a woman who had hypertension but no proteinuria before 20 weeks of gestation
   - Sudden exacerbation of hypertension, elevation of liver enzymes, decrease in platelet count (<100,000 mm^3), development of renal insufficiency (serum creatinine increasing to or above 1.1 mg/dL or doubling of serum creatinine levels in absence of renal disease) or sudden increase in protein excretion, appearance of symptoms such as right upper quadrant pain, headache or development of pulmonary edema in a woman who had hypertension or proteinuria before 20 weeks of gestation.

Q4. What are the special investigations you would like to order in this case apart from the routine antenatal investigations?

- Complete blood count including platelet count
- Urine albumin
  - An automated reagent strip can be used to detect proteinuria and if a result of 1+ or more is obtained, proteinuria should be quantified using a spot urinary protein: creatinine ratio or 24-hour urine collection
  - If urine protein: creatinine ratio is greater than 30 mg/mmol or a 24-hour urine collection shows greater than 300 mg protein, significant proteinuria is diagnosed

- Liver function test including enzymes aspartate transaminase (AST) and alanine transaminase (ALT) levels
- Kidney function tests including serum creatinine and uric acid levels
- Lactate dehydrogenase (LDH)
- Fundus examination
- Prothrombin time-international normalized ratio (PT-INR), if platelet count is abnormal.

Q5. What is the diagnosis and how will you manage this patient?

This patient should be investigated for the presence of end organ dysfunction and quantification of proteinuria is done. A diagnosis of gestational hypertension is made when there is no proteinuria or any feature suggestive of end organ dysfunction. Hospitalization is advisable at least initially for 48 hours to rule out severe hypertension. During this period, investigations and four hourly blood pressure measurements are performed. Patients with controlled blood pressure and normal investigations can be managed on outpatient basis. She should follow weekly in ANC OPD and should be explained about the importance of daily BP measurement at home and symptoms suggestive of end organ damage (blurring of vision, headache, epigastric pain) in which case they should immediately report to the hospital. The management of gestational hypertension is as follows:

Table 2: Management of gestational hypertension in pregnancy

Antihypertensive treatment	• Start oral labetalol as first line drug if BP ≥150/100 mm Hg • Aim is to keep diastolic BP between 80–100 mm Hg and systolic BP <150 mm Hg
BP measurement	At least twice daily
Urine albumin (Dipstick or urinary protein: creatinine ratio)	At each visit (weekly)
Blood investigations	Weekly CBC, KFT, electrolytes, serum bilirubin, transaminases
Fetal monitoring	• Daily fetal movement count • Fundal height measurement at each visit • Ultrasound for fetal growth and AFI and umbilical artery Doppler velocimetry every 3 weeks • NST weekly (The frequency of these tests may be modified based on subsequent clinical findings)

Abbreviations: BP, Blood pressure; CBC, Complete blood count; KFT, Kidney function test; AFI, Amniotic fluid index; NST, Nonstress test

Q6. When will we consider termination of pregnancy in patients with gestational hypertension?

Patients with gestational hypertension whose blood pressure is lower than 160/110 mm Hg, with or without antihypertensive treatment should be offered termination at 38 weeks of gestation if maternal and fetal surveillance remains normal.

CASE SCENARIO

A 26 years old lady, G2P1L1 with 36 weeks of period of gestation comes to casualty with complaint of headache. Her blood pressure is 170/110 mm Hg and urine albumin on dipstick is 2+. On examination fundal height is corresponding to the period of gestation and fetal heart is regular, 136 beats/minute.

Q1. What is the diagnosis?

The diagnosis of this patient is severe preeclampsia with impending eclampsia. If patient is a known case of hypertension or gives history of hypertension before 20 weeks of gestation, then it is preeclampsia superimposed on chronic hypertension. According to ACOG (2013) recommendations, preeclampsia is classified as severe when any of these findings are present:

- Systolic BP ≥160 mm Hg, or diastolic BP ≥110 mm Hg on two occasions at least 4 hours apart while the patient is on bed rest
- Thrombocytopenia (platelet count <100,000/mm^3)
- Elevated liver enzymes to twice the normal levels, severe persistant right upper quadrant or epigastric pain
- Pulmonary edema
- Progressive renal insufficiency (doubling of serum creatinine or serum creatinine >1.1 mg/dL in the absence of other renal disease)
- New-onset cerebral or visual disturbances.

Q2. What are the additional points to be noted in history and examination?

History

- Ask about headache, visual disturbances like scotoma, blurring of vision, epigastric pain or right upper quadrant pain
- History of excessive weight gain
- History of decreased urine output
- History of convulsion
- Any history of chest pain, breathlessness suggestive of pulmonary edema/impending cardiac failure.

Examination

- *Reflexes:* Brisk deep tendon reflexes occur as a result of nervous system irritability. In some cases, twitching of digits and clonus may also occur. It is unusual for preeclamptic patients to have seizures without first showing signs of nervous system irritability

- *Fundus:* Segmental vasospasm and increase in vein to artery ratio are common findings in severe preeclampsia. Presence of hemorrhage, exudates suggest chronic hypertension.

Q3. How will you manage this patient?

Our aims for the management of this patient are:
- Control of blood pressure by using antihypertensive agents
- Assessment for presence of risk factors for convulsions, i.e altered sensorium, headache, visual disturbances, epigastric or right upper quadrant pain
- Assessment for the presence of end organ damage and HELLP syndrome with the help of investigations
- Assessment of fetal well-being and maturity
- Termination of pregnancy with least possible trauma to the mother and the fetus.

To control blood pressure, intravenous labetalol in 20 mg dose is given followed by 40 mg → 80 mg → 80 mg after every 15–20 minutes till control of BP or maximum dose of 220 mg. Once blood pressure control is achieved, patient is started on oral labetalol or methyldopa or nifedipine. Investigations as discussed above are sent. Hourly BP monitoring and urine output charting is done. Magnesium sulfate prophylaxis for seizure prevention is started and as patient is at 36 weeks period of gestation, an immediate delivery is planned. If cervix is favorable (Bishop's score >6) amniotomy followed by oxytocin is used. If cervix is unfavorable (Bishop's score <6), *prostaglandin* E2 (PGE2) gel intracervically is inserted for cervical ripening.

Q4. What is the role of expectant management in severe preeclampsia? What are the indications of delivery in a patient with preeclampsia with severe features on expectant management?

Although definitive treatment for severe preeclampsia is the delivery of the fetus, expectant management has been tried in women remote from term without compromising maternal condition for better fetal outcome. It is useful between 28 to 34 weeks of gestation in a tertiary care center with intensive maternal and fetal monitoring. Antihypertensive agents are given for blood pressure control and a course of antenatal corticosteroids is given for fetal lung maturity. Prophylactic anticonvulsant therapy with magnesium sulfate may be required. Prompt delivery is indicated in the following conditions:

Maternal Indications
- Persistent severe headache or visual changes
- Uncontrolled hypertension despite maximum dose of two antihypertensive drugs

Table 3: Management of preeclampsia

	Preeclampsia without severe features	*Preeclampsia with severe features*
Admission to hospital	Yes	Yes
Antihypertensive treatment	• Oral labetalol is used as first line drug if BP ≥150/100 mm Hg • Aim is to keep diastolic BP between 80–100 mm Hg and systolic BP <150 mm Hg	• Oral labetalol is used as first line drug • Aim is to keep diastolic BP between 80–100 mm Hg and systolic BP <150 mm Hg
BP measurement	4 times a day	More than 4 times a day depending on clinical circumstances
Blood investigations	CBC, KFT, electrolytes, serum bilirubin, transaminases weekly	CBC, KFT, electrolytes, serum bilirubin, transaminases three times a week. Coagulation profile if platelet count is abnormal
Fetal monitoring	• Daily fetal movement count • Monitor symphysis fundal height and abdominal girth • Ultrasound for fetal growth, AFI and umbilical artery Doppler velocimetry every 2 weeks • NST twice weekly	
Delivery	At 37 weeks or earlier in case of: • Development of severe hypertension or eclampsia • HELLP syndrome • Abruptio placentae • Fetal growth restriction	At 34 weeks or earlier in case of maternal or fetal compromise • Magnesium sulfate prophylaxis should be given for seizure prevention • Corticosteroid therapy if delivery < 34 weeks

Abbreviations: BP, blood pressure; CBC, complete blood count; KFT, kidney function test; NST, nonstress test; HELLP, hemolysis elevated liver enzymes and low platelets, AFI, amniotic fluid index

- Progressive renal insufficiency (serum creatinine >1.1 mg/dL or doubling of serum creatinine in absence of other renal disease)
- Elevated liver enzymes with persistent severe epigastric pain or right upper quadrant pain
- Persistent thrombocytopenia or HELLP syndrome
- Eclampsia
- Pulmonary edema
- Abruptio placentae.

Fetal Indications
- Severe fetal growth restriction [estimated fetal weight (EFW) <5th percentile]
- Persistant oligohydramnios (maximum vertical pocket <2 cm)
- Reversed or absent umbilical artery end-diastolic flow
- Biophysical profile ≤4 on atleast two occasions 6 hours apart
- Recurrent variable or late decelerations during nonstress test (NST).

Q5. What are the different antihypertensive drugs used in pregnancy?

The objective of antihypertensive therapy is to prevent severe hypertension and associated maternal complications such as cerebrovascular hemorrhage and left ventricular failure. The role of antihypertensive therapy in mild to-moderate hypertension is controversial and is not recommended. Antihypertensive therapy may decrease progression to severe hypertension in such cases but overall maternal benefit is small and serious impairment of fetal growth can occur. National Institute of Health and Clinical Excellence (NICE) guidelines recommend treatment at BP levels of 150 mm Hg systolic and 100 mm Hg diastolic, or both.[3]

- *Labetalol (alpha-1 and nonselective beta blocker):* First line drug for management of hypertension in pregnancy. It acts by decreasing peripheral vascular resistance (PVR). The alpha to beta blockade ratio is 3:1 when given orally and 1 : 7 when given intravenously.
  - The drug is given intravenously for hypertensive emergencies in patients with severe preeclampsia. 20 mg initial dose, followed by 40–80 mg every 15–20 minutes until the therapeutic response is achieved. Maximum dose per treatment cycle is 220 mg.
  - When used orally, the initial dose is 100 mg twice daily which may be increased according to the patient's response to a maximum dose of 2400 mg/day
- *Methyldopa (Centrally acting adrenergic agonist):* Methyldopa induces the synthesis of alpha-methylnorepinephrine which stimulates alpha receptors and decrease the sympathetic outflow from central nervous system which reduces systemic vascular resistance. Its maximum effect is reached in 4–6 hours and its duration of action is 8 hours.
  - The usual starting dose is 250 mg thrice a day. The drug may be given up to a maximum of dose of 2 g/day
  - Postural hypotension, depression and excessive sedation are the common side effects. Positive Coomb's test and abnormal liver function tests are also reported.
- *Nifedipine (Calcium channel blocker):* It impedes the influx of calcium into vascular smooth muscle cells causing vascular relaxation and decrease in PVR.
  - It can be used in acute hypertensive situations, 10 mg initial oral dose followed by repeat dose if necessary after 30 minutes
  - The usual oral dose is 10–30 mg orally every 6 hours and can be increased to 20 mg every 4 hours up to a maximum of 90 mg/day
  - Facial flushing and headache are the common side effects
  - Sublingual nifedipine is contraindicated, as it causes sudden maternal hypotension and fetal distress due to placental hypoperfusion
- *Hydralazine (Peripheral vasodilator)*
  - In patients with hypertensive crisis, the drug is given as 5–10 mg IV and can be repeated after 15–20 minutes till desired BP level is attained. The maximum dose is 30 mg per treatment cycle.
  - Its side effects are tachycardia, hypotension, palpitations and it may cause uteroplacental insufficiency leading to fetal heart decelerations due to rapid fall in BP
- *Diuretics:* Potent loop diuretics cause depletion of intravascular volume, which is often already reduced in pregnancy induced hypertension and can further compromise placental perfusion. Therefore, diuretics are not used to lower blood pressure before delivery.[8] Diuretics during pregnancy are only given for the management of heart failure and pulmonary edema.

Q6. What is the mechanism of action of magnesium sulfate and what are the different regimens for prevention and treatment of seizure activity in patients with severe preeclampsia?

Mechanism of Action of Magnesium Sulfate
- Reducing presynaptic release of neurotransmitter glutamate
- Blocking glutamatergic N-methyl-D-aspartate receptors

- Increased mitochondrial calcium buffering and blockage of calcium entry through voltage gated channels
- Enhancement of adenosine action.

Various Regimens of Magnesium Sulfate

- *Pritchard regimen*
  - **Loading dose:** Magnesium sulfate 4 g is given IV slowly over 3–4 minutes as 20 mL of 20% solution, followed by 5 g in each buttock intramuscularly as 10 mL of 50% solution
  - **Maintenance dose:** Magnesium sulfate 5 g is given intramuscularly in alternate buttock 4 hourly as 10 mL of 50% solution. The following should be monitored before administration of maintenance dose:
    - Deep tendon reflexes
    - Urine output should be more than 30 mL/h
    - Respiratory rate should be >14/minute.

  Therapeutic level of magnesium is 4–7 mEq/L. Depression of patellar reflex occurs at serum levels of 8–10 mEq/L and is the earliest sign of magnesium toxicity. Respiratory depression occurs at serum levels of 12–14 mEq/L and cardiac arrest occurs at 25–30 mEq/L. If respiratory depression develops, stop magnesium sulfate and give calcium gluconate 10%, 10 mL IV slowly over 3 minutes. Magnesium sulfate is discontinued 24 hours after delivery or last seizure, whichever is late.

- *Zuspan regimen:* Loading dose of 4 g magnesium sulfate IV followed by IV infusion of 1 g/hour until 24 hours after delivery
- *Sibai regimen:* This regimen has been recommended by recent ACOG (2013) guidelines as it gives reliable blood magnesium levels and there is no risk of gluteal abscess. A loading dose of 6 g magnesium sulfate is given IV over 15–20 minutes followed by 2 gm/hour IV infusion as maintainence dose.
- *Dhaka regimen:* In this regimen a loading dose of 4 g magnesium sulfate is given IV over 15 minutes followed by 3 g magnesium sulfate intramuscularly 4 hourly in each buttock. This regimen is suitable for south-east Asian women with smaller body habitus and magnesium toxicity is lower. It is also useful in women with jeopardized renal function.

Q7. What is the etiopathogenesis of preeclampsia?

Abnormal Trophoblastic Invasion

Preeclampsia is a two stage disorder which includes "maternal and placental preeclampsia".

- Stage 1 is caused by incomplete trophoblastic invasion of spiral arteries with failure of secondary wave and deficient blood supply to the placenta.
- Stage 2 includes the effects of placental ischemia on both mother and the fetus. Diminished perfusion and a hypoxic environment lead to release of placental debris into the maternal circulation, thereby inciting systemic inflammatory response.

Immunological Factors

Dysregulation or loss of maternal immune tolerance to paternally derived placental and fetal antigens has also been implicated in the etiology of preeclampsia. Tolerance dysregulation also explains greater risk associated with increase in paternal antigenic load, that is, with two sets of paternal chromosome—a "double dose". For example, women with molar pregnancies have a higher incidence of early onset preeclampsia.

Endothelial Cell Activation

In response to worsening hypoxia at the uteroplacental interface, excessive amounts of antiangiogenic factors like soluble Fms-like tyrosine kinase 1 and soluble endoglin are generated. These along with other inflammatory mediators like interleukins (IL) and TNF alpha provoke endothelial cell injury. Cytokines like TNF alpha and interleukins also contribute to the oxidative stress by formation of free radicals and self-propagating lipid peroxides that injure endothelial cells, modify their nitric oxide production and interfere with prostaglandin balance. There is activation of microvascular coagulation manifesting as thrombocytopenia and increased capillary permeability manifesting as edema and proteinuria. Endothelial activation causes vasospasm with increased resistance and subsequent hypertension. Diminished blood flow leads to ischemia of the surrounding tissues leading to necrosis, hemorrhage and end-organ damage.

Genetic Factors

Preeclampsia is a multifactorial, polygenic disorder. There is 20–40% risk of preeclampsia in daughters of preeclamptic mother, 11–37% risk in sisters of preeclamptic women and 22–47% risk in twin sisters.[9]

Q8. What are the different organ systems involved in preeclampsia?

Cardiovascular System

Preeclampsia is characterized by contracted plasma volume and hemoconcentration. Hemoconcentration occurs as a result of generalized vasoconstriction that follows endothelial activation and leakage of plasma into interstitial space. Cardiac preload is decreased and there is decreased cardiac output due to increased peripheral resistance. Ventricular remodeling may occur leading to diastolic dysfunction in 40% of the cases.[10] Central venous pressure and pulmonary wedge pressure is reduced in preeclamptic women.

Hematological Changes

Most women with preeclampsia and eclampsia have normal coagulation profile. Thrombocytopenia is the most common hematological abnormality. Microangiopathic hemolytic anemia may occur due to increased erythrocyte destruction. There is increased factor VIII consumption, increased levels of D-dimers and of fibrinopeptides A and B and decreased levels of regulatory proteins—protein C, protein S and antithrombin III, but these aberrations are mild and seldom clinically significant.

Volume Homeostasis

Endothelial injury leads to expansion in extracellular fluid causing edema in patients with preeclampsia. In addition to edema and proteinuria, these women have reduced plasma oncotic pressure leading to further displacement of intravascular fluid into extravascular space. The levels of rennin, aldosterone and angiotensin II are increased in normal pregnancy but in patients with preeclampsia their concentrations are reduced to nonpregnant levels. Levels of vasopressin are normal and levels of atrial natriuretic peptide are increased in patients with preeclampsia.

Kidney

Due to reversible anatomical and pathophysiological renal changes occurring in patients with preeclampsia, renal perfusion and glomerular filtration is reduced and there is increase in blood urea, serum creatinine and proteinuria. There is glomerular enlargement. Endothelial cells are swollen, termed as glomerular capillary endotheliosis which block the capillary lumen. Subendothelial deposits of proteins and fibrin like material are also seen. Preeclampsia is associated with hyperuricemia due to reduced glomerular filtration and enhanced tubular reabsorption. In severe cases, acute tubular necrosis may occur leading to acute renal failure manifesting as oliguria and azotemia.

Liver

Due to vasospasm, endothelial damage, vasoconstriction and intravascular coagulation, various hepatic changes occur which include subcapsular and periportal hemorrhages, periportal fibrin deposition and areas of infraction and necrosis. Hemorrhages in the liver may extend beneath the Glisson's capsule causing subcapsular hematoma formation. In more severe cases hepatic rupture may also occur. Hepatic changes are seen in 10% cases of severe preeclampsia and are more common in presence of HELLP syndrome.

Brain

The changes in brain mainly affect the posterior hemisphere and following abnormalities have been identified:
- Intracerebral hemorrhage, hemorrhage in ventricles, cortical and subcortical petechial hemorrhages
- Cerebral edema
- Cerebral infracts and hemorrhages and infracts in basal ganglia.

With imaging studies, the changes are referred to as posterior reversible encephalopathy syndrome (PRES). The most frequently affected region is the parietiooccipital cortex and in most cases these lesions are reversible.

Visual Changes

Blurring of vision, diplopia and scotomata are common in patients with severe preeclampsia and eclampsia. Blindness is less common and reversible. It may occur due to vasogenic edema in occipital lobe. Blindness from retinal lesions is caused by retinal detachment or retinal infarction termed as Purtscher's retinopathy.

Uteroplacental Perfusion

There is vasospasm of uteroplacental vessels in preeclampsia leading to increased perinatal morbidity and mortality by causing fetal growth restriction, placental infraction, abruptio placentae and iatrogenic prematurity. Histopathological studies of placenta in preeclamptic women demonstrate areas of acute red and white infracts on maternal surface of placenta. Microscopic examination of villi shows excessive proliferation of cytotrophoblasts, syncytial degeneration, thickening of basement layer and end arteritis.

Q9. How can you identify a woman at risk of developing preeclampsia?

Prediction of preeclampsia may help in stratifying women into high risk category so that prophylactic therapies can be initiated and surveillance can be intensified. However, none of these tests are reliable in clinical practice for use as a screening test.

Uterine Artery Doppler Velocimetry

Uterine artery Doppler velocimetry at 22–24 weeks is useful to identify women at risk of early onset preeclampsia. Increased resistance to flow within the uterine arteries due to faulty trophoblastic invasion of the spiral arteries results in an abnormal waveform characterized by the presence of early diastolic notching (unilateral or bilateral) or pulsatility index above 95th percentile. These pregnancies are associated with six-fold increase in risk of preeclampsia.[11] Abnormal uterine artery Doppler has a sensitivity of 20–60% for predicting preeclampsia.

Provocative Pressor Tests

These tests assess blood pressure increase in response to a stimulus. The *roll-over test* measures hypertensive response in women at 28–32 weeks when she rolls over from left lateral decubitus position to the supine position. A positive test is considered as an elevation of 20 mm Hg or more in blood pressure. The *isometric exercise test* employs the same principle by squeezing a handball. The *angiotensin II infusion test* is performed by giving increasing doses intravenously, and hypertensive response is quantified. The sensitivities of all three tests range from 55 to 70% and specificity around 85%.

Mean arterial pressure (systolic+2 (diastolic)/3)(MAP)>90 mm Hg in second trimester is also one of the predictors of preeclampsia but it has low sensitivity and low positive predictive values.

Endothelial Dysfunction and Oxidant Stress

- *Fibronectin:* These high molecular weight glycoproteins are released from extracellular matrix and endothelial cells following endothelial injury. Patients with preeclampsia have elevated levels of plasma fibronectin.
- *Elevated serum homocysteine levels:* Hyperhomocysteinemia causes endothelial cell dysfunction and oxidative stress and is characteristic of preeclampsia. Although four-fold increased risk of preeclampsia was found in women with elevated serum homocysteine levels, these tests have not been shown to be clinically useful.
- Increased *soluble fms-like tyrosine kinase receptor-1* (sflt-1), decreased *placental growth factor* (PLGF) are other markers for prediction of preeclampsia.

Fetoplacental Unit Endocrine Dysfunction

Raised **Human chorionic gonadotropin (hCG), alpha-fetoprotein (AFP), placental protein-13**, low **Pregnancy-associated plasma protein (PAPPA)** and low **Inhibin - A** may also help in prediction of preeclampsia.

Tests of Renal Function

Urinary calcium: Hypocalciuria occurs early and persists throughout pregnancy in women with preeclampsia. Urinary calcium concentration ≤12 mg/dL in a 24 hour collection has positive and negative predictive values of 85 and 91% respectively for diagnosis of preeclampsia. Determination of calcium/creatinine ratio in a random urine sample is as accurate as 24-hour urine collection. In preeclampsia the ratio is less than 0.03.

Preeclampsia is associated with **microalbuminuria** and **hyperuricemia**. Hyperuricemia occurs due to reduced uric acid clearance from diminished glomerular filtration, increased tubular reabsorption and decreased secretion. It has sensitivity of 0–55% and specificity of 77–95%.

Others

Antithrombin III, cell-free fetal DNA.

Q10. What are the various strategies for prevention of preeclampsia?

Strategies to prevent preeclampsia have been studied extensively but no intervention has been proved to be effective.

Antiplatelet Agents

Preeclampsia is characterized by increase in thromboxane production and decrease in prostacyclin levels leading to vasoconstriction and platelet aggregation. Low dose aspirin irreversibly inhibits platelets thromboxane production but has minimal effects on vascular prostacyclin production. NICE recommends 75 mg aspirin daily to all women at moderate to high-risk for developing preeclampsia from 12 weeks to the birth of the baby.

Antioxidant Supplementation

Imbalance between oxidant and antioxidant activity may play an important role in the pathogenesis of preeclampsia. Thus, naturally occurring antioxidants like vitamin C and E may help in prevention of preeclampsia. However, large randomized, placebo-controlled trials did not find any benefit and administration of vitamin C and E for prevention of preeclampsia is not recommended.

Calcium

Calcium supplementation reduces the risk of preeclampsia in women with a diet deficient in calcium and is recommended in a dose of 1.5 g/day for prevention of preeclampsia in women with low calcium intake.

Dietary Salt Intake

Guidelines do not recommend salt restriction during pregnancy for prevention of preeclampsia

Lifestyle Modifications

It is suggested that restriction of physical activity or bed rest should not be used for prevention of preeclampsia.

Q11. What is the criterion for diagnosis of HELLP syndrome and what is the management?

The term HELLP syndrome is an acronym for the following presentation: Hemolysis, elevated liver enzymes and low platelet count.[12]

Hemolysis

- Abnormal peripheral blood smear (schistocytes, burr cells)
- Elevated bilirubin ≥1.2g/dL
- Low serum haptoglobin
- Raised serum LDH >600U/L (twice the upper limit of normal).

Elevated Liver Enzymes

Elevated AST, ALT > 40 IU/L.

Low Platelet Count (<150,000/mm^3)

The Mississippi classification categorizes the severity of HELLP syndrome into three categories according to maternal platelet count.[13]

- Class I (severe thrombocytopenia): Platelet count <50,000/mm^3, AST or ALT >70 IU/L, LDH >600 IU/L
- Class II (moderate thrombocytopenia): Platelet between 50,000 and 100,000/mm^3, AST or ALT >70 IU/L, LDH >600 IU/L
- Class III (mild thrombocytopenia): Platelet count between 1lakh and 1.5 lakh/mm^3, AST or ALT >40 IU/L, LDH >600IU/L.

Tennessee classification classifies HELLP syndrome into complete if all the three parameters are abnormal and incomplete or partial syndrome if one or two of the three parameters are abnormal.[14]

Differential Diagnosis

Idiopathic thrombocytopenic conditions, hemolytic uremic syndrome, viral hepatitis, acute fatty liver of pregnancy, renal disease, gallbladder disease and hyperemesis gravidarum.

Management

HELLP is associated with 1% risk of maternal mortality. Most of these deaths are due to acute renal failure, abruptio placentae, pulmonary edema and disseminated intravascular coagulation (DIC). Perinatal morbidity and mortality are also significantly increased due to prematurity, growth restriction and abruptio placentae. The diagnosis of HELLP syndrome is an indication for immediate delivery after 34 weeks of gestation or at any gestational age if pulmonary edema, renal failure, severe liver dysfunction, placental abruption, nonreassuring fetal status or uncontrolled hypertension is present. For women <34 weeks of gestation delivery may be delayed for 24-48 hours to complete a course of corticosteroids for fetal benefit if maternal and fetal condition remain stable. Platelet transfusion may be required for a platelet count less than 50,000/mm^3. Careful monitoring of input/output, periodic auscultation of lungs and pulse oximetry is necessary for assessment of pulmonary and renal condition. Data on maternal benefits of dexamethasone in patients with HELLP syndrome are conflicting and at present corticosteroids are not recommended for treatment of HELLP syndrome.

Q12. How do we manage a patient with eclampsia?

The basic principles of management are:
- Control of convulsion
- Control of hypertension
- Immediate delivery.

The first step is to maintain cardiorespiratory function and prevent maternal injury. Bedside rails should be elevated and patient is placed in lateral decubitus position to prevent aspiration. Padded tongue blade should be inserted between teeth to avoid injury to the tongue and oral secretions should be suctioned if needed to keep the airway clean. Oxygen should be supplemented by face mask at 8-10 L/minute. Magnesium sulfate is the drug of choice for control of convulsions. It should be continued till 24 hours after delivery or 24 hours after the last convulsion.

Antihypertensive should be used for blood pressure control. Labetalol is the first line antihypertensive drug followed by nifedipine. After inital stabilization of the patient, delivery should be planned. After a seizure, labor often ensues spontaneously, progresses fast or can be induced successfully. If cervix is favorable (Bishop's score >6) amniotomy followed by oxytocin is used. If cervix is unfavorable (Bishop's score <6), PGE2 gel intracervically is used. Cesarean section is done for obstetric indications like transverse lie, placenta previa or in the presence of prolonged fetal bradycardia, fetal growth restriction (FGR), unripe cervix, poor progress in labor, uncontrolled blood pressure and uncontrolled convulsions.

Q13. What is the risk of recurrence of hypertensive disorders of pregnancy?

- A woman who had gestational hypertension has 16-47% risk of developing gestational hypertension in future pregnancy and 2-7% risk of developing preeclampsia in future
- In women with preeclampsia in first pregnancy, the risk of recurrence is 16% in future pregnancy
- The risk of recurrence of HELLP syndrome ranges from 5-26% in subsequent pregnancy
- The risk of recurrence of eclampsia is 1.4%.

Q14. What is the risk of developing chronic hypertension in future?

The incidence of chronic hypertension is significantly increased, 5.2-fold in patients who had gestational hypertension, 3.5-fold after preeclampsia without severe features and 6.4-fold after severe preeclampsia.

CASE SCENARIO

A 36 years old lady comes to antenatal OPD with first trimester pregnancy with history of hypertension being treated with enalapril (ACE inhibitor).

Q1. How will you manage?

Enalapril belongs to angiotensin converting enzyme inhibitors group and causes cardiovascular and central nervous system (CNS) malformations and abnormal renal development in fetus. They also cause fetal growth restriction and maldevelopment of calvaria. These drugs should be stopped and patient should be admitted for inital work-up and blood pressure monitoring. Since there is spontaneous reduction in blood pressure in early second trimester, this patient may not require any antihypertensive drug. However, if BP is still high, this patient can be started on antihypertensives safe in pregnancy like labetalol or methyldopa.

Q2. What are the complications expected in this patient and what modified management besides those discussed earlier is needed?

Maternal Complications

- Superimposed preeclampsia
- Abruptio placentae
- Malignant hypertension
- Renal damage
- Cerebrovascular accidents.

Fetal Complications

- Fetal growth restriction
- Intrauterine death
- Prematurity.

Management

Preconceptionally these patients should be assessed for the severity of hypertension and renal function tests (or other organ specific tests in other causes of secondary hypertension). These associated medical conditions must be controlled before conception. One must look for structural defects in fetus if mother has been exposed to fetotoxic drugs early in pregnancy. Ultrasonography (USG) at 18–20 weeks must be done to rule out gross congenital anomalies. Patients are seen regularly in antenatal clinic and their BP and renal function are checked regularly. Blood pressure should be controlled with the help of labetalol, methyldopa or nifedipine. Any evidence of fetal growth restriction and superimposed preeclampsia must be looked for and managed.

REFERENCES

1. Khan KS, Wojdyla D, Say L, et al. WHO analysis of causes of maternal death: a systematic review. Lancet. 2006;367:1066.
2. Sibai BM, Hauth J, Caritis S, et al. Hypertensive disorders in twin versus singleton gestations. Am J Obstet Gynecol. 2000;182:938.
3. National Institute of Health and Clinical Excellence. Hypertension in pregnancy: The management of hypertensive disorders during pregnancy, CG No 107. London: National Institute of Health and Clinical excellence, 2010.
4. Scholten RR, Hopman MT, Sweep FC, et al. Co-occurrence of cardiovascular and prothrombotic risk factors in women with a history of preeclampsia. Obstet Gynecol. 2013;121(1):97.
5. Kraus D, Fent L, Heine RP, et al. Smoking and preeclampsia protection: cigarette smoke increases placental adrenomedullin expression and improves trophoblast invasion via the adrenomedullin pathway. Am J Obstet Gynecol. 2013;208(1):S26.
6. Cunningham FG, Leveno KJ, Hauth JC, Bloom SL, Rouse DJ, Spong CY. Pregnancy Hypertension.L. Williams Obstetrics. 23rd edition. New York: Mc Graw Hill Medical Publishing Division; 2010;705-56.
7. Podymow T, August P. Update on the use of antihypertensive drugs in pregnancy. Hypertension 2008;51;960-9.
8. Zeeman GG, Cunningham FG, Pritchard JA. The magnitude of hemoconcentration with eclampsia. Hypertens Pregnancy. 2009;28(2):127.
9. Ward K, Taylor RN. Genetic factors in the etiology of preeclampsia. In: Taylor RN, Roberts JM, Cunningham FG (Eds). Chesley's hypertensive disorders in pregnancy, 4th edition Amsterdam, Academic Press; 2014.
10. Melchiorre K, Sutherland G, Watt-Coote I, et al. Severe myocardial impairment and chamber dysfunction in preterm preeclampsia. Hpertens Pregnancy 2012;31(4):454.
11. Papageorghiou AT, Leslie K. Uterine artery Doppler in the prediction of adverse pregnancy outcome. Curr Opin Obstet Gynecol. 2007;19:103-7.
12. Weinstein L. Syndrome of hemolysis, elevated liver enzymes, and low platelet count: a severe consequence of hypertension in pregnancy. Am J Obstet Gynecol. 1982;142:159-67.
13. Martin-JN J, Magann EF, Blake PG. Analysis of 454 pregnancies with severe preeclampsia/eclampsia/ HELLP syndrome using the 3-class system of classification. Am J Obstet Gynecol. 1993;68:386-91.
14. Audibert F, Friedman SA, Frangieh AY, et al. Clinical utility of strict diagnostic criteria for the HELLP (hemolysis, elevated liver enzymes, and low platelets) syndrome. Am J Obstet Gynecol. 1996;175:460-4.

3
CHAPTER

Diabetes in Pregnancy

Krishna Agarwal, Aastha Raheja

CASE SCENARIO

Mrs X w/o Mr Y, 34 years old, a resident of Mustafabad, Delhi.
Gravida 5 Para 2 Live 2 Abortion 2
LMP: 13th November 2016, EDD: 20th August 2017, POG: 35 weeks 6 days.

Presenting Complaints

- Eight and a half months of amenorrhea.
- Admitted from antenatal clinic in view of high blood sugars and presence of sugar in urine.

History of Presenting Complaints

Patient first visited our hospital at 4 months of pregnancy in antenatal clinic. Patient was advised admission in view of presence of sugar in urine but did not get admitted and did not come for follow up. Second visit was at 8 ½ months of pregnancy when she was found to have increased blood sugar and was admitted in labour room.

- No history of excessive hunger, thirst or increased frequency of micturition.
- No history suggestive of recurrent urinary tract infections. No history of vaginal discharge.
- No history suggestive of skin infections.

History of Present Pregnancy

First Trimester

- Pregnancy was diagnosed by urine pregnancy test done at one month after the missed period.
- Had 2 antenatal visits at dispensary.
  - Took folic acid tablets
  - No history of fever/rash/X-ray exposure/drug intake
  - No history of hyperemesis
  - No history of bleeding P/V
  - No USG done

Second Trimester

Patient first visited our hospital at 4th month of pregnancy in antenatal clinic. Patient was advised admission in view of presence of sugar in urine but did not get admitted and did not come for follow up.

- 2 doses of tetanus toxoid taken at 4th and 5th month of pregnancy from dispensary.
- Oral iron and calcium taken regularly.
- Quickening felt at 5th month of amenorrhea.
- No history suggestive of polyphagia/polydipsia/polyuria.
- No history of headache/blurring of vision/pedal edema/epigastric pain/decreased urine output/swelling of feet.
- No history of bleeding per vaginum (P/V) or Leaking P/V or discharge P/V
- First USG done at 20 weeks, she was told by the sonologist that the report was normal.

Third Trimester

- Fetal movements were good
- No history of headache/blurring of vision/decreased urine output/epigastric pain/swelling of feet
- No history of bleeding P/V/leaking P/V
- Patient got USG done at 8th month of pregnancy and was told by the sonologist that liquor was increased, otherwise baby was alright
- Patient visited antenatal clinic at 8 ½ months amenorrhea when she was found to have increased blood sugar and was admitted in labor room.

Menstrual History

Cycles regular, no history of prolonged cycles.

Obstetrical History

G4P3L3

- Married for 13 years
- First pregnancy—11 years ago, booked pregnancy at district hospital, had a normal vaginal delivery (NVD), male child, birth weight 3.1 kgs, alive and healthy, no antepartum, intrapartum and postpartum complications.
- Second pregnancy—10 years ago, booked pregnancy at district hospital, NVD, male child, birthweight 3.2 kg, alive and healthy, no antepartum, intrapartum or postpartum complications.
- Third pregnancy and fourth pregnancy—She had two missed abortions, 3 and 4 years back, around two and a half month amenorrhea, diagnosed on USG, terminated medically.
- Patient had blood test for sugar and thyroid and was normal.

Past History

No history suggestive of tuberculosis/hypertension/thyroid illness or any prolonged surgical or medical illness.

Personal History

Normal sleep pattern. Normal bowel and bladder habits. No addictions.

Dietary History (24-Hour Recall Method)

- Calorie intake 2000 kcal/day
- Protein intake 70 gm/day
- Started on medical nutrition therapy/diabetic diet (MNT) with calorie intake of 1600 kcal since 3 days.

Family History

Not significant.

Socioeconomic History

Lower middle class family by modified Kuppuswamy scale.

General Examination

- Patient is conscious, cooperative, well-oriented in time, place and person
- *Height:* 152 cm
- *Weight:* 65 kg
- Body mass index could not be calculated as pre-pregnancy weight is not known
- General condition fair
- Hydration adequate
- Afebrile
- *PR:* 84/min in right radial artery, regular, rhythmic, good in volume, normal in character and bilaterally synchronous. No radio-radial or radio-femoral delay. All peripheral pulses were palpable.
- *BP:* 110/70 mm/Hg in right arm in sitting position
- *RR:* 16/min
- No pallor, icterus, cyanosis
- Orodental hygiene well maintained. No signs of nutritional deficiency
- No thyromegaly or dilated veins over the neck. No peripheral lymphadenopathy
- No clubbing/pedal edema
- Bilateral breast shows normal changes of pregnancy nipple areola complex is normal. No lump palpable
- *Respiratory system:* B/L air entry is equal, no added sounds
- *Cardiovascular system:* S1 and S2 is normal, no murmur, no added sounds.

Abdominal Examination

Inspection

- Abdomen is uniformly distended
- All quadrants moving well with respiration
- No dilated veins, scars
- Umbilicus central flat
- Striae gravidarum and linea nigra seen
- All hernial sites free.

Palpation

- Local temperature is not raised
- Abdomen is uniformly distended
- *Fundal height:* 36 weeks
- *Symphysio-fundal height:* 36 cm
- *Abdominal girth:* 36 inches

Grips

- *Fundal grip:* Soft broad irregular mass felt suggestive of breech
- *Right lateral grip:* Multiple knobby structures on right side suggestive of limbs
- *Left lateral grip:* Smooth curved structure on left side suggestive of back
- *Superficial pelvic grip:* Hard, round, globular mass felt suggestive of head, ballotable
- *Deep pelvic grip:* Converging: s/o non-engaged head

- Liquor appears to be adequate, estimated fetal weight is 2.6–2.8 kg
- FHS: Left spinoumbilical line, 136 bpm.

Per Speculum Examination

Cervix and vagina healthy, no abnormal discharge.

Diagnosis

G4P2L2A2 with 35 $^{+6}$ weeks of gestation with diabetes mellitus type 2.

Q1. Why do you label it as type 2 diabetes mellitus?

Since the patient presented with presence of sugar in urine in early pregnancy and with grossly deranged blood sugar values, it is high likely to be type 2 diabetes mellitus.

Q2. What investigations you will do?

- **Routine antenatal investigations**
  - Blood grouping and Rh typing, hemoglobin, hematocrit
  - VDRL, HIV, HbsAg, urine routine and culture.
- **Investigations specific for diabetes mellitus:**
  - 7 value blood sugar profile would be done one week after 5–10 days of starting diabetic diet.
  - If GTT is grossly deranged and gestation is more than 32 weeks then it should be done after 3 days of diabetic diet
  - Liver and kidney function tests
  - Fundoscopy
  - Glycosylated hemoglobin (HbA1c)
  - 24-hour urinary protein.
- **USG level II for biometry, liquor, placenta and gross congenital abnormalities.**

Q3. How will you manage this patient?

Maternal Monitoring

Patient should be started on diabetic diet (MNT) and advised isometric exercises. Blood sugar profile should be done after one week of diet.

- *Medical nutrition therapy:* Ideal dietary composition should consist of daily total calorie out of which 50–60% is contributed by carbohydrate, 20% by protein and 25% by fat, of which less than 10% is saturated fat.[1]

Table 1: Caloric requirement as per pre-pregnancy BMI

Pre-pregnancy BMI (kg/m^2)	Calories (kcal/kg/day)
<18.4	35
18.5–24.9	30
25–30	25

It is advisable to take three major and three minor meals so that there is no intermittent hypoglycemia.

Diabetic diet of 1600 kcal would be started for this patient as patient's height is 152 cm and weight of 65 kg and the BMI calculated is 28.1 kg/m^2 which comes out to be 25 kcal/kg/day.

- *Exercise:* Moderate physical activity for 30 minutes/day is recommended for all pregnant individuals. Exercise in conjunction with diet improves blood glucose control and reduces the need for insulin.[2]
- *Sugar profile:* Sugar profile (fasting, 2 hours post meals—post breakfast, post lunch and post dinner) would be done for the patient and if deranged she should be started on insulin and seven sample profile should be done (fasting, pre-meals, post-meals and 2 a.m.). Ideally sugar charting should be done after 1 week of diabetic diet but since the patient is near term therefore it should be done after 3 days.

Fetal Monitoring

- USG for fetal growth is done to detect macrosomia or FGR (diabetic vasculopathy).
- USG level II to rule out gross congenital abnormalities.
- Doppler velocimetry is done if FGR is present.
- Biophysical profile/non-stress test would be done twice weekly especially in patients with FGR with abnormal umbilical artery Doppler, increased BP records or suboptimal control of diabetes or vasculopathy.

Q4. With this profile of the patient what treatment you would start?

Since the women is near term with uncontrolled diabetes, insulin therapy would be started to achieve adequate and faster glycemic control.

Q5. Which insulin you would start and what is the aim?

Normally 3 or 4 divided doses of short acting insulin before each meal and 1 or 2 long or intermediate acting insulin per day is preferred.

However, usually 2 long acting or intermediate acting, one before breakfast and one before dinner is given as compliance is better.

Table 2: Target plasma glucose levels with insulin[1]

Fasting	60–90 mg/dL
Pre-meal	< 100 mg/dL
1 hour postprandial	<140 mg/dL
2 hour postprandial	<120 mg/dL
2 a.m.	60–120 mg/dL

(1 unit of insulin takes care of 30 mg rise in blood sugar levels in gm %)

- In type 1 diabetes mellitus generally requirement is 0.9 U/kg in first trimester, 1 U/kg in second trimester and 1.2 U/kg in third trimester. In type 2 diabetes mellitus requirement is 0.9 U/kg, 1.2 U/kg and 1.6 U/kg respectively.[3]
- In GDM patient requirement is 0.7–1 U/kg/day
- If insulin is planned start with regular insulin which is given before three major meals and once the daily total requirement is known, it is divided into 2/3rd morning dose and 1/3rd evening dose of long/intermediate acting insulin.

Q6. What are the preparations of insulin commonly available and used in your wards?

For GDM patients we routinely use plain insulin, mixtard and NPH.

Table 3: Types of insulin commonly used in GDM

- Plain insulin is short acting with onset of action of 30 minutes and duration of action of 6–8 hours. (*Source*: Human)
- NPH is intermediate acting insulin with onset of action of 1–2 hours and duration of action of 20–24 hours. (*Source*: Human)
- Mixtard is a combination of short acting regular and intermediate acting NPH insulin (30/70) with onset of action of 1–2 hours and duration of action of 24 hours. (*Source*: Human)
- In type 1 diabetes patients with not so good control of blood sugars even long acting insulin can be added. Insulin glargine is available with onset of action of 2 hours and duration of action of > 24 hours. (*Source*: Analog)

Different Types of Insulin Preparations

Type	Appearance	Onset (hr)	Peak (hr)	Duration (hr)
Rapid acting				
Insulin lispro	Clear	0.2–0.3	1–1.5	3–5
Insulin aspart	Clear	0.2–0.3	1–1.5	3–5
Insulin glulisine	Clear	0.2–0.4	1–2	3–5
Short acting				
Regular (soluble) insulin	Clear	0.5–1	2–3	6–8
Intermediate acting				
Insulin zinc suspension of lente	Cloudy	1–2	8–10	20–24
NPH or isophane insulin	Cloudy	1–2	8–10	20–24
Long acting				
Insulin glargine and insulin detemir	Clear	Glargine: 2–4 Detemir: 1–4	Glargine: – Detemir: –	Glargine: 24 Detemir: 201–224

Q7. What is the role of hypoglycemic agents in GDM?

The most commonly used oral hypoglycemic agents (OHA) in GDM are glibenclamide and metformin.

- Glibenclamide (Glyburide) is most common agent, belongs to sulfonylurea group of OHA. They act by increasing insulin secretion, induce better insulin sensitivity and suppress production of hepatic glucose. However, it is FDA **category B** drug and its side effects are hypoglycemia and can cause sudden intrauterine deaths near term.
  Starting dose is 2.5 mg in morning. Dose is changed every 3–5 days according to blood sugar profile. Dose is increased by 2.5 mg/week until 10 mg/day, and then switched to twice daily until maximum of 20 mg/day is reached.
- Metformin is most commonly used, belongs to biguanides group of OHA. It mainly acts on peripheral insulin sensitivity counteracting insulin resistance and it decreases hepatic glucose output. It is mainly excreted by kidneys. It is FDA **category B** drug and side effects are nausea, vomiting, flatulence and lactic acidosis. Dosage is 500–850 mg in beginning with maximum of 2000 mg/day in divided doses. About 7–20% of patients fail to achieve adequate glycemic control with diet and exercise alone, oral hypoglycemic/insulin are required for glycemic control. Both metformin and glibenclamide are effective treatment for gestational diabetes. Both cross the placenta, while no immediate safety concerns for the fetus have been demonstrated, potential long-term effects remain under investigation.

Q8. How will you monitor her sugar control when she is on insulin and what advice you will give her?

Seven times venous blood sugar testing will be done—fasting, 2 hours post-breakfast, pre-lunch, 2 hours post-lunch, pre-dinner, 2 hours post-dinner and 2 a.m.
- Patient would be explained about symptoms of hypoglycemia and to report immediately if any signs and symptoms of hypoglycemia occur.
- She is advised to keep glucose biscuits handy.

Q9. What are signs and symptoms of hypoglycemia?

Signs and symptoms of hypoglycemia include sweating, dizziness, confusion, hunger, headache, irritability, weakness, anxiety and poor concentration.

Q10. What is your plan for delivery?

Elective induction at 38 weeks would be done in this patient with diabetes controlled on insulin. It reduces the risk of shoulder dystocia from 10 to 1–4%.[4]

Q11. What will you do night prior to induction of labor and how will you monitor patients on insulin during labor?

Bedtime dose of insulin would be given. Morning dose of insulin would be omitted and fasting blood sugar levels and serum electrolytes will be done. If the cervical is unfavorable, cervical ripening with intracervical PGE2 gel would be done. Light snacks would be allowed till labor commences.

- Dextrostix and urine sugar and ketone monitoring would be done 4 hourly. CTG monitoring would be done in active labor and serum electrolytes would be monitored 12 hourly.
- Start 5 unit insulin in 500 mL of 5% dextrose at rate of 100 mL/hr once labor commences. If blood sugar >140 mg/dL, plain insulin would be given subcutaneously according to sliding scale
  - 140–180 mg%—4U
  - 180–250 mg%—8U
  - 250–400 mg%—12U
  - \>400 mg%—16U

If blood sugar is <80 mg/dL, then i would start 5% dextrose at the rate of 100 mL/hr.

Q12. What complications newborn may develop?

The newborn is at increased risk of hypoglycemia, hypocalcemia, hypomagnesemia, hyperbilirubinemia, hypothermia, polycythemia and respiratory distress syndrome. Therefore, babies of diabetic mother are kept under observation for 48–72 hours.

Q13. What contraceptive advice you would give to the patient?

I would advise her to go for postpartum CuT insertion which is MEC category 1. If she is exclusively breastfeeding then DMPA injection or progesterone only pills would be good for her and started after 3 months (MEC1). As my patient is a multiparous, sterilization would be advised after 6 weeks.

Q14. How will you monitor in postpartum period and when will you discharge her?

- In GDM, patients usually do not require insulin in postpartum period and blood sugar fasting and postprandial would be done on 3rd postpartum day and if deranged, OHA/insulin started accordingly.
- If sugars are normal on day 3, patient would be discharged and advised sugar fasting and postprandial at 6 weeks and 3 yearly assessments should be done thereafter.
- In type 2 diabetes mellitus, patients usually require no treatment as insulin requirement is reduced in postpartum period.
- Blood sugar charting is done 4 hourly and insulin is given according to sliding scale till the patient is not allowed orally (LSCS postoperative patient) and later 6 point sugar values are done and OHA/insulin started according to sugar profile.

CASE SCENARIO

A 30 years old weighing 65 kg G2P1L0 with previous one FTIUD at 9 months presented with single live fetus at 30 weeks estimated gestation age. On antenatal evaluation her GTT (Glucose tolerance test) (100 g) was deranged—109/190/160/150.

Q1. What are the screening methods of GDM?

ACOG (September 2011) recommends two-step technique—universal screening of patient history, risk factors. With 50 g one hour loading test at 24–28 weeks which if positive is followed by 100 g oral glucose tolerance test (OGTT). Diagnosis should be done on the basis of two or more positive values in 3 hours 100 g OGTT.[5]

- GCT—venous plasma glucose is measured 1 hr after administering 50 g of glucose.
- Cutoff value of >/= 140 mg/dL has a sensitivity of 80% while cutoff value of >/= 130 mg/dL has 90% sensitivity.
- GTT—The test should be performed in the morning after overnight fast of at least 8 hours but no more than 14 hours and after atleast 3 days of unrestricted diet (>150 gm of carbohydrate/day) and physical activity. The subject should remain seated and should not smoke during test.
- Two or more venous plasma glucose concentrations must be met or exceed for a positive diagnosis.

ACOG	Criteria	Fasting (mg/dL)	1 hour (mg/dL)	2 hours (mg/dL)	3 hours (mg/dL)
	Carpenter and Coustan criteria	95	180	155	140
	NDDG	105	190	165	145

Abbreviations: ACOG, The American College of Obstetricians and Gynecologists; NDDG, National Diabetes Data Group

WHO recommendation: The NICE guidelines of 2008 recommends that screening for GDM be done using risk factors in healthy population such as BMI>30 kg/m^2, previous baby>4.5 kg, first degree relative with diabetes and ethnicity. Test is done by 2 hours 75 g OGTT at 24–28 weeks. Women with previous history of gestational diabetes should be offered OGTT at 16–18 weeks and repeat testing at 24–28 weeks.[6]

WHO	Fasting (mg/dL)	2 hours (mg/dL)
75 g glucose load	≥ 126	≥ 140

American Diabetic Association (ADA) and The International Association of Diabetes and Pregnancy Study Group (IADPSD) 2011 recommends one step diagnostic 75 g 2 hours OGTT.

ADA/IADPSG	Fasting (mg/dL)	1 hour (mg/dL)	2 hours (mg/dL)
75 g glucose load	≥92	≥180	≥153

Diabetes in Pregnancy Study Group India (DIPSI)
- DIPSI recommends single step diagnostic procedure as universal screening. 75 grams glucose load is given orally irrespective of fasting status or timing of previous meal.
- GDM is diagnosed if post 2 hours blood glucose value is ≥ 140 mg/dL.
- Advantages of DIPSI are
  – It is both a screening and diagnostic procedure.
  – Patient need not to be fasting and it can be performed in the first visit of the patient and can be repeated in second and third trimester.

Q2. What pre-conceptional advice should have been given to such patient?
- Pre-conceptional counseling should be done prior to planning pregnancy to achieve optimal glycemic control. Till then contraception must be used to prevent unwanted pregnancy.
- Glucose is teratogenic at high levels and rate of congenital fetal anomalies are directly related to glycemic control in first trimester.
- Good glycemic control during organogenesis reduces rate of congenital malformations.
- Appropriate dietary measures, exercise, weight loss, drug therapy with oral hypoglycemic or insulin can help achieve optimal glycemic control. Renal, cardiovascular and retinal assessment must be done to detect end organ damage.
- All oral hypoglycemics except metformin and glibenclamide to be stopped before pregnancy and substituted by insulin.
- Other medications such as ACE inhibitors, angiotensin receptor antagonist and statins must be discontinued.

"Therapy must be targeted to achieve a pre-pregnancy HbA1c less than 6.1% (NICE guidelines, 2008). Those with HbA1c ≥10% should be advise to avoid pregnancy".

Q3. What is the effect of pregnancy on carbohydrate metabolism?
- Pregnancy is a diabetogenic state as human placental lactogen has anti-insulin and lipolytic effects.
- It increases glucose level in maternal plasma thus makes it more available to the fetus, also corticosteroids and progesterone have an anti-insulin effect.
- Some insulin is destroyed by the placenta. Thus pregnancy exacerbates the diabetic tendency of asymptomatic.[7]

Q4. What is the likely cause of IUD of previous baby in this patient?
- Patient may had preexisting diabetes/GDM in previous pregnancy which could have caused IUD.
- It may be linked to hyperglycemia mediated aberration in oxygen and fetal metabolites transport which is further accelerated by placental vasculopathy.
- Chronic hypoxia can cause sudden fetal demise.
- Another problem associated is ketoacidosis which increases the acidity of maternal blood, fetal enzymes can no longer function in high acidic environment.
- Other probable causes could be associated congenital defects or FGR.

Q5. What are the maternal complications associated with diabetes, during pregnancy?
- *Medical complications:* Diabetic ketoacidosis, hyperosmolar hyperglycemic nonketotic syndrome, infections, nephropathy, neuropathy, retinopathy, stroke, peripheral vascular disease, coronary artery disease and cardiomyopathy.
- *Obstetric complications:*
  – Antepartum—preeclampsia, preterm labor, premature rupture of membranes, polyhydramnios, chorioamnionitis.
  – Intrapartum—prolonged labor, uterine inertia, instrumental deliveries, perineal injuries, postpartum hemorrhage and cesarean section.
  – Postpartum—wound sepsis, puerperal sepsis, postpartum hemorrhage.

Q6. What is Somogyi and Dawn phenomenon?
- In early morning hours, hormones such as growth hormone, cortisol and catecholamines cause the liver to release large amount of sugar into the bloodstream. For most people, body produces insulin to control rise in blood sugar. In diabetics, body doesn't produce enough insulin causing blood sugar levels to rise in morning causing the dawn effect.
- If a diabetic person takes excess insulin at night or misses a bedtime snack, the blood sugar levels drops during night. Body responds to the low blood sugar by releasing hormones that raises the blood sugar level.

This may also present as high sugar level in morning causing the Somogyi effect.
- To sort out whether an early morning rise is caused by dawn or Somogyi phenomenon, blood sugar levels should be checked at around 2 a.m. Presence of night time hypoglycemia confirms Somogyi effect and requires reduction in dose of bedtime insulin.

Q7. When do you plan termination of pregnancy in a patient with GDM?

GDM controlled on diet or OHA can be taken up to 40 weeks awaiting spontaneous onset of labor while GDM controlled on insulin needs termination at 38 weeks of gestation.[4]

Q8. How will you manage a patient who presents to emergency after missing a dose of insulin with uneasiness, tachycardia and large urine sugar and ketones?

The patient is likely to be in diabetic ketoacidosis. Diagnosis of ketoacidosis is made when:
- Blood glucose ≥250 mg/dL but may occur at low levels in pregnancy
- Arterial pH <7.3
- Ketone bodies in blood and urine
- Serum bicarbonate <15 mEq/L
  - Cornerstone of management is vigorous rehydration with crystalloid solution of normal saline or ringer lactate.
  - Periodic monitoring of pulse, blood pressure, input and output and fetal heart to be done.
- Laboratory assessment—obtain arterial blood gases to assess degree of acidosis present, measure blood glucose, ketones and serum electrolytes at 1–2 hour intervals.
- Insulin—0.2–0.4 U/kg intravenous bolus followed by 2–10 U/hour in normal saline as maintenance dose. If the blood glucose does not drop by 30% in first 3 hours then drip rate is doubled. Once the glucose is between 200 mg/dL 250 mg/dL, normal saline is changed to 5% dextrose.
- Fluids—Severe dehydration may result in a large fluid deficit. The estimated deficit of 4–6 liters must be replaced in first 12 hours. In the first hour, 1 liter of normal saline is infused followed by 500–1000 mL/hour for 2–4 hours and then 250 mL/hour till 80% is replaced.
- Potassium—Hypokalemia generally occurs with diabetic ketoacidosis. Level of Potassium should be maintained above 5 mEq/L.
  - Below 5 mEq/L—20 to 30 mEq potassium/L iv fluid should be given
  - If levels are < 3.3 mEq/L—Insulin should be stopped and it should be started only after potassium correction.
- Bicarbonate administration is required if pH falls below 6.8.
- Antibiotics can be considered if suspicion of infection is there.

Q9. How do you manage shoulder dystocia?

- Extra help should be sought, mouth and nose of the baby should be cleared and no traction is to be applied over the baby head, fundal pressure should never be kept light as it may cause further impaction of fetal shoulder.
- Wide mediolateral episiotomy should be performed to provide adequate space posteriorly, pediatrician and anesthetist should be available.
- *Mac Robert's maneuver:* Abduct the maternal thighs and sharply flex them unto her abdomen, there is rotation of symphysis pubis upwards and decrease in angle of pelvic inclination. It straightens the sacrum in relation to lumbar vertebra.
- *Woods maneuver:* General anesthesia is administered, posterior shoulder is rotated to anterior position by cork screw movement by inserting 2 fingers in posterior vagina, simultaneous suprapubic pressure is applied, this pushes the bisacromial diameter from antero-posterior to oblique diameter which helps its easy entry to the pelvic inlet.
- *Extraction of the posterior arm:* The operators hand is inserted into the vagina along the fetal posterior humerus. The arm is then swept across the chest and thereafter delivered by gentle traction. It may cause fracture humerus or clavicle or both.
- When the above maneuvers fail cleidotomy or Zavanelli maneuver (pushing the fetus back into the uterus and delivering by LSCS) are done.

Q10. Which method do you use for sugar testing?

In our set up, glucose oxidase method is used for blood glucose estimation.

Method

Glucose oxidase catalyze the oxidation of Beta-D-glucose present in plasma to D-glucono-1,5-lactone with formation of hydrogen peroxide. The hydrogen peroxide produced is then broken down to oxygen and water by a peroxidase enzyme. Oxygen reacts with an oxygen acceptor such as ortho-toluidine which is converted to a colored compound that can be measured colorimetrically.

Q11. What is the difference between venous plasma sugar and venous blood sugar levels?

Venous plasma sugar levels are 10–12% higher than venous blood sugar levels.[8]

REFERENCES

1. Cunningham, Leveno, Bloom, et al. Williams obstetrics.24th edition. New York. Mc Graw Hill.2014.
2. Garcia-Patterson A, Martin E, Ubeda J, et al. Evaluation of light exercise in treatment of gestational diabetes. Diabetes Care. 2001;24(11):2006-7.
3. Diabetes in pregnancy. National Institute for Health and Clinical Excellence (NICE) 2008.
4. Galerneau F, Inzucchi SE. Diabetes mellitus in pregnancy. Obstet Gynecol Clin North Am. 2004;31(4):907-33.
5. Committee opinion no. 504: Screening and diagnosis of gestational diabetes mellitus. Obstet Gynecol. 2011;118:751-3.
6. NICE clinical guideline 63, March 2008. Management of diabetes and its complications from preconception to postnatal period. Available at: www.nice.org.uk/CG063
7. Lain KY, Catalano PM. Metabolic changes in pregnancy. Clin Obstet Gynecol. 2007;50(4):938-48.
8. World Health Organisation: Definition, diagnosis and classification of diabetes mellitus and its complications. Report of WHO consultation. Part 1: diagnosis and classification of diabetes mellitus.1999, genebra WHO.

Fetal Growth Restriction

Simar Kaur, Sangeeta Gupta

Fetal growth restriction (FGR) is associated with significantly increased perinatal mortality as well as immediate and long-term morbidity. Moreover, according to pregnancy audits, most instances of avoidable stillbirth are related with a failure to antenatally detect FGR.[1] One of the most challenging aspects of this condition is the ability to accurately define and adequately diagnose it in order to determine appropriate clinical management.

CASE SCENARIO

Mrs X, 22 years, booked case, married for 1.5 years, G3A2 at 33+1 weeks period of gestation came to OPD for a routine absolute neutrophil count (ANC) visit.

Last menstrual period (LMP)—9/12/2016, Estimated date of delivery (EDD)—16/9/2017, previous cycles regular, sure of dates, pregnancy was confirmed by urine pregnancy test (UPT) at 10 days overdue. First scan done at 9w6d showed a crown-rump length (CRL) corresponding to 9 weeks. Dual marker at 12 weeks was low risk for trisomies. First trimester of pregnancy was uneventful. In second trimester, patient had regular oral hematinic intake. Quickening was appreciated at 20 weeks. Anomaly scan at 20 weeks was corresponding with no gross congenital anomalies. Blood pressure (BP) readings were within normal limits. OGTT done was normal. Thyroid stimulating hormone (TSH) was normal. Clinically growth of the baby had been normal till the previous visit. Weight gain in present pregnancy until now was 7 kg. Patient had adequate daily fetal movement count.

Past Obstetric History

- G1—spontaneous abortion at 2 months of gestation. Medically managed.
- G2—spontaneous abortion at 2.5 months of gestation, followed by D and E.
- No significant family history.

On Examination

No pallor, no pedal edema, BP—120/80 mm Hg, PR—82/min.

Systemic Examination

Normal.

Per Abdomen

Uterus—30 weeks of gestation, SFH—31 cm, cephalic presentation, FHS +, 130 bpm, clinically FFW ~ 1.4 kg baby, liquor adequate.

Investigations

- Routine blood test and biochemistry was within normal limits.
- Ultrasound (33w1d)—Single live intrauterine fetus (SLIUF), Cephalic presentation, BPD—32 w6d, HC 33 w, AC—30 w2d, FL—33 w1d, EFW—1.45 kg, liquor adequate, UA Doppler PI—1.4 (>95th centile), S/D—3.7, placenta—upper segment, grade 3.

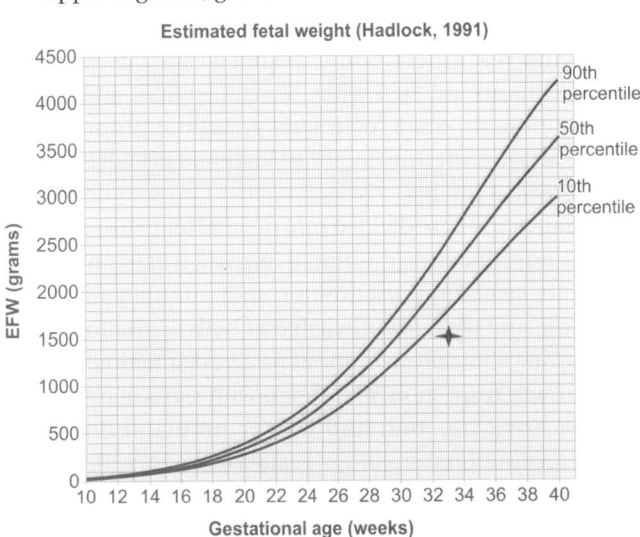

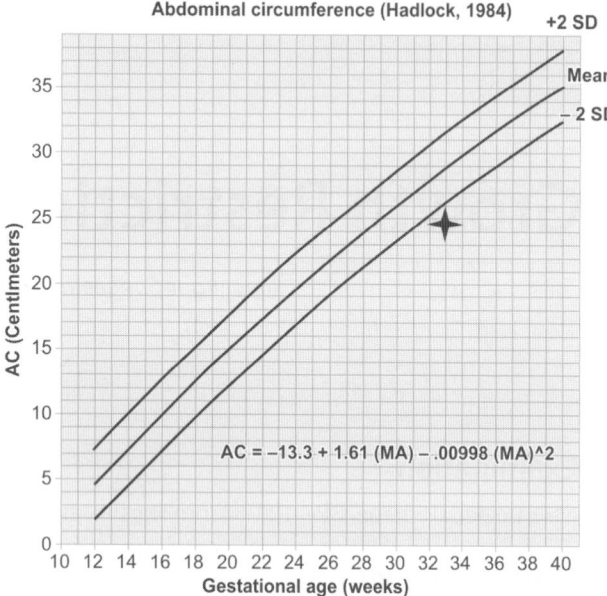

Q1. How will you define 'fetal growth restriction'?

Fetal growth restriction (FGR) is defined as pathological inhibition of fetal growth and failure of the fetus to attain its growth potential.[2] Placental dysfunction is the leading cause of this condition, which affects approximately 3% of the pregnancies.[3] A major clinical challenge of FGR is the ability to accurately identify the truly growth restricted fetus.

Q2. What do you understand by 'small for gestational age' (SGA) fetus?

Small for gestational age birth is defined as an estimated fetal weight (EFW) or abdominal circumference (AC) less than the 10th centile and severe SGA as an EFW or AC less than the 3rd centile. Fetal growth restriction (FGR) is not synonymous with SGA. Some, but not all, growth restricted fetuses/infants are SGA while 50–70% of SGA fetuses are constitutionally small, with fetal growth appropriate for maternal size and ethnicity.[4] The likelihood of FGR is higher in severe SGA infants.

Small fetuses are divided into normal (constitutionally) small, nonplacenta-mediated growth restriction, for example; structural or chromosomal anomaly and fetal infection, and placenta-mediated growth restriction.[4]

The first clinically relevant step is the distinction of 'true' fetal growth restriction, associated with signs of abnormal fetoplacental function and poorer perinatal outcome, from constitutional small-for-gestational age, with a near-normal perinatal outcome.

Q3. How will you differentiate a constitutionally small fetus from a fetus with true FGR? Is the fetus mentioned in above case constitutionally small or has true FGR?

Fetuses with true FGR are at higher risk of in utero deterioration, stillbirth and overall poorer perinatal outcome as compared with normally grown fetuses. FGR is associated with Doppler signs suggesting hemodynamic redistribution as a reflection of fetal adaptation to placental dysfunction.[5] On the contrary, SGA fetuses do not show any Doppler changes and have virtually normal perinatal outcome. The fetus in the above case has true growth restriction as there are Doppler changes in umbilical artey suggesting increased resistance to blood flow.

Q4. What are the causes of fetal growth restriction?

The causes of FGR are fetal, maternal, environmental, and placental.[6]

Fetal

- Aneuploidy (trisomy 13, 18 and 21, triploidy, uniparental disomy)
- Fetal malformations (heart disease)
- Multiple gestation
- Infection (toxoplasmosis, rubella, cytomegalovirus, herpes).

Maternal

- Gestational hypertension, pre-eclampsia, chronic hypertension
- Diabetes with vasculopathy
- Chronic kidney disease
- Hypoxia (pulmonary disease, cardiac disease)
- Systemic lupus erythematosus, antiphospholipid syndrome
- Thrombophilia (Factor V Leiden heterozygote, prothrombin gene G20210A heterozygote, *MTHFR* heterozygote).

Placental

- Placenta previa
- Placental tumors
- Mosaicism.

Environment

- Low socioeconomic status
- Malnutrition
- Smoking
- Alcohol
- Drugs (cocaine, heroin).

Q5. What is the normal rate of fetal growth in utero?

Fetal growth in utero depends on two components—genetic potential and substrate supply. The genetic potential is derived from both parents and is mediated through growth factors such as insulin like growth factor. An adequate substrate supply is essential to achieve the genetic potential. This supply is derived from the placenta which is dependent on uterine and placental vascularity.

Fetal growth accelerates from about 5 g per day at 14–15 weeks to 10 g per day at 20 weeks, peaks at 30–35 g per day at 32–34 weeks, after which the growth rate decreases.

Q6. Elaborate the important points in history taking of a patient with suspected FGR.

History of Present Pregnancy

- Determining the period of gestation with accuracy is crucial for diagnosing FGR
- Date of last menstrual period, surety of dates, and history of regular cycles or any prolonged or irregular cycles prior to conception
- An ultrasound in first trimester with pregnancy dated by crown-rump length (CRL) would help to date the gestation more accurately.

First Trimester

- History of fever with or without rash to rule out infections like rubella, herpes, chickenpox, malaria which can lead to FGR if transmitted to the fetus in utero.
- History of exposure to drugs or radiation.

Second/Third Trimester

- History of poor weight gain
- History of excessive swelling of feet as in preeclampsia
- History of perceiving fetal movements.

Obstetric History

- History regarding outcomes in previous pregnancies, including birth weight of previous babies
- Any complications like preeclampsia, previous growth restricted babies, history of previous still births.

Q7. What are the maternal risk factors that can lead to development of FGR?

Maternal Characteristics

Extremes of maternal age, nulliparity or grand multiparity, history of FGR in previous pregnancy and low pre-pregnancy maternal weight contribute to an increased risk of FGR.

Maternal Diseases

Uteroplacental insufficiency resulting from medical complications such as hypertension, renal disease, autoimmune disorders, thyroid disorders or long-term insulin dependent diabetes with vasculopathy place the fetus at an increased risk of FGR. These conditions influence fetal growth primarily by reducing blood supply via the uterine arteries, depriving substrate supply to the fetus.

Congenital heart disease, particularly cyanotic heart disease is associated with growth restricted infants. Maternal respiratory diseases such as asthma and bronchiectasis also affect fetal growth.

Thrombophillias

Antiphospholipid antibody syndrome and hereditary thrombophillias are also associated with growth restriction. The likely mechanisms are placental thrombosis and impaired trophoblastic function.

Smoking, Alcohol and Drugs

Active and passive smoking, especially in the second and third trimesters, is an important cause of FGR. Mothers who smoke during pregnancy generally deliver infants weighing 100–300 g less than children born to nonsmoking mothers.

Excessive alcohol intake can result in fetal alcohol syndrome when consumed in early pregnancy and FGR during second and third trimester. Cocaine and opiates are potent vasoconstrictors. Their use in pregnancy has influence on the uterine vasculature to cause fetal growth constriction. Therapeutic medications such as warfarin, anticonvulsants, etc. are also implicated in growth restriction.

Nutritional Deficiency

Nutritional deficiency in pregnancy is also one of the common causes of FGR.

Q8. Elaborate important points in the examination of a patient with FGR.

General Build and Nutritional Status of Mother

- Height, weight and body mass index (BMI) of mother—a constitutionally small mother may have a constitutionally small fetus
- Blood pressure
- Pallor, cynaosis, pedal edema
- Thyroid swelling
- Jugular venous pressure.

Systemic Examination

Cardiovascular and respiratory system.

Per Abdomen Examination

Fundal height in weeks and SFH in cms, abdominal girth in inches
- Clinical estimation of fetal weight and liquor
- Auscultation of fetal heart rate.

Q9. What are the clinical methods to detect a growth restricted fetus?

Clinically, the most commonly used method of detecting FGR is the serial measurement of fundal height, symphysiofundal height and abdominal girth.

A lag in fundal height of 4 weeks is suggestive of moderate FGR, while a lag of over 6 weeks suggests severe FGR. However, this method has low sensitivity when used alone because of variables such as maternal habitus, amount of amniotic fluid and examiner bias.

Symphysiofundal height is measured from upper border of symphysis pubis to the level of uterine fundus. It is expressed in centimeters and corresponds to period of gestation in weeks. It increases by approximately 1 cm per week between 14 and 32 weeks.

Abdominal girth is measured at the level of umbilicus and is expressed in inches. It is about 30 inches at 30 weeks in an averagely built woman. It increases on an average by 1 inch per week after 30 weeks.

All three parameters—fundal height, symphysiofundal height and abdominal girth should be checked every weekly while monitoring a patient with fetal growth restriction.

Q10. Can abdominal examination alone diagnose FGR in all patients?

Abdominal examination alone has a limited role in the diagnosis of FGR. Abdominal palpation has a sensitivity of 30% for detecting SGA fetuses.[6] The symphysis-fundal distance has a sensitivity of 65% and specificity of 80–93% for detecting SGA, with variations depending on the methodology used and the presence of factors like high maternal BMI, uterine tumors (leiomyoma) or multiparity.

Q11. What are the various ultrasound parameters used for fetal growth assessment?

Commonly used parameters for calculating estimated fetal weight include biparietal diameter, head circumference, abdominal circumference and femur length.
- *Biparietal diameter (BPD):* It is measured in the transthalamic plane of head which includes thalami, cavum septum pellucidum and midline falx. It is measured at the level of thalami from the outer border of the proximal calvarium to inner border of the distal calvarium.
- *Head circumference (HC):* It is also measured in the transthalamic plane by measured the outer circumference of the calvarial margin.
- *Abdominal circumference (AC):* It is measured in a transverse section at the level of birfurcation of main portal vein into right and left branch (boomerang appearance). AC is the most affected parameter in fetuses with growth restriction.
- *Femur length (FL):* It is measured by measuring the diaphysis of femur, leaving the epiphyseal ends.

Fetal weight is calculated by a variety of formulae—Hadlock, Ott, Shepherd using ultrasound parameters like BPD, HC, AC and FL.

Q12. What are the various ultrasound parameters used for assessment of gestational age?

An accurate determination of the gestational age is fundamental for the management of pregnancies with fetal growth restriction.

Mean Sac Diameter (MSD)

In the early first trimester, when no structures are visible within the gestational sac, gestational age may be estimated from the sac diameter. A common method is to measure the mean sac diameter, by calculating the mean of the 3 sac diameters. An alternative simpler method is to add 30 to the sac size in millimeters, to give GA in days. By the time the embryo becomes visible on ultrasound the sac diameter is no longer accurate in estimating gestational age.

Crown Rump Length (CRL)

Measurement of CRL in first trimester of pregnancy is the most accurate method to determine gestational age. The crown-rump length is the longest straight line length of the embryo from the outer margin of the cephalic end to the rump.

Biparietal Diameter (BPD)

The BPD is the most accurate measurement to determine the gestational age in the second trimester of pregnancy. It is measured in a transverse plane of the head at the level of the thalamus. If the fetal head looks flattened or elongated, it is necessary to measure the cephalic index which is the ratio of BPD divided by occipitofrontal diameter (OFD).

Head Circumference (HC)

The HC is measured in the same transverse plane as is used to measure the BPD and is not altered by brachycephaly or dolicocephaly of the head.

Femur Length (FL)

The FL is an excellent parameter to calculate the gestational age, because it is not significantly affected by alterations in the fetal growth.

Transverse Cerebellar Diameter (TCD)

It is often measured as an additional fetal biometric parameter. It is measured as the maximal diameter between the cerebellar hemispheres on an axial scan. The value of the transverse cerebellar diameter in mm's is considered roughly equivalent to the gestational age in week (particularly between the 14–26 weeks of gestation). The TCD is not altered by the presence of FGR.

Q13. What is the accuracy of various ultrasound parameters for estimating gestational age?

Ultrasound parameter	Error[7]
MSD	4–11 days
CRL	3–8 days
BPD (1st trimester)	3–8 days
BPD (2nd trimester)	7–12 days
FL	7–17 days

Abbreviations: MSD, mean sac diameter; CRL, Crown-lump length; BPD, biparietal diameter; FL, femur length

Q14. What is symmetrical and assymetrical FGR?

The main differences between the two include:[8]

Symmetrical FGR	Asymmetrical FGR
Incidence—20–30%	70–80%
Growth inhibition occurs early in pregnnacy	Onset late in pregnancy, usually after 32 weeks
Hyperplastic stage is affected	Hypertrophic stage is affected
Reduced number of cells	Reduced cell size
Causes: Intrauterine infections; TORCH Chromosomal abnormalities Fetal structural anomalies Early onset severe preeclampsia	Cause: Uteroplacental insufficiency Associated with chronic hypertension, renal disease, etc.
All parameters (BPD, HC, AC, FL) are below the 10th centile for gestational age	Only AC is below the 10th centile Liver size reduced due to diminished glycogen stores
Normal ponderal index	Low ponderal index

Abbreviations: BPD, biparietal diameter; HC, head circumference; AC, abdominal circumference; FL, femur length

Q15. What are the various parameters used for assessment of fetal well-being?

Fetal well-being tests and indices can be roughly classified as chronic or acute. Whilst the former become progressively abnormal due to increasing hypoxemia and/or hypoxia, the latter correlate with acute changes occurring in advanced stages of fetal compromise, characterized by severe hypoxia and metabolic acidosis, and usually precedes fetal death in a few days.

Various parameters monitored are:
- Doppler: Umbilical artery, middle cerebral artery, cerebroplacental ratio, ductal venosus, aortic isthmus
- Biophysical profile
- Fetal heart rate analysis by conventional and computerized cardiotocography
- Amniotic fluid index.

Q16. What are the various Doppler parameters used for management of FGR fetuses?

Commonly used Doppler assessment in SGA fetus encompasses that of the umbilical artery (UA), middle cerebral artery (MCA), uterine artery and ductus venosus (DV). More specialized and uncommonly performed Dopplers include that of the umbilical vein (UV) and aortic isthmus.

Umbilical Artery Doppler

Umbilical artery (UA) Doppler is most commonly used for the monitoring and timing of delivery of the fetus compromised by FGR. UA Doppler is the only measure that provides both diagnostic and prognostic information for the management of FGR.[9] Increased UA Doppler PI or S/D has a great clinical value for the identification of FGR. The progression of UA Doppler patterns to absent or reverse end-diastolic flow correlates with the risks of injury or death. The PI becomes abnormal when placenta is working less than 50% of its capacity and absence and reversal appear at 70% and 90% deficit respectively. Pattern of absent end diastolic flow (AEDF) appears to be present 12 days preceding acute fetal deterioration.[10] Figures 1A to C demonstrate normal and abnormal UA Doppler waveforms.

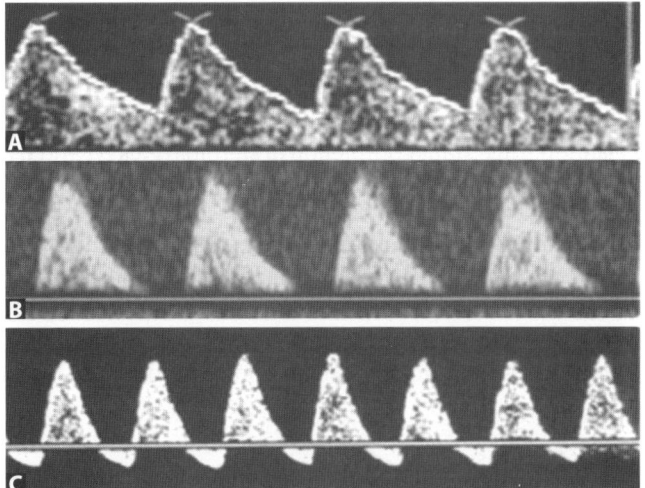

Figs 1A to C: UA Doppler waveform with: (A) Normal diastolic flow; (B) Absent end-diastolic flow (AEDF); (C) Reversal of diastolic flow (REDF)[11]

UA Doppler	Frequency of monitoring[5]
Normal	Every 14 days
Reduced diastolic flow	Weekly
AEDF	Biweekly
REDF	1–2 days

Abbreviations: UA, umbilical artery; AEDF, absent end-diastolic flow; REDF, reversal of diastolic flow

Middle Cerebral Artery (MCA) Doppler

In the presence of fetal hypoxemia, central redistribution of blood flow results in increased blood flow to the brain, heart, and adrenal glands, and a reduction in flow to the peripheral circulations. This blood flow redistribution, known as the brain-sparing reflex, is characterized by increased end-diastolic flow velocity (reflected by low Doppler indices) in the middle cerebral artery. MCA Doppler is particularly valuable for the identification of late onset FGR, independently of the UA Doppler, which is often normal in these fetuses.[12] Current role of MCA Doppler in late onset FGR is to guide termination of pregnancy at 37 weeks, if MCA Doppler is deranged.

Ductus Venosus (DV) Doppler

The DV Doppler acts as a marker of cardiovascular deterioration in response to FGR, specifically in cases of early-onset FGR, where the DV typically becomes abnormal after an elevation of the PI in the UA. RCOG recommends that DV Doppler should be used for the surveillance and timing of delivery of the preterm growth-restricted fetus with absence or reversal of EDF on UA Doppler, provided that the fetus is viable and steroids have been administered.[4]

Absent-reversed velocities during atrial contraction are associated with perinatal mortality independently of the gestational age at delivery with a risk ranging from 40% to 100% in early onset FGR.[13] Thus, this sign is normally considered sufficient to recommend delivery at any gestational age, after completion of steroids (Figs 2A and B).

Uterine Artery

Uterine artery has been mainly used as a screening tool for prediction of FGR, but now its role in diagnosis of late onset FGR is being established. Increased uterine artery resistance (uterine artery PI > 95th centile) is being used as parameter to predict adverse outcomes among SGA fetus with normal UA PI.[14]

Aortic Isthmus

The aortic isthmus is the segment of the aorta located between the origin of the left subclavian and the connection of the ductus arteriosus to the descending aorta. Abnormal aortic isthmus Doppler is an important step between placental insufficiency and cardiac decompensation. The aortic isthmus (AoI) Doppler is associated with increased fetal mortality and neurological morbidity in early-onset FGR. Reverse AoI flow is a sign of advanced fetal deterioration and precedes DV abnormalities by 1 week.[15]

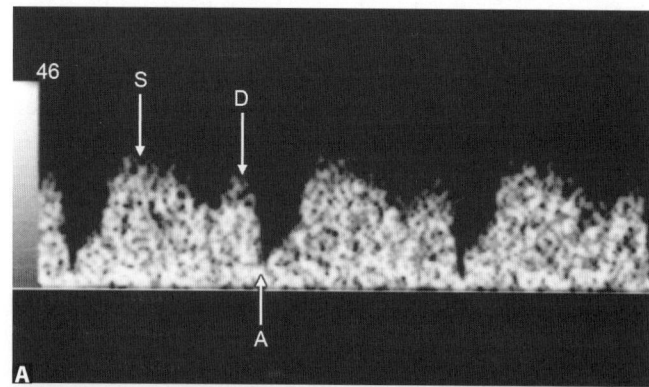
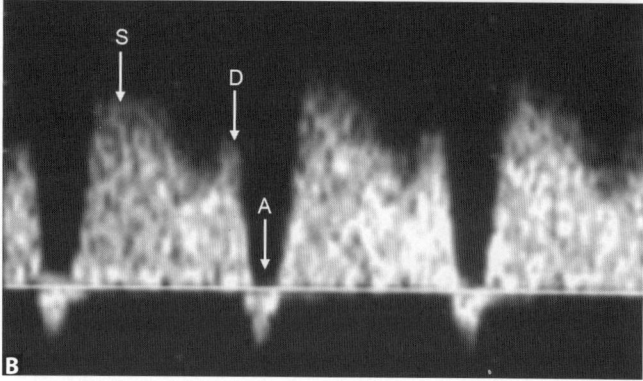

Figs 2A and B: Ductus venosus doppler waveform: (A) Normal waveform; (B) Reversal of a wave. S—ventricular systole ; D—ventricular diastole; A—atrial contraction

Q17. What are the various Doppler indices used in the assessment of uteroplacental blood flow?

The parameters used in the assessment of uteroplacental blood flow include:
- **S/D:** Systolic/Diastolic ratio
- **PI:** Pulsatility index
- **RI:** Resistive index.

Systolic/Diastolic (S/D) Ratio

This is calculated by:
- Peak systolic velocity/end diastolic velocity.

Pulsatility Index (PI)

This is calculated by the following equation:

$$PI = (peak\ systolic\ velocity - end\ diastolic\ velocity)/time\ averaged\ velocity = (PSV - EDV)/TAV$$

Resistive index (RI)

This is calculated by the following equation:

RI = (PSV-EDV)/PSV = (peak systolic velocity—end diastolic velocity)/peak systolic velocity

Among these parameters PI is the recommended parameter for assessment of Doppler changes. In cases of AEDV, S/D ratio cannot be calculated. Hence, PI is considered better.

Q18. What is the sequence in which various Doppler changes occur in an FGR fetus?

Though this is the sequence of Doppler changes occurring in FGR fetuses most of the times, we may not always find this exact sequence of alterations.[16]

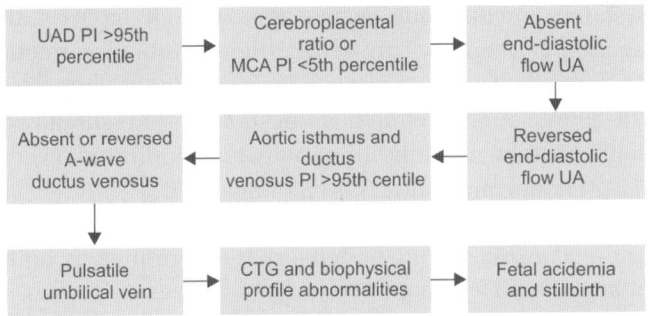

Abbreviations: UAD PI, umbilical artery Doppler pulsatility index; MCAPI, middle cerebral artery pulsatility index; CTG, Cardiotocography; UA, umbilical artery

Q19. What is the role of cardiotocography (CTG) in management of FGR?

Spontaneous decelerations on conventional CTG represent a very late event preceding fetal demise, and therefore measures that allow earlier identification and delivery must be used. A main limitation of conventional CTG is the subjective interpretation of the FHR, which is extremely challenging in very preterm fetuses with a physiologically reduced variability.

Computerized CTG (cCTG) has provided new insights into the pathophysiology and management of FGR. cCTG evaluates short-term variability (STV) of the FHR, an aspect that subjective evaluation cannot assess. cCTG is sensitive to detect advanced fetal deterioration, and it provides a value similar to DV reverse atrial flow for the short-term prediction of fetal death.[17]

Q20. What is the role of biophysical profile (BPP) in management of FGR?

Biophysical profile (BPP) has a high false-positive rate of 40% to 50%. Fetal heart rate variability decreases first followed by fetal breathing. Loss of fetal movements and tone are late events. Changes in BPP occur much later than changes in Doppler. Consequently, whenever Doppler expertise and/or cCTG are available, the use of BPP is questionable. It may be more useful when UA Doppler is abnormal as it has a high negative predictive value in high-risk cases.

Amniotic fluid volume is believed to be a chronic parameter. In fact, among the components of BPP, it is the only parameter that is not considered to indicate acute asphyxia. Because of the limited evidence, the inclusion of oligohydramnios in the management protocols of SGA/FGR is doubtful.[14]

Q21. What do you understand by cerebroplacental ratio (CPR)?

Cerebroplacental ratio is the ratio of MCA PI and UA PI. This index reflects in a combined fashion mild increases in placental resistance with mild reductions in fetal brain vascular resistance. CPR is more sensitive to hypoxia than its individual components and correlates better with adverse outcome in pregnancy.[18]

Q22. Constitutionally small fetuses can be distinguished from fetuses with true FGR by Doppler velocimetry. Which is the best Doppler parameter for the same?

For almost 20 years, UA Doppler has been widely accepted as the standard to identify true FGR. However, current evidence demonstrates that constitutionally small fetus, as defined by a normal UA PI, contains a large proportion of fetuses with worse perinatal outcomes than normally grown fetuses. Thus, UA Doppler cannot be used as a standalone criterion to differentiate the two. The CPR improves the sensitivity of UA and MCA alone because it is already decreased when its individual components are still within normal range. The cerebroplacental ratio (CPR), which combines the pulsatility index of the MCA and UA, is affected in about 25% of small fetuses at term. The CPR is more sensitive to hypoxia than its individual components and it correlates better with adverse outcome.[15]

Q23. SGA fetus with normal UA PI can be reclassified as true FGR based on cerebroplacental ratio. What are the other new criteria proposed for the same?

Aside from CPR, the uterine artery Doppler PI (UtA PI) can be abnormal in the presence of a normal UA Doppler in small fetuses and predicts a poorer outcome in small fetuses. Another predictor of poor outcome is a very small EFW. Among fetuses below the 10th centile, those with an EFW <3rd percentile have a much higher risk of adverse perinatal outcome irrespective of the CPR and UtA Doppler indices.[15]

Q24. What is stage-based classification of FGR?

Stage[5]	Pathophysiological correlate	Criteria (any of)
I	Mild placental insufficiency	EFW <3rd centile UA PI > p95 MCA PI < p5 CPR <p5 Ut A PI >p95
II	Severe placental insufficiency	UA AEDV
III	Low-suspicion fetal acidosis	UA REDV DV PI >p95
IV	High-suspicion fetal acidosis	DV reversal a wave cCTG <3 ms FHR decelerations

Q25. How frequent fetal monitoring should be done for an FGR fetus and what is the ideal gestational age for delivery?

The frequency of fetal monitoring and gestational age for delivery will depend on the stage of FGR.[5]

Stage	Pathophysiological correlate	Monitoring	Gestational age
I	Mild placental insufficiency	Weekly	37 weeks (IOL)
II	Severe placental insufficiency	Biweekly	34 weeks (CS)
III	Low-suspicion fetal acidosis	1–2 days	30 weeks (CS)
IV	High-suspicion fetal acidosis	12 hours	26 weeks

Stage I fetal growth restriction (mild placental insufficiency): UtA, UA or MCA Doppler, or the CPR are abnormal. In the absence of other abnormalities, evidence suggests a low risk of fetal deterioration before term. Labor induction beyond 37 weeks is acceptable, but the risk of intrapartum fetal distress is increased.[19] Weekly monitoring seems reasonable.

Stage II fetal growth restriction (severe placental insufficiency): This stage is defined by UA absent-end diastolic velocity (AEDV). Delivery should be recommended at 34 weeks. The risk of emergent cesarean section at labor induction exceeds 50% and, therefore, elective cesarean section is a reasonable option. Monitoring twice a week is recommended.

Stage III fetal growth restriction (advanced fetal deterioration, low-suspicion signs of fetal acidosis): The stage is defined by reverse absent end-diastolic velocity (REDV) or DV PI >95th centile. There is an association with a higher risk of stillbirth and poorer neurological outcome.

However, since signs suggesting a very high risk of stillbirth within days are not present yet, it seems reasonable to delay elective delivery to reduce as possible the effects of severe prematurity. Delivery is recommended by cesarean section after 30 weeks. Monitoring every 24–48 hours is recommended.

Stage IV fetal growth restriction (high suspicion of fetal acidosis and high risk of fetal death): There are spontaneous FHR decelerations, reduced STV (<3 ms) in the cCTG, or reverse atrial flow in the DV Doppler. Spontaneous FHR deceleration is an ominous sign, normally preceded by the other two signs, and thus it is rarely observed, but if persistent it may justify emergency cesarean section. cCTG and DV are associated with very high risks of stillbirth within the next 3–7 days and disability. Deliver after 26 weeks by cesarean section at a tertiary care center under steroid treatment for lung maturation. Intact survival exceeds 50% only after 26–28 weeks, and before this threshold parents should be counseled by multidisciplinary teams. Monitoring every 12–24 hours until delivery is recommended.

In cases with associated maternal morbidity like pre-eclampsia, timing of delivery is determined by both maternal and fetal parameters.

Q26. How will you manage the pregnancy in the case scenario? What is the ideal time to deliver and mode of delivery?

The above-mentioned patient is 33 weeks pregnant with SFH of 30 weeks, EFW less that 10th centile (1.4 kg), UA PI >95th centile. These findings suggest that this is a case of true FGR (late onset type), with mild placental insufficiency (stage I).

The patient should be admitted and monitored weekly for fundal height, SFH, abdominal girth and maternal weight gain. Though, her BP is currently normal, daily BP monitoring should be done, as there could be coexisting hypertensive disorder. Corticosteroids should be administered for fetal lung maturity. Twice weekly biometry for estimated fetal weight should be done and plotted on a growth chart to assess the fetal growth. Fetus should be monitored weekly with UA Doppler, biophysical profile (BPP), amniotic fluid volume. If there is absence or reversal of end-diastolic flow on UA Doppler or BPP <4 consider termination of pregnancy. If these changes do not occur, pregnancy can be continued up to 37 weeks. Plan a vaginal delivery at 37 weeks, by inducing labor.

Fetal Growth Restriction

Q27. Draw a flowchart to depict stage-based decision algorithm for the management of FGR.

Flowchart 1: Stage-based decision algorithm for the management of fetal growth restriction

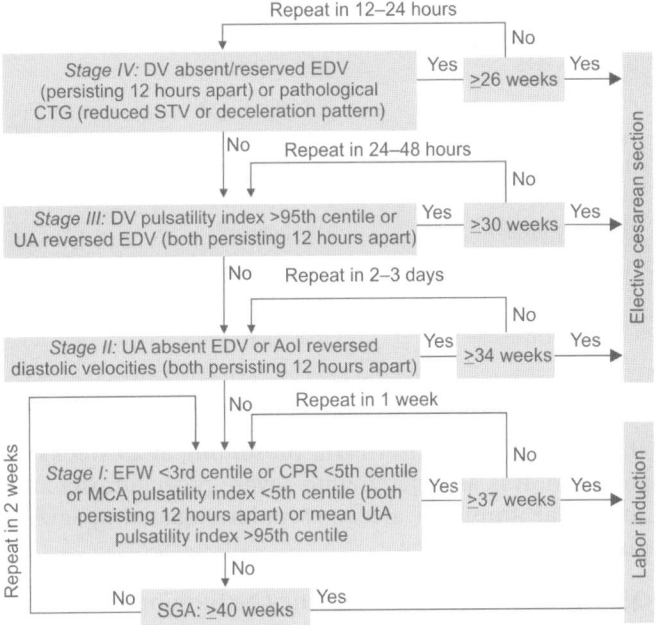

Abbreviations: DV, ductus venosus; EDV, end-diastolic velocity; UA, umbilical artery

CASE SCENARIO

Mrs N, 28 years, primigravida referred from a private hospital at 28 weeks period of gestation in view of severe pre-eclampsia with blood pressure records of 150/100–160/110 with a urine albumin of 1+.

Married for 9 months, LMP–16/4/2016, EDD–23/1/2017, previous cycles regular, sure of dates, pregnancy confirmed by a scan at 6 weeks which showed a CRL of 5w5d. She was started on regular folic acid intake. Nuchal translucency scan at 12w5d was normal and corresponding. Dual marker at 12 weeks showed a low PAPP A, however, there was no overall increase in the risk for trisomies. First trimester was uneventful. In second trimester, she had regular oral hematinic intake. Quickening was appreciated at 20 weeks. Anomaly scan at 18 weeks was normal and corresponding. OGTT at 24 weeks was normal. BP readings had been normal until 28 weeks period of gestation. At 28 weeks she was found to have two high blood pressure readings of 150/100 and 160/110. Urine albumin was 1+. Patient had complaints of slight headache, but no complaints of blurring of vision, nausea, and vomiting or epigastric pain. She was appreciating fetal movements well.

No significant past or family history.

On Examination

- No pallor, pedal edema +
- BP—160/110 mm hg, PR—80/min
- Cardiovascular system and respiratory examination was within normal limits.

Per Abdomen Examination

Uterus—26 weeks, SFH—27 cm, cephalic, relaxed, FHR—132 bpm, clinically fetus—1 kg

Per Vaginal Examination

- Cervix long, os closed, Vertex—3
- Urine albumin (By Dipstick 1+)

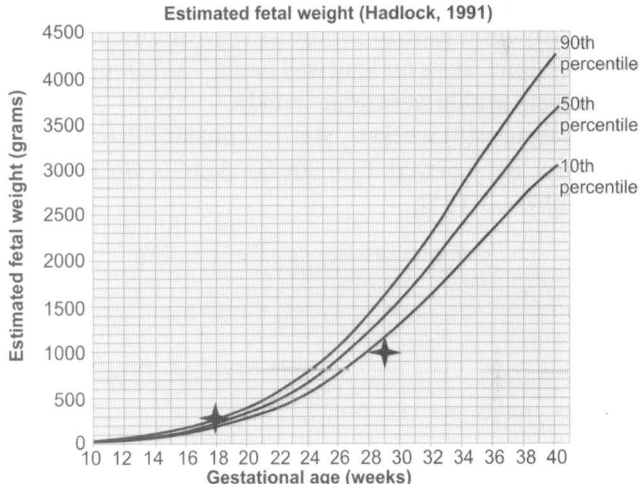

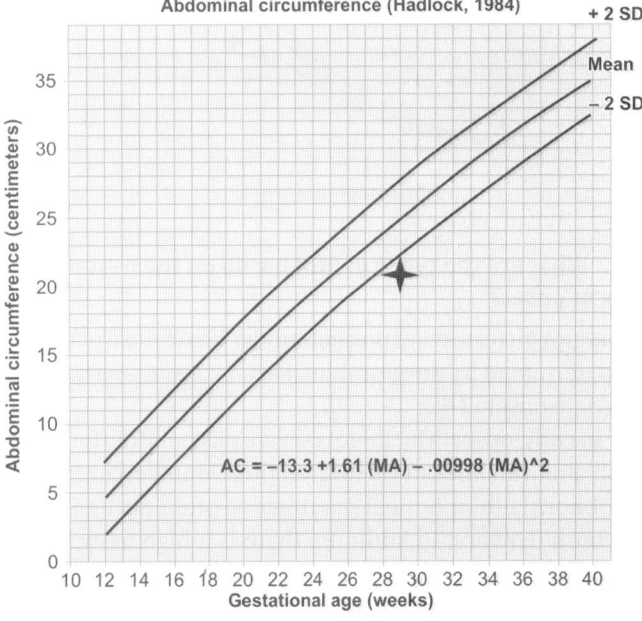

Investigations

- CBC—WNL, RFT/LFT—WNL, 24 hours urine protein—450 mg/24 hours, Fundus—normal
- Ultrasound (29 weeks)—SLIUF, cephalic presentation, BPD—29w1d, HC—29 w, AC—26w1d, FL—28w5d, placenta posterior grade 2, AFI—8, EFW—1 kg
- UA Doppler—S/D—3.6, PI—1.5 (> 95th centile).

Course in Hospital

Patient was admitted. Injection labetalol 20 mg IV stat given. BP checked after 20 minutes—130/94 mm Hg, patient was started on T Labetalol 200 mg TDS. Injection $MgSO_4$ was started prophylactically as per Pritchard's regimen.

BP readings were controlled on oral labetalol. Weekly monitoring of Hb, platelets, renal and liver function was done.

Weekly fetal growth monitoring with fundal height SFH was done. Tests for fetal well being— UA Doppler and biophysical profile were done weekly.

Ultrasound (31 weeks)—SLIUF, cephalic, BPD—30w2d, HC—31w, AC—27w2d, FL—30w5d, AFI—5, UA Doppler AEDV, EFW—1.16 kg.

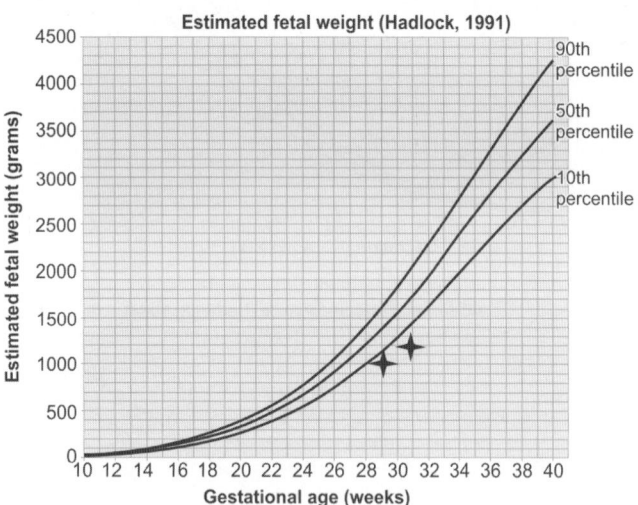

Q1. What are the types of FGR based on the gestational age at onset?

Fetal growth restriction presents under two clinical patterns, as determined by the gestational age at onset—early onset and late onset FGR.

In early-onset FGR, there is severe placental dysfunction with abnormalities in UA and venous Doppler parameters to abnormal biophysical parameters, often necessitating preterm delivery. In addition, there is a high association with PE and perinatal mortality. In contrast, late-onset FGR is normally associated with less severe placental disease and normal or minimally elevated UA Doppler indices but abnormal CPR and no obvious cardiovascular adaptation beyond the cerebral circulation.[5]

Early-onset FGR	Late-onset FGR
GA <32 weeks	GA >32 weeks
Prevalence: 1%	Prevalence: 3–5%
Severe placental disease: UA Doppler abnormal, high association with pre-eclampsia	Mild-placental disease: UA Doppler may be normal, low association with pre-eclampsia
Severe hypoxia	Mild hypoxia
High mortality and morbidity	Low mortality (but common cause of late still birth)
Challenge: Management	Challenge: Diagnosis

Q2. Is this a case of early-onset or late-onset FGR?

This case of early-onset FGR, presenting at 29 weeks of gestation. It is associated with severe preeclampsia and abnormal umbilical artery Doppler suggesting severe placental insufficiency.

Q3. When should this pregnancy be terminated?

As per the stage-based classification of FGR, this is a case of severe placental insufficiency with AEDV on UA Doppler. Once there is AEDV on UA Doppler in a preterm fetus, the risk of still birth increases. However, at the same time fetus has a high risk of neonatal death due to prematurity if pregnancy is terminated. DV Doppler should be done in these cases to decide the time of termination of pregnancy. As per RCOG guidelines.[4]

- In the preterm FGR fetus with umbilical artery AEDV detected prior to 32 weeks of gestation, delivery is recommended when DV Doppler becomes abnormal provided the fetus is considered viable and after completion of steroids.
- Even when DV Doppler is normal, delivery is recommended by 32–34 weeks of gestation.

However, since there is coexisting severe preeclampsia in this case, pregnancy might have to be terminated earlier in case of uncontrolled BP records, eclampsia, HELLP (hemolysis, elevated liver enzymes, and low platelet count) syndrome or abruption.

Q4. What will be the ideal mode of delivery in this case?

The ideal mode of delivery in this case will be by an elective cesarean section at 34 weeks. In preterm fetuses with unfavorable cervix with serious fetal compromise like AEDV, BPP <4, delivery is ideally recommended by a cesarean section.

Q5. Is there a role of therapeutic measures in management of pregnancies with FGR?

Many interventions have been tried to treat FGR, but there is no evidence from randomized controlled trials that any specific antenatal treatment is beneficial. The only interventions likely to be useful include treatment of the undrerlying causes such as hypertension, cessation of smoking and protein supplementation in poorly nourished women.

Bed rest in left lateral position is commonly advised in an attempt to increase uteroplacental blood flow. However, there is paucity of good evidence to draw any conclusion for or against the role of bed rest.[20]

Maternal nutritional supplementation with high caloric and protein diets various mineral and vitamins have all been tried to prevent and treat FGR. There is not enough evidence to recommend routine supplementation of any nutrients except probably protein energy supplements to poorly nourished women.[21]

Maternal Oxygen Therapy

Recent Cochrane review concluded that there is not enough evidence to evaluate the benefits and risks of maternal oxygen therapy for fetal growth restriction.[22]

Pharmacologic Therapy

There is no concrete evidence to support the use of various pharmacological agents like aspirin, beta mimetics, calcium channel blockers for management of FGR.

Q6. What is the role of sildenafil in FGR?

Sildenafil citrate is a phosphodiesterase inhibitor which augments the vasodilatory effects of nitric oxide (NO). Evidence suggests sildenafil citrate as a therapeutic strategy to improve uteroplacental blood flow, fetal growth, and meaningful outcomes in FGR pregnancies. Sildenafil administered at 25 mg 3 times a day in patients with early onset FGR has been shown to be associated with improved fetal growth velocity, as assessed by serial AC measurement by ultrasound.[23] At present the STRIDER (Sildenafil Therapy In Dismal prognosis Early-onset intrauterine growth Restriction) trial is under way to establish with certainty the true health benefits of sildenafil in FGR.[24]

Q7. What is the role of uterine artery Doppler in predicting FGR?

Uterine artery Doppler reflects trophoblastic invasion and identifies impedance on maternal side of placental circulation. It has been extensively evaluated as a screening tool for prediction of FGR with variable results.

At 20–24 weeks of gestation, uterine artery Doppler can detect a fetus at high risk of growth restriction, though its sensitivity is low. Women with an abnormal uterine artery Doppler at 20–24 weeks (defined as a PI >95th centile) and/or notching should be referred for serial ultrasound measurement of fetal size and assessment of wellbeing with umbilical artery Doppler commencing at 26–28 weeks of pregnancy.

In high-risk populations, uterine artery Doppler at 20–24 weeks of pregnancy has a moderate predictive value for a severely SGA neonate. However, screening an unselected population seems to be of limited value.[25] The predictive ability of uterine artery Doppler improves when used in combination with maternal characteristics, previous history and biomarkers. Hence, screening with uterine artery Doppler may be done in pregnancies at high risk of developing FGR.

Q8. What is the role of biochemical markers in prediction of FGR?

Numerous studies have also shown that some maternal biochemical markers [e.g. pregnancy associasted plasma protein-a (PAPP-A); alfa-fetoprotein (AFP); human chorionic gonadotropin, (hCG); inhibin A] are associated with placental function and fetal growth, and their levels are altered in FGR pregnancies. A low level (<0.4 MoM) first trimester PAPP-A should be considered a major risk factor for delivering a SGA neonate. The combination of uterine artery Doppler and maternal serum markers appears promising for improving prediction of SGA fetus, although predictive values are still poor.[26]

Q9. What are the different types of growth charts?

- Population-based growth chart
- Customized growth chart

Population growth charts are based on the analysis of large samples of fetuses starting from the principle that all the fetuses have the same growth potential.

However, there is a possibility that fetal size is influenced by race, ethnicity, sex, parity, maternal size and genetic factors. Customized growth charts were designed to identify the growth potential for individual fetuses. They were customized for maternal characteristics including height, weight, ethnic origin and parity.[27]

The use of customized growth charts is purported to increase the antenatal detection of fetal growth restriction, improving the distinction between normal and abnormal growth, but whether this improves clinical outcomes still has to be demonstrated. Customization is questioned by intergrowth 21st according to which growth patterns in healthy pregnancies are not considered to be modulated by ethnic and environmental conditions.[28]

Q10. What is growth restriction intervention trial (GRIT)?

It was a multicentric randomized controlled study which included 587 FGR fetuses between 24 weeks and 36 weeks of gestation, when the obstetrician was uncertain, whether or not to deliver. Recruited patients were randomized into "deliver now" 'and "defer delivery" groups until it could safely be delayed no longer. The interventions considered were immediate delivery within 48 hours or delay until the obstetrician was no longer uncertain. The delayed delivery group was associated with a delay of 4 days. There was no difference in the total number of deaths before discharge from the hospital (9% versus 10%), although it was associated with higher still birth and lower mortality rate. At 2 years, the overall rate of death or severe disability was similar in both groups (16% vs 19%).[29]

CASE SCENARIO

Mrs X, 29 years, unbooked case, G2P1L0, referred at 37 weeks of gestation, in view of previous bad obstetric history, for further management.

Married for 4 years, LMP—5/9/2016, EDD—12/6/2017, regular cycles, sure of dates.

Pregnancy was confirmed by an ultrasound at 8 weeks which showed CRL corresponding to 7w5d, excellent dating. First trimester was uneventful. In second trimester, patient was on regular oral hematinic intake. Anomaly scan at 20 weeks revealed no gross congenital anomalies. BP readings during pregnancy were normal. OGTT done was normal. At 37 weeks patient was referred for further management in view of previous bad obstetric history. Patient was appreciating fetal movements well.

Past Obstetric History

- First pregnancy (2 years back)—booked case. Antenatal period uneventful. No history of high BP readings or impaired sugars in pregnancy. History of decreased fetal movements for one day at 38 weeks, diagnosed to have antepartum still birth, induced vaginal delivery, 2.3 kg, female baby, fresh still born, no gross anomalies.
- No significant family or past history.

On Examination

- Normal built
- No pallor, no edema

- BP—110/80 mm Hg, PR—80/min
- CVS and respiratory system—within normal limits.

Per Abdomen Examination

Uterus ~34–36 weeks, cephalic presentation, relaxed, FHS—130 bpm, clinically EFW ~ 2.2 kg, liquor appeared adequate.

Per Vaginal Examination

Multiparous os, Uneffaced, Vertex—3, pelvis adequate

Investigation

- Routine blood investigations—within normal limits
- Ultrasound (37 weeks)—SLIUF, cephalic presentation, BPD—36w, HC—36w3d, AC—34w5d, FL—36w1d, EFW—2.36 kg, AFI—7, placenta—grade 3 fundal
- UA Doppler—S/D 2.27, PI —1.1 (< 95th centile), MCA Doppler—PI - 0.8 (< 5th centile), CPR <1 (<5th centile).

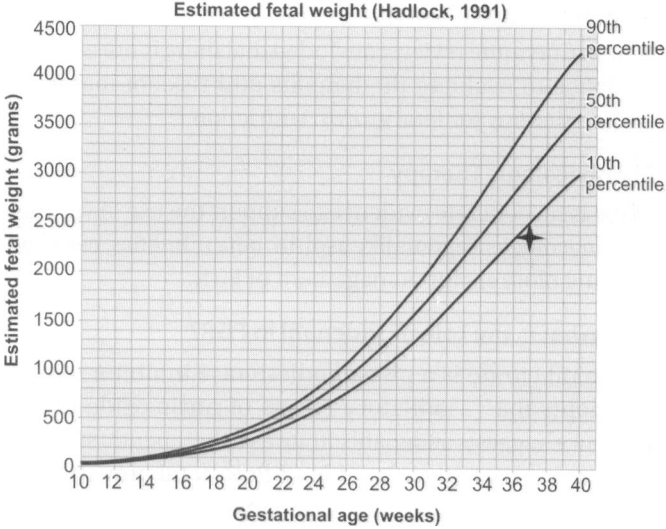

Q1. What could be the cause of still birth in previous pregnancy in this case?

In the previous pregnancy patient was a booked case. There is no history of any antepartum risk factors like pre-eclampsia, etc. which can cause sudden still birth. There were no congenital anomalies in the baby. However, since the birth weight is only 2.3 kg, probably the feus had a true growth restriction. Since the mother is well built, the possibility of fetus being constitutionally small is less likely. Late onset FGR was probably the cause of this unexplained still birth.

Q2. Is this fetus constitutionally small or there is true growth restriction?

This fetus has an estimated fetal weight less than 10th centile with normal UA artery Doppler flow. However, the cerebroplacental ratio is less than the 5th centile. CPR has an improved sensitivity over UA and MCA Doppler individually in detecting FGR. A reduced CPR may be seen even when UA and MCA Doppler PI are normal and helps in predicting adverse outcome.

Q3. What will be the further management in this pregnancy?

Since, this case of true FGR and patient is already 37 weeks of gestation; termination of pregnancy should be planned. The patient already has an unexplained still birth in previous pregnancy possibly due to late onset FGR. This pregnancy warrants strict vigilance. Preferable mode of delivery is vaginal in this case and induction of labor can be planned depending on the Bishop's score. Strict fetal heart rate monitoring with continuous CTG should be done in labor.

Q4. What are the immediate and long-term consequences of fetal growth restriction?

In the antepartum period FGR has been found to be associated with an increased incidence of still births. In a population based study, evidence of FGR was found in 52% of unexplained still births.[30] Growth restricted fetuses have a higher incidence of meconium aspiration, fetal distress and acidosis during labor. In the neonatal period, the incidence of hypoxic ischemic encephalopathy is increased. They have difficulty in temperature regulation because of absent brown fat and small body mass relative to the surface area. Lack of glycogen stores predisposes these babies to hypoglycemia, and chronic intrauterine hypoxia may lead to polycythemia, necrotizing enetrocolitis and other metabolic abnormalities.

In childhood, low birth weight is linked to mortality from causes such as infectious diseases and congenital anomalies. Higher risk if cerebral palsy and impairment in cognitive performance have been reported in these children.

Long-term implications of fetal growth restriction include increased risk of coronary heart disease, hypertension, type 2 diabetes mellitus, dyslipidemia and stroke. Chronic lung disease or bronchopulmonary dysplasia is also more common in FGR infants. Therefore, it is important to optimize the timing of delivery, avoid intrapartum hypoxia and provide skilled neonatal care at birth.

Q5. What is the role of TORCH profile and karyotype in cases of FGR?

The management of FGR must be individualized for each patient. A detailed sonogram should be performed to search for fetal anomalies. Presence of any structural anomalies or soft markers on ultrasound such as ventriculomegaly, increased nuchal fold thickness, etc. should alert the clinician regarding the possibility of an aneuploid fetus and may warrant an amniocentesis for karyotype. Aneuploid fetuses usually have a symmetrical type of growth restriction which is early in onset during pregnancy. Growth restriction in aneuploid fetuses is commonly associated with polyhydramnios instead of oligohydramnios, which is seen in FGR fetuses with placental insufficiency.

Symmetrical FGR also has association with TORCH infections. Sonographic features like ventriculomegaly, periventricular calcifications, intrahepatic calcifications, etc. with symmetrical FGR indicate the possibility of TORCH infection. TORCH testing is recommended in these patients.

REFERENCES

1. Richardus JH, et al. Differences in perinatal mortality and suboptimal care between 10 European regions: results of an international audit. BJOG. 2003;110:97-105.
2. Mandruzzato G, Antsaklis A, Botet F, et al. Intrauterine growth restriction (IUGR). J Perinat Med. 2008;36(4):277-81.
3. Monaghan C, Thilaganathan B. Fetal growth restriction (FGR): How the differences between early and late FGR impact on clinical management? J Fetal Med. 2016;3:101-10.
4. The investigation and management of the Small for Gestational age fetus. RCOG GreenTop Guideline No. 31 January 2013.
5. Figueras F, Gratacós E. Update on the diagnosis and classification of fetal growth restriction and proposal of a stage-based management protocol, Fetal Diagn Ther. 2014;36:86-98.
6. Bamfo J, Odibo A. Diagnosis and management of fetal growth restriction. J Pregnancy. 2011;2011:640715.
7. Butt K, Lim K. Determination of gestational age by ultrasound: In response. J Obstet Gynaecol Can. 2016;38(5):432.
8. Militello M. Obstetric management of IUGR. J Prenat Med. 2009;3(1):6-9.
9. Oros D, et al. Longitudinal changes in uterine, umbilical and fetal cerebral Doppler indices in late-onset small-for-gestational age fetuses. Ultrasound Obstet Gynecol. 2011;37:191-5.
10. Ferrazzi E, et al. Temporal sequence of abnormal Doppler changes in the peripheral and central circulatory systems of the severely growth-restricted fetus. Ultrasound Obstet Gynecol. 2002;19:140-6.
11. Berkley E, Chauhan SP, Abuhamad A. Doppler assessment of the fetus with intrauterine growth restriction. AJOG. 2012;206(4):300-8.

12. Hershkovitz R, Kingdom JC, Geary M, et al. Fetal cerebral blood flow redistribution in late gestation: identification of compromise in small fetuses with normal umbilical artery Doppler. Ultrasound Obstet Gynecol. 2000;15:209e12.
13. Cruz-Lemini M, Crispi F, Van Mieghem T, et al. Risk of perinatal death in early-onset intrauterine growth restriction according to gestational age and cardiovascular Doppler indices: a multicenter study. Fetal Diagn Ther. 2012;32:116e22.
14. Ghosh GS, Gudmundsson S. Uterine and umbilical artery Doppler are comparable in predicting perinatal outcome of growth-restricted fetuses. BJOG. 2009;116:424-30.
15. Figueras F, Gratacos E. An integrated approach to fetal growth restriction. Best Practice and Research Clinical Obstetrics and Gynaecology. 2017;38:48e58.
16. Mone F, McAuliffe FM, Ong S. The clinical application of Doppler ultrasound in obstetrics. The Obstetrician & Gynaecologist 2014; DOI:10.1111/tog.12152
17. Hecher K, Bilardo CM, Stigter RH, et al. Monitoring of fetuses with intrauterine growth restriction: a longitudinal study. Ultrasound Obstet Gynecol. 2001;18:564e70.
18. Bahado-Singh RO, Kovanci E, Jeffres A, et al. The Doppler cerebroplacental ratio and perinatal outcome in intrauterine growth restriction. Am J Obstet Gynecol. 1999;180:750e6.
19. Cruz-Martinez R, et al. Fetal brain Doppler to predict cesarean delivery for non-reassuring fetal status in term small-for-gestational-age fetuses. Obstet Gynecol. 2011;117:618-26.
20. Gülmezoglu AM, Hofmeyr GJ. Bed rest in hospital for suspected impaired fetal growth. Cochrane Database Syst Rev. 2000;(2):CD000034.
21. Villar J, Merialdi M, et al .Nutritional interventions during pregnancy for the prevention or treatment of maternal morbidity and preterm delivery: an overview of randomized controlled trials. J Nutr. 2003;133(5 Suppl 2):1606S-25S.
22. Say L, Gülmezoglu AM, Hofmeyr GJ. Maternal oxygen administration for suspected impaired fetal growth. Cochrane Database Syst Rev. 2003;(1):CD000137.
23. Von Dadelszen P, et al. Sildenafil citrate therapy for severe early-onset intrauterine growth restriction. BJOG. 2011;118(5):624-8.
24. Ganzevoort W, Alfirevic Z, von Dadelszen P, et al. STRIDER: Sildenafil Therapy In Dismal prognosis Early-onset intrauterine growth Restriction--a protocol for a systematic review with individual participant data and aggregate data meta-analysis and trial sequential analysis. Syst Rev. 2014;3:23. doi: 10.1186/2046-4053-3-23.
25. Utero–placental Doppler ultrasound for improving pregnancy outcome. Cochrane Database Syst Rev 2010;(9):CD008363.
26. Nicolaides KH. First-trimester biochemical markers of aneuploidy and the prediction of SGA fetuses. Obstetrical & Gynaecolgical Survey. 2009;64:370-2.
27. Gardosi J, Mongelli M, Wilcox M, Chang A. An adjustable fetal weight standard. Ultrasound Obstet Gynecol. 1995;6:168-174.
28. Resnik R. To customize or not to customize: that is the question. Paediatr Perinat Epidemiol. 2011;25:17-9.
29. GRIT study group. A randomised trial of timed delivery for the compromised preterm fetus: short-term outcomes and Bayesian-interpretation. BJOG. 2003;110(1):27-32.
30. Frøen JF, Gardosi JO, Thurmann A. Restricted fetal growth in sudden intrauterine unexplained death. Acta Obstet Gynecol Scand. 2004;83(9):801-7.

CHAPTER 5

Multifetal Pregnancy

Renu Tanwar, Shristi

CASE SCENARIO

G2P1L1 with 8 months amenorrhea with pain lower abdomen for two hours with discharge per vaginum (P/V), with twin pregnancy came to gyne casualty.

Q1. What are the important points to be asked in history?

- *Age:* Increasing age increases the rate of twinning. Women with advanced maternal age are more likely to undergo assisted reproductive technologies.
- *Parity:* Increasing parity increases the rate of twinning.
- *Race:* Racial variation has been implicated in increasing the rate of twinning in certain population.
- This has been attributed to the higher basal follicle stimulating hormone (FSH) levels in the certain population.
- *Heredity:* Maternal family history is more important as compared to the paternal family history.
- *Assisted reproductive technique (ART):* History of ovulation induction should be enquired. The incidence of twins is increased to 10% and triplets 1%.[1] Higher the number of embryos transferred, higher would be the chance of multifetal pregnancy.

Trimester-wise History

First Trimester

- Hyperemesis is more common in multifetal pregnancy due to higher β human chorionic gonadoptropin (β HCG) levels in these patients.
- Folic acid intake should be enquired about.
- History of bleeding/spotting per vaginum should be enquired about. It may be due to fetal loss or due to improper implantation.
- Any record of chorionicity to be checked.

Second Trimester

- History of easy fatiguability, breathlessness (history suggestive of anemia).
- Excess weight gain/swelling in lower limbs not relieved by rest should be checked.
- History of headache, blurring of vision, epigastric pain, vomiting (suggestive of hypertensive disorder).
- History of polyuria, polyphagia, polydipsia, recurrent infections, discharge P/V, history suggestive of urinary tract infection should be asked (history suggestive of diabetes).
- History of bleeding/leaking P/V should be taken.

Third Trimester

History similar to 2nd trimester along with history of pain lower abdomen (tend to go in preterm labor), and discharge P/V.

Q2. Describe the clinical conditions where fundal height is greater than the period of gestation?

- Wrong dates
- Multiple gestation
- Polyhydramnios
- Large for gestation
- Molar pregnancy
- Pregnancy associated with uterine fibroid or adnexal mass.

Q3. What is the incidence of multiple gestation?

- Difference in overall incidence of twinning are due to variable frequencies in the prevalence of dizygotic twins. Dizygotic twinning varies from 4–50 per thousand births, depending upon ethnicity, age, height, weight, parity and availability of assisted reproduction facilities.[2]
- The prevalence of naturally conceived monozygotic twins is relatively constant worldwide with a frequency of approximately 3–5 per 1000 live births.[3]
- Hellin's law—twins 1 in 80, triplets 1 in 80,[2] quadruplets 1 in 80.[3]

- Multiple pregnancies arise more frequently from fertilization of two separate oocytes (1.2 % pregnancies; dizygotic twinning), than from a single fertilized oocyte that subsequently divides into two identical structures (0.4% monozygotic twinning).[4]

Q4. What are the types of twinning?

Dizygotic Twinning
- Twinning which occurs because of fertilization of two separate oocyte is called as dizygotic twinning.
- Mothers of dizygotic twins have significantly higher basal FSH concentration and FSH pulse frequency.[4] This is accompanied by elevation of follicular phase estradiol, inhibin and luteinizing hormone (LH) concentration, hence higher number of follicles are available for fertilization.

Monozygotic Twinning
- Twinning in which a single fertilized oocyte subsequently divides into two identical structures is known as monozygotic twinning.
- The division of one fertilized ovum into two does not result into equal division of protoplasmic material. They may actually be discordant for genetic mutations because of post zygotic mutations and marked variability in expression.

Outcome and incidence[5] of the monozygotic twinning depends on the timing of division.

0–72 hours	Diamniotic dichorionic twins, occurs in 29% of cases
4–7 days	Diamniotic monochorionic twins, occurs in 70% of cases
8–12 days	Monoamniotic monochorionic twins, occurs in 1% of cases
13–16 days (incomplete division)	Conjoint twins, extremely rare

Vanishing Twin
- Incidence of twin in first trimester is much higher than incidence of twins at birth.
- In around 10–40% cases one twin is lost or 'vanishes' before the second trimester called as vanishing twin.[6]
- The incidence is higher in setting of assisted reproductive technology (ART). It has been seen that 1 in 8 pregnancies begin multifetal followed by spontaneous reduction of one or more embryos or fetus and thus resulting in 1 in 80 births as multifetal.[7]

Superfecundation: Refers to fertilization of two ova within the same menstrual cycle but not at same coitus, not necessarily by sperm from same male.

Q5. How do we diagnose twin pregnancy on clinical examination?
- Fundal height is more than the period of gestation.
- Three fetal poles are palpable and multiple fetal parts can be felt.
- The presence of more than one fetal heart sounds with difference of at least 10 beats per minutes and at a distance of at least 10 cm (auscultated by two persons simultaneously) will confirm the clinical diagnosis.

Q6. What is the role of ultrasonography in twin pregnancy?

Perinatal management and outcome in multiple pregnancy is largely driven by chorionicity, the accurate assignment of which is therefore of clinical importance. Hence chorionicity and amnionicity should be determined at the earliest opportunity. This is best achieved before 14 weeks of gestational age.

Different signs are:
- Two yolk sac—seen as early as 6–8 weeks, confirms diamnionicity.
- Two separate placenta—indicates dichorionic placenta.
- Twin peak or lambda sign—has 100% sensitivity and 86% specificity.[8]
- Lambda sign refers to triangular projection of trophoblastic tissue, isoechoic with the placenta is seen in dichorionic twins. T sign is found in monochorionic twins.
- Measurement of membrane thickness and counting the number of layers[9] of the intertwin membrane—visualization of intertwin membrane is a reliable sign of diamnionicity.
- A well-defined hyperechoic membrane of > 2 mm thickness and 4 layers (amnios-chorion-chorion-amnios) is a predictor of dichorionicity, but it is more reliable at less than 26 weeks of period of gestation. In monochorionic twin, the inter twin membrane is < 2mm and has 2 layers only (aminos-aminos). These techniques are of limited value in determining chorionicity in second and third trimester.

Twin labeling is necessary for monitoring twins, describing the highest number possible of sonographic finding, reciprocal position of fetuses, correlation with cervix and correlation with the placenta.

Q7. Why there is a need for first trimester screening in multifetal pregnancy?
- It is assumed that structural malformations are more common in multiple pregnancies and twins have a

two to three-fold greater risk than singletons, mainly because of the higher incidence of abnormalities (about 50%) in monozygotic twins compared with dizygotic twins.[10,11]
- There is little evidence for increased risks in dizygotic twins. Defects may be concordant or discordant but 80-90% are discordant regardless of zygosity.

Q8. When to do first trimester screening in multifetal pregnancy?
- Screening should be carried at crown-rump length (CRL) 45 mm to 84 mm (11–13^{+6} weeks)
- In twin pregnancies combined screening should be offered.
- First trimester serum screening combined with nuchal translucency is highly effective and should be offered to all women with twin pregnancies. Integrated screening (NT plus first and second trimester biochemical screening) is an option in twin pregnancies which improves the detection rates and reduces false positive rates.[12]
- In triplet pregnancies, nuchal thickness (NT) and maternal age should be used for screening trisomy 21. Second trimester serum screening should not be used in triplets, as it has not been validated.[13]

Q9. What is the sensitivity and specificity of combined screening?
In a 2014 systematic review of first trimester combined risk assessment (nuchal translucency and maternal serum analytes) in twin pregnancies, test sensitivity in dichorionic twins was 86% (95% CI 73–94) and test sensitivity in monochorionic twins was 87% (95% CI 53–98).[14]

Q10. What are the routine investigations done in multiple gestation ?
- *Routine:* Blood grouping and Rh typing, hemogram, urine routine and culture, oral glucose tolerance test, human immunodeficiency virus (HIV), HBs Ag, VDRL and ultrasonography.
- *Specific:* Other investigations should be advised depending upon the complications and comorbidities—kidney function test, liver function test, total protein, serum albumin.
- *USG:* The frequency of ultrasonography depends upon the complications suspected.

Q11. Why there is a need of detailed anomaly scan?
- Risk of gross congenital anomaly and early anomaly is high in multifetal pregnancy in comparison to the singleton pregnancy. A detailed ultrasonological evaluation for gross congenital anomaly (GCA) is recommended at 18–20 weeks.
- An early anomaly scan at 16 weeks may also be advised in monochorionic twins.

Q12. How to follow a twin pregnancy in the antenatal period?
- Early registration.
- Routine investigations.
- Early scan for dating and chorionicity—largest baby is taken as reference to estimate the gestational age in twin and triplet pregnancies.[15]
- Combined screening should be offered.
- Detailed anomaly ultrasonography at 18–20 weeks.
- Hypertension, gestational diabetes mellitus (GDM), and anemia is contributed by twin pregnancy therefore should be looked for and diagnosed early to prevent complications.
- Fetal echocardiography at 19–21 weeks (risk of cardiac anomalies is higher in monochorionic twins (2% in noncomplicated,5% in twin to twin transfusion syndrome (TTTS)[16]
- Cervical length should be measured by transvaginal sonography (TVS) at 20–24 weeks of gestation to evaluate the risk of spontaneous preterm delivery. The cut off value at this gestation is 25 mm.
- Growth scan 4 weekly in dichorionic twin pregnancy and 2 weekly in monochorionic twin pregnancy.
- Regular ANC visits—4 weekly till 28 weeks followed by 2 weekly from 28 weeks till 34 weeks and then followed by weekly visits (can be individualized according to complication).
- Antenatal steroids at 34 weeks.
- Biophysical profile should be done twice a week after 30 weeks for monochorionic monoamniotic twins, and weekly from 34 weeks onwards for monochorionic diamniotic twin pregnancy and 36 weeks onwards for dichorionic diamniotic twin pregnancy (can be individualized according to complication).

Q13. How to do USG monitoring in a monochorionic twin pregnancy?
- Approximately 30% are complicated by:
    - Twin to twin transfusion syndrome (TTTS)
    - Selective intrauterine growth restriction (sIUGR)
    - Twin anemia-polycythemia sequence (TAPS)
    - Concordant or discordant congenital defects
    - Intrauterine fetal death.[17]

- USG examination between 16–24 weeks is devoted for the detection of TTTS and following 24 weeks, fortnightly monitoring is done to detect sIUGR. It involves:
  - Anatomic
  - Biometric measurement
  - Doppler velocimetry
  - Amniotic fluid evaluation.

Q14. What are the complications specific to monochorionic twin pregnancy?

- Complications arise due to anatomical sharing of two fetal placenta. Vascular anastomoses occur in around 90% monochorionic pregnancies and do not usually harm the fetuses. Artery to artery anastomoses are most common and are found in around 75% of cases. Vein to vein and artery to vein and artery to artery communications are found in approximately half of the cases.
- *Twin oligo-polyhydramnios sequence (TOPS):* In as many as 35% of cases involving monochorionic twins, one will experience marked polyhydramnios and the other will be stuck in oligohydramnios.[18] In TOPS ultrasonographic findings are marked growth discordance, with weight discordance of 20% or more.
- *Twin to twin transfusion syndrome (TTTS):* It is seen in about 10–15%[19] of monochorionic twins. TTTS, however, is responsible for as much as 17%[20] of prenatal mortality.
  - With increasing resistance to placental perfusion in an asymmetrically small placental portion, gradual transplacental interfetal transfusion develops between the umbilical artery of the restricted fetus (donor) and the umbilical vein of the larger twin (recipient).[20]
  - The donor is growth restricted, hypovolemic and anemic, and in the umbilical artery there is increased vascular resistance due to the lack of placental vasculature.
  - The recipient, on the other hand, is hypervolemic and plethoric, and vascular resistance changes gradually. The recipient may have circulatory overload from heart failure to severe hypervolemia and hyperviscosity.
  - Polycythemia in the recipient twin may lead to kernicterus and brain damage.

Diagnosis is based on Two Criteria–It is Staged by Quintero Staging System (1999)

- Presence of monochorionic diamniotic pregnancy and hydramnios.
- Staging of TTTS based on sonographic and Doppler findings (Quintero et al.).[21]

Stage	Poly/oligohydramnios	Absent bladder in the donor	Doppler abnormalities	Hydrops	Death
I	+	–	–	–	–
II	+	+	–	–	–
III	+	+	+	–	–
IV	+	+	+	+	–
V	+	+	+	+	+

Stage I—benign form of TTTS with polyhydramnios of the recipient (deepest vertical pocket 8 cm) and oligohydramnios of the donor twin (deepest vertical pocket 2 cm)

Stage V—fetal demise of one or both twin.

- Treatment modalities of TTTS:
  - *Endoscopic laser ablation*—treatment of choice for TTTS between 16 and 26 weeks of gestation,[22] survival rate is 50–70%, with both twins alive in 35–73% and only one survival in 16–38%)[23] and has significantly better neurological outcome.
  - Ultrasonic monitoring should be done on weekly basis including examination of EDF of umbilical artery and PSV of MCA in both twins.
  - *Therapeutic amniocenteses*—when TTTS is diagnosed after 26 weeks, to decrease polyhydramnios and early delivery in case of worsening of fetomaternal conditions.[24]
- Twin anemia polycythemia sequence (TAPS): The spontaneous form complicates 3–5% and it occurs in up to 13% of pregnancies after laser photocoagulation. Defined as finding of MCA-PSV > 1.5 MoM in one twin and < 0.8 MoM in the other twin at 26–28 weeks[25] (in case of growth discordance and FGR, to be managed accordingly).
- Acardiac twinning (twin reversed arterial perfusion syndrome)—rare anomaly 1 in 35,000 births, occurs in 1% of monozygotic twins and is the extreme manifestation of TTTS.[26]
  - The acardiac twin exists as a parasite, depending on normal donor called as pump twin for its blood supply via transplacental anastomoses and retrograde perfusion of acardiac umbilical cord. In an acardiac fetus, cardiac structures are absent or nonfunctioning, and the head, upper body and upper extremities are poorly developed.
  - The lower body and lower extremities are almost normal.

Acardiac anomalies can be divided into four categories:
- Acardius acephalus—most common type, lacking a head, though it may have arms. Thoracic organs are generally absent.
- Acardius anceps—the acardius has most body parts, including a head with a face and incomplete brain. Organs are crudely formed.
- Acardius acormus—this type has no apparent body. Umbilical cord is attached to neck. It occurs due to embryopathy.
- Acardius amorphous—extreme form, lacks a head and limbs and internal organs. It consists of tissue with blood vessels and umbilical cord.

Pump twin has 50-70% mortality rate due to CHF, polyhydramnios and preterm delivery.

Q15. How do we manage acardiac twin pregnancy?

In acardiac twins we aim to disrupt the vascular channel between the twins. Around 90% survival rate has been found with second trimester radiofrequency ablation.[27] Strict monitoring is required as the mortality of normal twin is 50%.

Q16. What is the mechanism of conjoined twins?

Conjoined twins also called as Siamese twins are the least common form of monozygotic twinning and are always associated with monochorionic monoamniotic twins. They result from incomplete division of inner cell mass at thirteen days after the fertilization.

Distribution by type of union[28]	
Distribution of ventral reunion	Relative incidence
Cephalopagus	11%
Thoracopagus	19%
Omphalopagus	18%
Ischiopagus	11%
Parapagus (pelvis and variable trunk)	28%
Distribution by dorsal reunion	
Craniopagus	5%
Rachipagus (vertebral column)	2%
Pygopagus (sacrum)	6%

Q17. How to do monitoring of sIUGR twins?

- It affects 10% of monochorionic twins.[29] This complication develops due to disparity in the placental territory. It should be diagnosed when:
  - estimated fetal weight is <10th percentile in one fetus
  - abdominal circumference discrepancy is >10%
  - birth weight discordance is >25%. This is confirmed after two successive measurements performed at one or two weeks interval.
- sIUGR can potentially be diagnosed during the 11-14 weeks screening examination on the basis of a CRL discrepancy of >11% or >12 mm
- sIUGR are classified in three types according to the umbilical artery Doppler flow in the growth retarded twin.[30]
- Type I—positive end diastolic flow and prognosis is usually good
- Type II—absent or reversed end diastolic flow constantly observed during all the examinations
- Type III—intermittent AREDF, defined as the observation of periods of AREDF alternating with periods of positive diastolic flow
- Type II and Type III carry high risk of preterm delivery, IUD and neurological sequelae
- Management is not universally recognized. A strict and individualized USG monitoring is suggested. In early and severe sIUGR—cord occlusion of the growth retarded twin could protect the survival of the larger twin. In late sIUGR, early delivery is indicated.

Q18. Discuss the role of nutrition in twin pregnancy?

The current literature supports the benefits of BMI specific weight gain guidelines specific for twin gestation for improved twin birth weight gain. Practice may be aimed to track the maternal weight gain and supplementation accordingly. Supplementation with iron, calcium and folate is recommended. Increased attention to specific nutritional needs in twin—specific prenatal care settings have been associated with improved neonatal outcomes.[31]

Daily energy intake is divided over three meals and three snacks, with 20% of calories from protein, 40% of calories from low-glycemic index carbohydrates, and 40% of calories from fat.

Q19. How do we manage multifetal pregnancy during labor?

- Management of labor and delivery is the same for dichorionic and monochorionic diamniotic twins.[32-34]
- Oxytocin for augmentation or induction of labor appears to be effective,[35-38] if indicated.
- Monitor both twins continuously during labor. Intermittent auscultation/continuous CTG monitoring (if available) has to be done.
- After the delivery of the first baby, do fetal heart rate monitoring and check the lie of the second twin and

if longitudinal lie, wait for the presenting part to be engaged and then ARM to be done. In case of inadequate contractions augmentation with oxytocin can be done.
- Placenta should be thoroughly examined after delivery. Strict watch for postpartum hemorrhage.
- Morbidity and mortality tend to be lower in first born than second born twins, regardless of route of delivery. A systematic review of observational studies reported the overall neonatal morbidity of first and second twins was 3.0% and 4.6% respectively (OR 0.53, 95% CI 0.39–0.70), and overall neonatal mortality was 0.3 and 0.6%, respectively (OR 0.55, 95% CI 0.38–0.81).[39]

Q20. How to manage transverse lie of the second twin after the delivery of the first twin?

After the delivery of first twin the second twin may assume transverse lie, irrespective of the original position of the fetus.
- External cephalic version can be done in between the contractions and if the lie becomes longitudinal, vaginal delivery is allowed.
- Internal podalic version to breech presentation and breech extraction of the second twin. This procedure should be performed in OT under general anesthesia immediately after delivery of first twin while the cervix is fully dilated and the membranes are still intact.[40]
- There are no prospective trials that provide strong evidence of relative merits of internal versus external version versus cesarean delivery of second twin in transverse lie.
- But in lack of the expertise, LSCS is the preferred way of delivery.

Q21. What are the recommendations for delivery timing for multifetal pregnancy?

Timing of Delivery[41]
- Elective delivery of uncomplicated dichorionic diamniotic twins at 38 to 38+6 weeks of gestation.
- For uncomplicated monochorionic diamniotic twins, delivery is suggested at 36–37 weeks of gestation.
- For monoamniotic twins, 32 weeks after steroid cover.

Q22. What is the mode of delivery for twins?

Vaginal delivery is recommended in the absence of standard indications for cesarean delivery:
- Uncomplicated twins (cephalic- cephalic)
- Uncomplicated cephalic—noncephalic twin pregnancy
- Previous cesarean section with first twin with vertex presentation.

Q23. What are the indications for cesarean section in twin pregnancy?
- Monoamniotic twins (the risk of entrapment is too great to permit elective vaginal delivery)
- First twin nonvertex presentation
- Previous cesarean with first nonvertex presentation.
- Conjoined twins other than gestation remote from term
- Indications as for singleton pregnancies.

Q24. Discuss about role of epidural analgesia in labor.

Epidural analgesia/anesthesia is generally recommended because it provides good pain relief, does not cause neonatal depression, and is a suitable anesthetic, if uterine manipulation (e.g. version) or operative delivery (e.g. forceps, cesarean) are needed.

Q25. What is the role of induction of labor in twin pregnancy after 36 weeks of pregnancy?

The studies have found no statistical dfference in patients with twin pregnancy who underwent labor induction and those with spontaneous labor regarding parity, chorionicity, history of previous cesarean delivery and cervical dilatation at admission as well as maternal and neonatal morbidity. There was significant difference in the cesarean section rate in the group which underwent induction of labor.[42]

Q26. How to monitor monochorionic monoamniotic twin pregnancy?
- Monochorionic monoamniotic twin placentation is found in 1% of all twin gestation and high mortality rates (up to 50%) are attributed to cord entanglement, knots and twists, congenital anomalies and prematurity.
- Sonographic diagnostic features—absence of dividing amniotic membrane, presence of single placenta, both fetuses of same gender, adequate amniotic fluid surrounding each fetus, both fetuses moving freely within the uterine cavity.
- Color Doppler—Recognition of the entangled cords starting from the first trimester.
- *Ultrasound monitor*ing—Fortnightly surveillance from 16 to 24–28 weeks and then intensive monitoring every week or twice a week.
- Elective delivery by cesarean section at 32 weeks after giving corticosteroids.[16]

Q27. How to manage single fetal demise in twin pregnancy?

IUD of One Twin Occurs in 2–7% of Twin Pregnancy
- Intrauterine death of one twin in a monochorionic pregnancy can cause acute hypotension, anemia, and

ischemia in the co-twin due to exsanguination into the low pressure vascular system of the deceased twin, leading to morbidity or death of the co-twin.
- In dichorionic pregnancy, death of one twin may reflect an adverse intrauterine environment and place the co-twin at risk, but the risk is much lower.
- The type and magnitude of these risks were illustrated in a 2011 systematic review of 22 studies that evaluated the prognosis of the co-twin following a single twin death in various clinical settings.[43] Following intrauterine demise of one twin:
  - The rates of fetal demise of the co-twin in monochorionic and dichorionic pregnancies were 15 and 3%, respectively [odds ratio (OR) 5.24, 95% CI 1.75–15.73].
  - The rates of preterm birth in monochorionic and dichorionic pregnancies were 68% and 54%, respectively (OR 1.10, 95% CI 0.34–3.51).
  - The rates of abnormal postnatal cranial imaging in monochorionic and dichorionic pregnancies were 34% and 16%, respectively (OR 3.25, 95% CI 0.66–16.1).
  - The rates of neurodevelopmental impairment of the co-twin in monochorionic and dichorionic pregnancies were 26% and 2%, respectively (OR 4.81, 95% CI 1.39–16.64).

Management
- **Dichorionic twins:** In dichorionic twins, death of one twin is not, by itself, a strong indication for delivery of the surviving twin. However, if a condition affecting both twins is present (e.g. pre-eclampsia, chorioamnionitis), then close surveillance and timely delivery of the surviving twin are indicated to prevent a second fetal loss.
- **Monochorionic twins:** Death of one twin of a monochorionic pair may have harmful effects on the survivor because of intertwin vascular anastomoses. The hemodynamic changes are immediate; therefore, prompt delivery after death to prevent damage to the survivor appears to be futile.[44]
  - Anemia should be evaluated by monitoring the peak systolic velocity (PSV) of middle cerebral artery in the survivor.
  - Anti D prophylaxis has to be given.
  - A prenatal MRI 2–3 weeks following the fetal death is recommended as it is able to detect ischemic lesions in the survivor earlier than USG.[45]
  - It is not necessary to monitor for maternal coagulopathy since it is rare, although a platelet count and fibrinogen level are desirable prior to delivery.
  - Delivery generally occurs within 3 weeks of fetal demise, thus antenatal corticosteroid for survivor lung maturity should be considered.

Q28. What is selective fetal reduction?
Embryo reduction techniques were developed initially to carry out selective feticides in cases of fetuses affected by some malformation or genetic disorder. Later the technique was employed to the reduction of one or more fetuses in cases of higher order multiple pregnancies.[46]
- Procedure is variously named—selective abortion, selective reduction, multifetal reduction.
- Selective fetal reduction is the removal of one or several fetuses in a pregnancy that has greater than one fetus with the intent to achieve a pregnancy with twin fetuses or one fetus.[47]
- It is now recognized safe and effective method to improve outcome in multiple pregnancies, without doubt in triplets, quadruplets and higher order pregnancies.
- Selective termination of one fetus due to abnormality in the fetus is different from that of multifetal pregnancy reduction.
- Fetuses affected by a genetic, chromosomal, or anatomical abnormalities would be preferentially selected for reduction.
- Multiple fetal pregnancy reduction (MFPR) is when the indication is solely the fetal number without an apparent fetal defect.[48] The fetus(es) to be reduced are chosen on the basis of technical considerations, such as which is most accessible to intervention.

Q29. How is the procedure performed?
- Under USG guidance
- At 9–12 weeks gestation
- By injecting into the heart of fetus 1–2 mL of KCl
- Transabdominal and transvaginal route are prefered[48]
- For any starting number of embryos, the fewest losses occur for a pregnancy reduced to two fetuses.

Q30. What are the neonatal complications and risk factors associated with multifetal pregnancy?
Complications associated with multifetal births include:
- Increased risk of prematurity
- Abnormal fetal growth including discordant growth
- Increased risk of congenital anomalies.

Preterm Birth

The most common risk is spontaneous preterm delivery, which is associated with increased perinatal mortality and short-term and long-term morbidity due to complications associated with immaturity.[49-52] These include hypothermia, respiratory abnormalities, patent ductus arteriosus, intracranial hemorrhage, hypoglycemia, necrotizing enterocolitis, infection, and retinopathy of prematurity.

Fetal Growth

Growth of twins is not significantly different from that of singletons in the first and second trimesters. It appears that the rate of growth after 30 weeks gestation of twins of uncomplicated pregnancies is slower than that of singleton fetuses.

Fetal (Intrauterine) Growth Restriction

The higher rate of fetal growth restriction (FGR) is due to uterine crowding, and uteroplacental insufficiency. In particular, there is a risk of discordant growth, especially in monochorionic twins who share a common placenta.

Discordant Growth

Increasing discordant growth is associated with increasing risk of fetal and neonatal death, and neonatal morbidity.[53-56]

Discordant growth is most commonly defined as the difference in weight between the largest and smallest infants calculated as a percentage of the birth weight of the larger infant.[57] Using this definition, the distribution for twin births is 75% with <15% discordance, 20% with 15% to 25% discordance (mild), and 5% with severe discordance (>25%).

Congenital Anomalies

Congenital anomalies are more common in multiple births, primarily due to increased risk in monozygotic (MZ) twins, and is classified as follows:[58]
- Malformation sequences including conjoined twins.
- Anomalies due to abnormal placental vascular anastomoses.
- Deformations due to uterine crowding that occur in both monozygotic and dizygotic multifetal pregnancies.

Early Malformations

The following malformations that occur early in gestation are more common in MZ twins. This suggests that they are caused by the same factor that results in MZ twinning.[58]
- Anencephaly.
- Holoprosencephaly.
- Exstrophy of the cloaca malformation sequence.
- VATER association (a constellation of malformations, including vertebral, anal, cardiac, tracheoesophageal, renal, and limb defects).
- Sacrococcygeal teratoma.
- Sirenomelia.
- Conjoined twins.

Only one twin is affected by the malformation in the majority of cases. In the 5–20% of cases in which twins are concordant for the defect, one twin often is more severely affected.[59]

Q31. What is first trimester discordance?

In twin pregnancies, CRL discordance at 11 to 14 weeks is associated with adverse pregnancy outcomes, but alone has low accuracy to predict outcomes, such as fetal loss ≥24 weeks and preterm delivery <34 weeks or birth weight discordance.[60]

Q32. How to diagnose discordant twins?

It develops in 15% of twin gestation. Discordance in dichorionic twins results from various factors—different genetic potential, separate placenta (may have suboptimal implantation site), placental pathology. Discordancy in monochorionic twins is because of placental vascular anastomosis that cause hemodynamic imbalance between the twins.

Diagnosis

- Size discordance can be determined sonographically in several ways. Sonographic fetal biometry can be used.

$$\text{Percentage discordance} = \frac{\text{weight of larger twin} - \text{weight of smaller twin}}{\text{Weight of larger twin}}$$

- Another method—difference in AC of > 20 mm.
  Mild discordance—15–25%
  Severe discordance—>25%.

Implications—incidence of respiratory distress, interventricular hemorrhage, seizures, periventricular leukomalacia, sepsis, necrotizing enterocolitis increases directly as the discordance increases. The relative risk of fetal death increased significantly to 5.6, if there was more than 30% discordancy.

Monochorionic twins need more frequent follow-up. Patients with discordance are managed as inpatient basis. Nonstress testing, biophysical profile scores, and umbilical artery Doppler assess have all been recommended in management of twins, but none have been validated.

All patients with discordance > 25% or more undergo daily monitoring as inpatient.

Q33. What about triplet pregnancy?

The rate of triplet and higher-order multiple births is higher than the spontaneously occurring rate due in vitro fertilization and controlled ovarian hyperstimulation with gonadotropins. They are associated with significantly increased risks of maternal and neonatal morbidity compared with twin and singleton gestations, as almost all triplets are born preterm and at an earlier mean gestational age (mean gestational age of delivery for triplets, twins, and singletons: 31.9, 35.3, and 38.7 weeks, respectively.[61,62] Determination of chorionicity is to be done in first trimester. Surveillance of triplet pregnancies includes frequent ultrasound examinations and office visits, particularly after 20 weeks of gestation.

Q34. What are the maternal complications in multifetal pregnancy?

- *Maternal hemodynamic changes*: Twin pregnancy results in greater maternal hemodynamic changes than singleton pregnancy.[63-66] Women carrying twins have a 20% higher cardiac output and 10–20% greater increase in plasma volume than women with singleton pregnancy, which increases their risk of pulmonary edema when other risk factors are also present.[63,64] Physiological anemia is common in multifetal pregnancy.
- *Gestational hypertension and pre-eclampsia*: Gestational hypertension and preeclampsia are more common in women carrying twins.[67,68]
- *Gestational diabetes mellitus*: Increased risk of gestational diabetes mellitus is seen in multifetal pregnancy.
- *Other important diseases whose incidence is increased in multifetal pregnancy are*: Acute fatty liver of pregnancy, pruritic urticarial papules and plaques of pregnancy (PUPPP), intrahepatic cholestasis of pregnancy, iron deficiency anemia, hyperemesis gravidarum, and thromboembolism.[69,70]

REFERENCES

1. Wright VC, Chang J, Jeng G, et al. Assisted reproductive technology surveillance—Unites States 2005. MMWR. 2008;57(5):1-11.
2. Luke B, Martin JA. The rise in multiple birth in United States: who, what, when, where and why. Clin Obstet Gynecol. 2004;47:118-33.
3. Multiple gestation pregnancy. The ESHRE capri workshop group. Human Reproduction. 2000;15(8):1856-65.
4. Lambalk CB, Boomsma DI, De Boer L, et al. Increased levels and pulsatility of FSH in mothers of hereditary DZ twins. J Clin Endocrinol Metabol. 1998;83:481-6.
5. Corner WG. The observed embryology of human single-ovum twins and other multiple births. Am J Obstet Gynaecol. 1955;70:933-51.
6. Brady PC, Correria KF, Missmer SA, et al. Early β- human chorionic gonadotropin trends in vanishing twin pregnancies. Fertile Steril. 2013;100(1):116.
7. Corsello G, Piro E. World of twins: An update. J Matern Fetal Neonatal Med. 2010;23(S3):59.
8. Wood SL, Onge RS, Connors G, et al. Evaluation of the twin peak or lambda sign in determining chorionicity in multiple pregnancy. Obstet Gynecol. 1996;88:6-8.
9. Monteagudo A, Timer Tritsch IE, Sharma S. Early and simple determination of chorionic and amniotic type in multifetal gestation in first fourteen weeks by high frequency transvaginal ultrasonography. Am J Obstet Gynaecol. 1994;170(3):824-9.
10. Edwards MS, Ellings JM, Newman RB, et al. Predictive value of antepartum ultrasound examination for anomalies in twin gestations. Ultrasound Obstet Gynecol. 1995;6:43-9.
11. Schinzel AA, Smith DW, Miller JR. Monozygotic twinning and structural defects. J Pediatr. 1979;95:921-30.
12. Audibert F, Gagnon A. Genetics committee of the Society of Obstetricians and Gynaecologists of Canada; Prenatal Diagnosis Committee of Canadian College of Medical Geneticists. Prenatal screening for and diagnosis of aneuploidy in twin pregnancies. J Obstet Gynaecol Can. 2011;33(7): 754-67.
13. Committee Opinion No. 640: Cell-Free DNA Screening for Fetal Aneuploidy. Obstet Gynecol. 2015;126:e31. Reaffirmed 2017.
14. Prats P, Rodríguez I, Comas C, et al. Systematic review of screening for trisomy 21 in twin pregnancies in first trimester combining nuchal translucency and biochemical markers: a meta-analysis. Prenat Diagn. 2014;34:1077.
15. Royal college of obstetricians and gynaecologists. Multiple pregnancy: the management of twin and triplet pregnancies in the antenatal period. September 2011. pg 14.
16. Royal College of Obstetricians and Gynaecologist. Management of monochorionic twin pregnancy. Decemeber 2008.
17. Acosta-Rojas R, Becker J, Munoz-Abellana B, et al. Twin chorionicity and the risk of adverse perinatal outcome. Int J Gynaecol Obstet. 2007;96:98-102.
18. Mahony BS, Petty CN, Nyberg DA, et al. The stuck twin phenomenon: ultrasonographic finding, pregnancy outcome and management with serial amniocentesis. Am J Obstet Gynaecol. 1990;163:1513-22.
19. Mosquera C, Miller RS, Simpson LL. Twin-twin transfusion syndrome. Semin Perinatol. 2012;36:182-9.
20. Bruner JP, Andrson TL, Rosenmond RL. Placental pathophysiology of the twin oligohydramnios- polyhydramnios sequence and the twin-twin transfusion syndrome. Placenta. 1998;19:81-6.
21. Quintero RA, Morales WJ, Allen MH, et al. Staging of twin to twin transfusion syndrome. J Perinatol. 1999;19:550-5.
22. Rossi AC, D'Addario V. The efficacy in quintero staging system to assess severity of twin twin transfusion syndrome treated with laser therapy: a systematic review with meta-analysis. Am J Perinatol. 2009;26:53-44.

23. Akkermans J, Peeters SH, Klumper FJ, et al. Twenty-five years of fetoscopy laser in TTTS: systematic review. Fetal Diagn Ther. 2015;38;241-53.
24. Twin-to-twin transfusion syndrome. Recommendations and guidelines for perinatal practice. J Perinatal Med. 2011;39: 107-12.
25. Simpson LL. Ultrasound in twins: dichorionic and monochorionic: Semin Perinatol. 2013;37(5): 348.
26. Jeong-Ah Kim, Jeong YC, et al. Complications arising in twin pregnancy: findings of perinatal ultrasongraphy. Koreon J Radiol. 2003:4:54-60.
27. Lewi L, Valencia C, et al. The outcome of twin reversed arterial perfusion sequence diagnosed in the first trimester. Am J Obstet Gynaecl. 2010;293(3):e1.
28. Baken L, Rousian M, Kompanje EJ, et al. Diagnostic techniques and criteria for first-trimester conjoined twin documentation: A review of the literature illustrated by three recent cases. Obstet Gynecol Surv. 2013;68:743.
29. Munoz-Abellana B, Hernande-Andrade E, et al. Hypertrophic cardiomyopathy like changes in monochorionic twin pregnancy with selective intrauterine growth restriction and intermittent AREDF in umbilical artery. Ultrasound Obstet Gynaecol. 2007;30:977-82.
30. Gratecos E, Lewi L, Munoz B, et al. Classification system for selective intrauterine growth restriction in monochorionic pregnancies according to umbilical artery Doppler flow in smaller twin. Ultrasound Obstet Gynaecol. 2007;30:28-34.
31. Goodnight W, Newman R. Optimal nutrition for improved twin pregnancy outcome. Obstet Gynecol. 2009;114:1121.
32. Silver RK, Haney EI, Grobman WA, et al. Comparison of active phase labor between triplet, twin, and singleton gestations. J Soc Gynecol Investig. 2000;7:297.
33. Schiff E, Cohen SB, Dulitzky M, et al. Progression of labor in twin versus singleton gestations. Am J Obstet Gynecol. 1998;179:1181.
34. Leftwich HK, Zaki MN, Wilkins I, et al. Labor patterns in twin gestations. Am J Obstet Gynecol. 2013;209:254.e1.
35. Fausett MB, Barth WH Jr, Yoder BA, et al. Oxytocin labor stimulation of twin gestations: effective and efficient. Obstet Gynecol. 1997;90:202.
36. Neimand KM, Gibstein A, Rosenthal AH. Oxytocin in twin gestation. Am J Obstet Gynecol. 1967;99:533.
37. Fleming AD, Rayburn WF, Mandsager NT, et al. Perinatal outcomes of twin pregnancies at term. J Reprod Med. 1990;35:881.
38. Leroy F. Oxytocin treatment in twin pregnancy labour. Acta Genet Med Gemellol (Roma). 1979;28:303.
39. Rossi AC, Mullin PM, Chmait RH. Neonatal outcomes of twins according to birth order, presentation and mode of delivery: a systematic review and meta-analysis. BJOG. 2011;118:523.
40. Rabinovici J, Barkai G, Reichman B, et al. Internal podalic version with unruptured membranes for the second twin in transverse lie. Obstet Gynecol. 1988;71:428.
41. Committee on Practice Bulletins—Obstetrics, Society for Maternal-Fetal Medicine. Practice Bulletin No. 169: Multifetal Gestations: Twin, Triplet, and Higher-Order Multifetal Pregnancies. Obstet Gynecol. 2016;128:e131.
42. Tavares MV, Domingues AP, Nunes F, et al. Induction of labour vs. spontaneous vaginal delivery in twin pregnancy after 36 weeks of gestation. J Obstet Gynaecol. 2017;37(1):29-32.
43. Hillman SC, Morris RK, Kilby MD. Co-twin prognosis after single fetal death: a systematic review and meta-analysis. Obstet Gynecol. 2011;118:928.
44. Karageyim Karsidag AY, Kars B, Dansuk R, et al. Brain damage to the survivor within 30 min of co-twin demise in monochorionic twins. Fetal Diagn Ther. 2005;20:91.
45. Righini A, Salmona S, et al. Prenatal magnetic resonance evaluation of ischemic brain lesions in the survivors of monochorionic twin pregnancies: report of three cases. J Comput Assist Tomogr. 2004;28:87-92.
46. Maymon R, Herman A, Shulman A, et al. First rimester embryo reduction: a medical solution to iatrogenic problem. Hum Reprod. 1995;10:668-73.
47. Bidgoli AZ, Ardbili FA. Permissibilty of multifetal pregnanc reduction from the Shiite point of view. Int J Fertil Steril. 2017;10(4):380-9.
48. Rath S, Kumar S, Sharma R, et al. Multifetal pregnancy reduction. Medical Journal, Armed Forces India. 2004;60(1):67-68.
49. Spellacy WN, Handler A, Ferre CD. A case-control study of 1253 twin pregnancies from a 1982-1987 perinatal data base. Obstet Gynecol. 1990;75:168.
50. Roberts WE, Morrison JC, Hamer C, et al. The incidence of preterm labor and specific risk factors. Obstet Gynecol. 1990;76:85S.
51. Bodeau-Livinec F, Zeitlin J, Blondel B, et al. Do very preterm twins and singletons differ in their neurodevelopment at 5 years of age? Arch Dis Child Fetal Neonatal Ed. 2013;98:F480.
52. Mieth RA, Ersfeld S, Douchet N, et al. Higher multiple births in Switzerland: neonatal outcome and evolution over the last 20 years. Swiss Med Wkly. 2011;141:w13308.
53. Hartley RS, Hitti J, Emanuel I. Size-discordant twin pairs have higher perinatal mortality rates than nondiscordant pairs. Am J Obstet Gynecol. 2002;187:1173.
54. Demissie K, Ananth CV, Martin J, et al. Fetal and neonatal mortality among twin gestations in the United States: the role of intrapair birth weight discordance. Obstet Gynecol. 2002;100:474.
55. Branum AM, Schoendorf KC. The effect of birth weight discordance on twin neonatal mortality. Obstet Gynecol. 2003;101:570.
56. Victoria A, Mora G, Arias F. Perinatal outcome, placental pathology, and severity of discordance in monochorionic and dichorionic twins. Obstet Gynecol. 2001;97:310.
57. Blickstein I, Kalish RB. Birthweight discordance in multiple pregnancy. Twin Res. 2003;6:526.
58. Schinzel AA, Smith DW, Miller JR. Monozygotic twinning and structural defects. J Pediatr. 1979;95:921.
59. Branum AM, Schoendorf KC. The effect of birthweight discordance on twin neonatal mortality. Obstet Gynecol. 2003;101:570
60. Salomon LJ, Cavicchioni O, Bernard JP, et al. Growth discrepancy in twins in the first trimester of pregnancy. Ultrasound Obstet Gynecol. 2005;26:512.

61. Luke B, Brown MB. Maternal morbidity and infant death in twin vs triplet and quadruplet pregnancies. Am J Obstet Gynecol. 2008;198:401.e1.
62. Ballabh P, Kumari J, AlKouatly HB, et al. Neonatal outcome of triplet versus twin and singleton pregnancies: a matched case control study. Eur J Obstet Gynecol Reprod Biol. 2003; 107:28.
63. Kametas NA, McAuliffe F, Krampl E, et al. Maternal cardiac function in twin pregnancy. Obstet Gynecol. 2003;102:806.
64. Rao A, Sairam S, Shehata H. Obstetric complications of twin pregnancies. Best Pract Res Clin Obstet Gynaecol. 2004; 18:557.
65. Kuleva M, Youssef A, Maroni E, et al. Maternal cardiac function in normal twin pregnancy: a longitudinal study. Ultrasound Obstet Gynecol. 2011;38:575.
66. Ghi T, degli Esposti D, Montaguti E, et al. Maternal cardiac evaluation during uncomplicated twin pregnancy with emphasis on the diastolic function. Am J Obstet Gynecol. 2015;213:376.e1.
67. Sibai BM, Hauth J, Caritis S, et al. Hypertensive disorders in twin versus singleton gestations. National Institute of Child Health and Human Development Network of Maternal-Fetal Medicine Units. Am J Obstet Gynecol. 2000;182:938.
68. Francisco C, Wright D, Benk Z, et al. Hidden high rate of pre-eclampsia in twin compared with singleton pregnancy. Ultrasound Obstet Gynecol. 2017;50:88.
69. Gonzalez MC, Reyes H, Arrese M, et al. Intrahepatic cholestasis of pregnancy in twin pregnancies. J Hepatol. 1989;9:84.
70. Hall MH, Campbell DM, Davidson RJ. Anaemia in twin pregnancy. Acta Genet Med Gemellol (Roma). 1979;28:279.

6 CHAPTER

Pregnancy with Intrauterine Demise

Madhavi M Gupta, Sparsha

Stillborn is a baby with no signs of life at or after 28 weeks of gestation. Definition of stillbirth varies between countries and even between studies conducted in the same country. Although, most of the studies defining stillbirth have used a gestational age of between 20 and 28 weeks as a cut-off point, only 11% of the included studies used the standard World Health Organization (WHO) definition of ≥22 weeks gestation or weight of ≥500 grams. The WHO definition for international comparison, is ≥28 weeks of gestation or ≥1000 grams.[1]

An estimated 2.6 million stillbirths occur annually, of which 98% occur in low-income and middle-income countries and 75% in sub-Saharan Africa and south Asia. Half of all stillbirths occur during labor and birth, about 1.3 million each year. India ranks first in having highest number of stillbirths (5,92,000).[2]

CASE SCENARIO

Mrs X, 22 years old lady, G2P1L0, a city resident, presented to the gynecology casualty with complaints of:
- Reduced fetal movements—3 days
- Pain lower abdomen—1 day
- Last menstrual period (LMP)—30/11/16
- Expected date of delivery (EDD)—6/9/17.
- Period of gestation—30 weeks and 2 days on admission.

Patient was a booked case in Lok Nayak Hospital, New Delhi since her 3rd month of pregnancy and carrying her pregnancy well. Three days back, she experienced reduced fetal movements followed by pain starting from the back and radiating to thighs, intermittently, progressively increasing in intensity, not associated with any bleeding or leaking per vaginum. The patient reported to the gyne casualty where, on examination, the fetal heart could not be auscultated. Patient was admitted to the labor room and the ultrasound confirmed the absence of fetal cardiac activity.

History of itching all over the body since 7 months amneorrhea not associated with yellow sclera, high colored urine or clay colored stools.

Obstetric History

- Married for 3 years.
- G2P1L0.

First Pregnancy

1 1/2 year back:
- Registered at a government hospital with poor antenatal follow-up
- At 8 month amenorrhea—Presented with preterm labor and absent fetal heart
- Delivered a macerated male baby weighing 1750 g.
- History of itching since 7 month of amenorrhea never reported to any healthcare facility

Past History

Not significant.

Family History

Mother—hypertensive, on treatment.

Q1. What are the various risk factors associated with stillbirth?

Advanced maternal age
- Gestational age at birth
- Multiparity
- Lack of or inadequate antenatal care
- Multiple gestation
- Consanguinity
- Smoking, alcohol intake and drug abuse

- Low socioeconomic status
- Lack of education
- History of previous stillbirth.

Q2. What is the best investigation to confirm the diagnosis of IUFD?

- Only auscultation and cardiotocography should not be used to investigate suspected intrauterine fetal death (IUFD)
- Auscultation of the fetal heart by Pinard stethoscope or Doppler ultrasound is insufficient for diagnosis as auscultation can give false reassurance and maternal pelvic blood flow can result in an apparently normal fetal heart rate pattern with external Doppler
- Real-time ultrasonography is neccessary for the accurate diagnosis of IUFD
- Mothers should be prepared for the possibility of passive fetal movement. If the mother reports passive fetal movement after the scan to diagnose IUFD, a repeat scan should be offered.

Q3. Is there any role of daily fetal movement count? If yes, what are the different methods for fetal movement count?

Decreased fetal movement count is an indicator of decreased placental perfusion and fetal acidosis.[3]

Methods of Fetal Movement Count

Cardiff 'Count 10' Technique

- Developed by Pearson and Weaver
- Requires counting till 10 movements perceived
- To report if <10 movements perceived over 12 hours on 2 successive days OR no movement over 12 hours in a single day.

Daily fetal movement count:

- Counting thrice for 1 hour duration each (postmeal: recommended)
- Total daily count over 12 hours (sum of postmeal counts multiplied by 4) should be >10 in 12 hours.

Q4. What ultrasound findings will you expect in a stillborn baby?

The features are:
- Absent fetal heart beat
- Absent fetal movements
- Occasional findings
  - Overlapping of skull bones (Spalding sign)
  - Gross distortion of fetal anatomy (maceration)
  - Soft tissue edema: Skin >5 mm
  - Echogenic amniotic fluid (fetal demise fragments)
- Uncommon findings
  - Thrombus in fetal heart
  - Gas shadow in fetal heart (Robert's sign).

Q5. What precautions are required if the mother is Rh negative?

Women who are rhesus D (RhD)-negative should be advised to have a Kleihauer test to detect large fetomaternal hemorrhage (FMH) that may have occurred a few days earlier. Anti-RhD gammaglobulin should be administered as soon as possible in this condition.[8]

If there has been a large FMH, the dose of anti-RhD gammaglobulin should be adjusted upwards and the Kleihauer test should be repeated at 48 hours to ensure that the fetal red cells have cleared. It is important to know the baby's blood group but if no blood sample could be obtained from the baby or cord, RhD typing should be done using free fetal DNA (ffDNA) from maternal blood taken just after birth.

Q6. In antepartum stillbirth what is the role of expectant management?

More than 85% of women with an IUFD go in labor spontaneously within three weeks of diagnosis.

- If the woman is physically well with membranes intact and there is no evidence of preeclampsia, infection or bleeding (abruption), the risk of expectant management for 48 hours is low
- Women who opt for prolonged expectant management should be told that the value of postmortem may be reduced and the appearance of the baby may deteriorate.

Q7. What is the risk of coagulation abnormality in case of expectant management?

- There is a 10% moderate risk of disseminated intravascular coagulation (DIC) within 4 weeks from the date of fetal death increasing to 30% thereafter
- This can be tested by coagulation studies, blood platelet count and fibrinogen measurement. When expectant management is chosen for longer than 48 hours these tests should be repeated twice weekly.

Q8. What is the prefered mode of delivery in these patients?

- Vaginal birth is the recommended mode of delivery for most women, but cesarean birth to be considered sometmes if there is any contraindication to vaginal delivery
- More than 90% will deliver vaginally within 24 hours of induction of labor for IUFD.[4]

Q9. What are methods for induction of labor in stillbirths?

Unscarred Uterus
- A combination of mifepristone and a prostaglandin (misoprost) preparation is recommended as the first-line for induction of labor.[4]
  - It has been found that addition of single dose of mifepristone 200 mg decreases duration of labor by 7 hours.
- Misoprostol alone:
  - <26 weeks: 200 µg pervaginal (PV)/sublingual (SL)/buccal (bucc) every 4–6 hours
  - 27–28 weeks: 100 µg pv/sl/bucc every 4 hours
  - >28 weeks: 25 µg pv every 6 hours or 25 µg PO every 2 hours (FIGO guidelines 2017).[5]

Scarred Uterus
- The discussion regarding safety and benefits of induction of labor should be undertaken by a consultant obstetrician.
- Trial of vaginal birth after cesarean delivery (VBAC) can be given but there are very less studies to define the safety of VBAC in IUFD with scarred uterus. However, VBAC is not recommended for women with:
  - Three previous cesarean sections
  - Previous uterine rupture
  - Upper segment incisions.
- Women undergoing VBAC should be monitored for features of scar rupture (maternal tachycardia, atypical pain, vaginal bleeding, hematuria on catheter specimen and maternal collapse).
- Oxytocin augmentation can be used for VBAC, but the decision or its use should be made by consultant obstetrician and monitored very closely.
- Mifepristone can be used alone to increase the chances of labor within 72 hours (avoiding the use of prostaglandin). Dosage: 200 mg three times a day for 2 days or 600 mg once daily for 2 days.[6,7]
- Mechanical methods: Mechanical methods of induction have been found to increase the risk of ascending infection in the presence of IUFD[8] hence should not be used routinely.

Q10. Is there any need for routine intrapartum antimicrobial therapy?
- Only women with sepsis should be given intravenous broad-spectrum antibiotic therapy
- Routine antibiotic prophylaxis is not recommended.

Q11. How to differentiate a fresh from a macerated stillborn?
- A "macerated" fetus shows skin and soft-tissue changes (skin discoloration or darkening, redness, peeling, and breakdown) suggesting death was well before delivery (prepartum).
- A "fresh" fetus lacks such skin changes and is presumed to have died much more recently. Time duration of 8 hours is taken as cut-off after which signs of maceration starts appearing.[9]

Q12. What are the various options for suppression of lactation in these patients?
The options[10] are as follows:
- A single dose of cabergoline (1 mg) within 24 hours of the delivery of a stillborn
- Bromocriptine (2.5 mg twice daily) for 14 days
- Cabergoline is preferred as it is simpler to use and has significantly lower rates of rebound breast activity and adverse events
- Tablet Pyridoxine 200 mg TDS for 7 days used in patients with hypertensive disorders where Dopamine agonists are contraindicated.

Q13. What postpartum complications are anticipated in a patient with intrauterine fetal death?
- Postpartum hemorrhage
- Post-traumatic stress disorder
- Endometritis
- Puerperal sepsis
- Retained placenta.

Q14. What is the risk of recurrence of stillbirth?
The risk of recurrence of stillbirth in future pregnancies will depend on the clinical circumstances and investigation results.
- In low-risk women with unexplained stillbirth, the risk of recurrent stillbirth after 20 weeks is estimated at 7.8–10.5/1,000 with most of the risk occurring before 37 weeks of gestation.
- The risk of recurrent stillbirth after 37 weeks is very low at 1.8/1,000.

Q15. What samples should be sent after delivery of baby so that the cause of IUD and any recurrent condition can be identified?

Fetal and placental microbiology: For fetal infections
- Fetal blood
- Fetal swabs
- Placental swabs

For aneuploidy and single gene disorders
- Fetal and placental tissues
  - Deep fetal skin
  - Fetal cartilage
  - Placenta.

Q16. What tests are recommended for evaluation of a stillbirth?

- The most important tests in the evaluation of a stillbirth are fetal autopsy; examination of the placenta, cord, and membranes; and karyotype evaluation
- No specific cause is found in ~50% of stillbirths.

REFERENCES

1. Cousens S, Lawn JE, Blencowe H, et al. National, regional, and worldwide estimates of stillbirth rates. The Lancet. 2011;378(9794):873-4.
2. Ministry of Home Affairs, Govt. of India, Sample Registeration System statistical report, 2012:chapter4:81.
3. Heazell AE, Frøen JF. Methods of fetal movement counting and the detection of fetal compromise. J Obstet Gynaecol. 2008;28(2):147-54.
4. Wagaarachchi PT, Ashok PW, Narvekar NN, et al. Medical management of late intrauterine death using a combination of mifepristone and misoprostol. BJOG. 2002;109:443-7.
5. WHO Clinical Practice Handbook for Safe Abortion, 2014.
6. British Medical Association and Royal Pharmaceutical Society of Great Britain. British National Formulary (BNF) 58 .London: BMJ Publishing Group Ltd and RPS Publishing; 2009.
7. Cabrol D, Dubois C, Cronje H, et al. Induction of labor with mifepristone (RU 486) in intrauterine fetal death. Am J Obstet Gynecol. 1990;163:540-2.
8. Boulvain M, Kelly A, Lohse C, et al. Mechanical methods for induction of labour. Cochrane Database Syst Rev. 2001;(4):CD001233. DOI: 10.1002/14651858.CD001233.
9. Gold KJ, Abdul-Mumin ARS, Boggs ME, et al. Assessment of "fresh" versus "macerated" as accurate markers of time since intrauterine fetal demise in low-income countries. Int J Gynaecol Obstet. 2014;125(3):223-7.
10. European Multicentre Study Group for Cabergoline in Lactation Inhibition. Single dose cabergoline versus bromocriptine in inhibition of puerperal lactation: randomised, double blind, multicentre study. BMJ. 1991;302:1367-71.

CHAPTER 7

Rh Negative Pregnancy

Sudha Prasad, Meenakshi Goel

Most cases of severe fetal anemia requiring antenatal transfusion are attributable to anti-D, anti-Kell, or anti–c alloimmunization. The use of anti-D immunoglobulin has led to a decline in the incidence of Rh alloimmunization from 5–1.7% in last five decades but still it is the most common cause of hemolytic disease of the newborn (HDFN).

CASE SCENARIO

A young primigravida with 5 month's amenorrhea came to antenatal OPD with complain of spotting per vaginum. On blood investigations, her blood group was O negative.

26 years old, Mrs F, wife of Mr M, R/o Karolbagh, a housewife, came to gyne casualty on 4/3/17 with complaints of:
- Amenorrhea: 5 months
- Spotting per vaginum: 1 hour back
  Her LMP was 16/10/16 so her POG was 19 weeks and 6 days on 4/3/2017.

HOPI
- Patient was an unbooked case with no prior antenatal visits at any hospital or dispensary
- She complained of spotting per vaginum 1 hour back which was unprovoked with no prior history of trauma or coitus. It was dark colored associated with mucoid discharge per vaginum which was non foul smelling.
- Patient had superficial staining of one pad only
- No complains of pain lower abdomen or backache or leaking per vaginum

Course in the Hospital
- She was admitted to the septic labor room, received few injections in her buttocks and monitored for abdominal pain and bleeding per vaginum
- An ultrasound was done to confirm fetal cardiac activity, gestational age, cervical length and placental localization and everything was normal.

Examination
General physical examination—unremarkable.

Abdominal Examination
Inspection—nothing remarkable.

Palpation
Fundal height—20 weeks, Uterus—relaxed, non-tense non-tender.

Perineal Examination
External genitalia normal, no active bleeding and no leaking observed.

Per Speculum Examination
- Os closed, cervix long
- Minimal dark altered blood mixed discharge seen
- No active bleeding or leaking seen.

Per Vaginal Examination
Not done

Diagnosis after Examination
Primigravida with 19 weeks and 6 days POG with Rh negative pregnancy with threatened abortion.

Q1. How does the blood group of mother being Rh negative affect her management in this case?
- Rh factor is an antigen present on red cell membrane which can stimulate an immune response in an individual who is Rh factor negative. This phenomenon is called alloimmunization.

- Fetal RBCs (red blood cells) can enter into maternal circulation anytime during pregnancy, delivery or postpartum period.
- When Rh negative maternal blood is exposed to Rh positive fetal blood (RBCs), IgM antibodies are formed in maternal circulation after 6 weeks to 12 months. These IgM antibodies cannot cross the feto-placental barrier and donot harm the fetus.
- If the mother subsequently gets exposed to Rh positive cells, her immune system rapidly produces IgG antibodies which cross the placenta. This leads to destruction of fetal RBC's leading to hemolytic disease in the fetus and newborn. This is the first sensitized pregnancy.[1]
- So, all the potential sensitizing events (events leading to fetomaternal bleed) can lead to alloimmunization.

Q2. What are the possible causes of maternal alloimmunization?

- Blood transfusion (Rh mismatched)
- Fetomaternal hemorrhage—ante/intrapartum
- Ectopic pregnancy
- Abortion—therapeutic/spontaneous/threatened
- Abdominal trauma
- Obstetric procedures:
  - Amniocentesis
  - Chorionic villus sampling
  - Cordocentesis
  - External cephalic version
- Intrauterine death
- Multiple pregnancy
- Cesarean section
- Manual removal of placenta
- Infection with needles contaminated by Rh positive blood.

Q3. Can a nulliparous female with no prior history of blood transfusion or any other potential sensitizing event still develop alloimmunization?

Yes, this is because:
- In almost all pregnancies, small amounts of maternal blood enters the fetal circulation
- Thus, it is possible for a Rh D-negative female fetus exposed to maternal Rh D-positive red cells to develop sensitization
- When such an individual reaches adulthood, she may produce anti-D antibodies even before or early in her first pregnancy
- This mechanism is called the *grandmother theory* because the fetus in the current pregnancy is jeopardized by maternal antibodies that were initially provoked by his or her *grandmother's* erythrocytes.

Q4. Enumerate factors affecting development of alloimmunization?

Fetomaternal hemorrhage (FMH) occurs during delivery in almost all Rh negative patients but causes sensitization only in 10–15% of cases. This may be due to:
- Maternal inborn responsiveness—one-third of Rh negative woman are immunogenic nonresponders
- Strength of the antigenic stimulus—Rh D is the most potent Rh antigen.
- Amount of the FMH
- Coexistence of ABO incompatibility—reduces the risk of sensitization by 50–70% as ABO incompatible fetal cells are rapidly cleared from the maternal circulation making the fetal Rh antigen non-immunogenic.
- Inter pregnancy interval—Longer interval between primary and secondary sensitizations is associated with increased production of antibodies with greater avidity
- Du (weak D) positive individual—individuals who are Rh positive but D expression is weak.

Q5. What are other relevant investigations in this case?

- Husband's blood group and Rh factor.
- Nothing needs to be done if husband is Rh negative and paternity is certain.

Q6. How do you detect maternal alloimmunization?

It is detected by measuring the amount of anti-D antibodies in the maternal serum by the following methods:
- Indirect Coomb's test (human antiglobulin titer)
  - Most sensitive and reliable method
  - A titer value of 1:4 indicates alloimmunization.[2]
- Autoanalyzer—directly measures level of anti-Rh antibodies. Levels > 4 IU/mL are suggestive of alloimmunization.

Q7. How do you monitor a Rh negative non-sensitized pregnancy?

- Indirect Coomb's test (ICT) should be done 4 weekly starting from 1st ANC visit. If ICT is negative routine antenatal anti-D is administered at 28 weeks or earlier in events of fetomaternal hemorrhage
- If ICT is positive, ICT titers to be done to detect level of alloimmunization.
- Since incidence of Rh alloimmunization is <1% in antenatal period, screening for antibodies by ICT every 4 weeks is not universally accepted

- Mostly, ICT is done at first antenatal visit and at 28 weeks prior to anti-D administration to identify alloimmunized mothers.

Q8. What is RAADP?

Routine antenatal anti-D prophylaxis (RAADP) involves administration of anti-D to all non-sensitized women at 28 weeks in doses of 300 µg (1500 IU) sufficient to neutralize fetomaternal hemorrhage (FMH) of 15 mL fetal RBCs or 30 mL fetal blood.[3] The aim is to prevent antepartum sensitization by giving anti-D to take care of the silent bleeds which may occur in the antenatal period.

- Before the 28-week dose—repeat antibody screening is recommended to identify individuals who have become alloimmunized.
- As the risk of sensitization is <0.1% before 28 weeks, RAADP is not recommended before 28 weeks of gestation.
- After anti-D, ICT may be positive but the titer values do not go beyond 1:4
- Since the half-life of anti-D is 26 days, one dose negates sensitivity for 12 weeks
  So, one dose at 28 weeks and postpartum prophylaxis within 72 hours of delivery is recommended.
- Anti-D should also be given after any sensitizing event in pregnancy.

Q9. If a woman is weak D or Du individual, does she require RAADP?

- Du individuals are those who either have reduced numbers of normal Rh D antigens or express abnormal Rh D antigens
- Few cases of severe Rh D alloimmunization have been reported in Du phenotype women
- Diagnosing Du is not required in Rh D negative individual for transfusion[4]
- Similarly, if these individuals are pregnant, they are considered as candidates for anti-D immunoglobulines.

Q10. How does Rh immunoglobulin work?

Rh immunoglobulin (RhIg) is an antibody preparation, used for the prevention of Rh alloimmunization. It can be monoclonal or polyclonal.

- Mechanism of action—exact mechanism is not known
  - Masking of the Rh D antigenic sites by the antibodies
  - Partly through down regulation of B lymphocytes by Fc dependant mechanism before triggering an immune response
  - Another proposed mechanism is—rapid macrophage mediated clearance of anti-D coated RBCs
- Polyclonal antibody is the standard recommended prophylaxis—It is given deep intramuscular in the deltoid muscle. Injection in gluteus muscle is not given as it only reaches the subcutaneous tissue and absorption is delayed.

Q11. Are there any alternatives to Rh immunoglobulins?

- There are recent trials involving generation of recombinant Rh D immunoglobulins but none of them is commercially available as of now.
- A monoclonal antibody (Roledumab) and a recombinant antibody mixture (Rozrolimupab) are under phase II trials designed to prevent HDN.[5,6]

Q12. Are there any adverse consequences of Rh immunoglobulins?

- As its source is human plasma, potential risk of blood born infections are there
- Few reports of hepatitis C virus infections are there with contaminated immunoglobulins
- More advanced techniques of microfiltration reduces the risk to none.

Q13. How will you prevent alloimmunization in your case?

- A dose of 50 µg of anti-D is recommended for prophylaxis following all sensitizing events up to 12 weeks of pregnancy
- After 12 weeks, 300 µg or 1500 international units (IU) of anti-D should be given
- Thus I will administer 300 µg of anti-D to my patient in this case
- If FMH is > 4 mL-red cells and an additional anti-D should be given as required.

Q14. What is the dose of anti-D required in other antepartum potential sensitizing events?

- First trimester spontaneous/induced abortion—50 µg (Anti-D is not required in a case of first trimester spontaneous abortion without sugical evacuation).
- Ectopic pregnancy/molar pregnancy—50 µg.
- Chorionic villus biopsy—50 µg (<12 weeks) or 300 µg (> 12 weeks)
- Second trimester spontaneous/threatened/induced abortion—300 µg.
- Fetal blood sampling/amniocentesis—300 µg
- Abdominal trauma/external cephalic version—300 µg
- Antepartum hemorrhage—300 µg or more depending upon amount of FMH.

Anti-D should be given within 72 hours of the sensitizing event.

Q15. Does a patient with molar pregnancy require anti-D?

- Theoretically, there is no risk of Rh D alloimmunization in cases of classic complete molar pregnancy because organogenesis does not occur and thus Rh antigens are not present on trophoblasts
- In partial molar pregnancies, there may be some erythrocyte production making maternal exposure to the Rh D antigen possible.[7]
- However, since the diagnosis of partial versus complete molar pregnancy is completely based on histopathology, it is recommended to administer anti-D to all Rh D-negative women who are suspected of molar pregnancy and undergo uterine evacuation.

Q16. Had your patient been 11 weeks pregnant with threatened abortion, would you still administer anti-D?

- The Rh D antigen can be found on fetal erythrocytes as early as 5 weeks from fertilization and although rare, but cases of fetomaternal bleed have been seen in women with threatened abortion between 7 to 12 weeks of gestation
- It should be administered in late first trimester.

Q17. Does your patient require repeat Rh immunoglobulins? If Yes, When?

Yes, Because the half-life of anti-D is 26 days and so, the 300 µg dose provides protection only for 12 weeks.

- If the patient continues to bleed—it is advisable to assess FMH and administer required dose of anti-D accordingly or another dose of 300 µg may be repeated at six weekly intervals
- No more than 5 units (300 µg = 1 unit) of anti-D can be given in 24 hours by intramuscular route and if more dose is required in event of large FMH, intravenous route is preferred
- If using an intravenous preparation, 2 ampoules totaling 600 µg may be given every 8 hours
- To determine if the administered dose was adequate the ICT may be performed
- A positive results indicates excess of anti-D immunoglobulins suggesting the dose was sufficient.

Q18. What are the important considerations to be kept in mind during the delivery of a Rh negative mother?

- One should be gentle during delivery and cesarean and avoid blood mixing
- Early cord clamping to be done to minimize fetal blood mixing to mother
- Active management of the third stage should be withheld
- For any postpartum hemorrhage—avoid ergometrine
- The cord to be kept as long as possible—at least 10–15 cm to facilitate catheterization and exchange transfusion. (For alloimmunized pregnancy)
- Cord blood to be sent for blood grouping and Rh typing, hematocrit, bilirubin and direct Coomb's test
- Manual removal of placenta to be avoided as far as possible
- Baby should be attended by the neonatologist as baby may require resuscitation. Specially if the pregnancy is alloimmunized and the baby is affected
- O Rh negative blood should be made readily available
- The hematocrit and serum bilirubin concentrations are monitored at 6 hourly intervals in affected newborns.

Q19. What is postnatal immunoprophylaxis?

- A standard postnatal dose of 300 µg or 1500 IU is given to the mother intramuscularly within 72 hours of delivery if the baby is Rh positive and direct Coomb's test on umbilical cord blood is negative
- This decreases the incidence of Rh sensitization from 15 to 1-2%.

Q20. If you forget to administer postnatal anti-D in 1st 72 hours, does it have any role on day 4 postpartum?

- Although the ideal time to administer anti-D is within 72 hours of sensitizing event but it can be given up to 13 days after exposure
- Postpartum prophylaxis can be given up to as late as 28 days though protection provided against alloimmunization is suboptimal.[8,9]

Q21. Should a Rh negative woman undergoing postpartum sterilization still be administered anti-D?

Yes. Even though anti-D is given to prevent alloimmunisation and reduce risk to future pregnancies, still women undergoing sterilization should receive anti-D because:

- Sterilization failure can occur
- Alloimmunization complicates cross matching of blood products in the future.[10]

Q22. What methods are used to detect fetomaternal hemorrhage?

Fetomaternal hemorrhage can be detected through tests which either detect RhD antigen or cells with fetal hemoglobin.

- **Kleihauer Betke test**
- **Flow cytometry**
- **Rosetting test.**

Q23. What precautions are to be kept in mind to minimize ante/intra/postpartum fetomaternal hemorrhage?

- Abdominal palpation should be gentle in all cases of antepartum hemorrhage.
- External cephalic version should not be done under general anesthesia
- All invasive procedures during pregnancy should be performed under ultrasound guidance.
- Avoid Rh mismatched blood transfusions
- Avoid blood spillage during cesarean section
- Avoid prophylactic ergometrine at time of delivery to prevent postpartum hemorrhage
- Do not attempt manual removal of placenta.

Q24. Are there any contraindications to breastfeeding in a Rh negative mother?

No.

CASE SCENARIO

A young G2P1L1 with 32 weeks pregnancy came to antenatal OPD referred from district hospital in view of her blood group being O negative and ICT positive. Her previous pregnancy was uneventful. She had not received anti-D in her previous pregnancy.

Q1. What are the important points to be highlighted while history taking?

The important points to be noted while history taking are disscused below:

- *Possible sensitizing events during present pregnancy:*
  - Any history of any bleeding per vaginum, history of undergoing any procedure like chorionic villus sampling (CVS) or amniocentesis or history of any abdominal trauma
  - History of receiving anti-D after any such event
  - History of any blood transfusion in this pregnancy
- *Possible sensitizing events in previous pregnancy:*
  - History of any abortion/ectopic in the past
  - Any bleeding per vaginum/invasive procedures/ intrauterine manipulations/manual removal of placenta/blood transfusions in the previous antenatal period
  - Previous pregnancy outcome—baby with hydrops/ low birthweight/intrauterine death/baby born with jaundice or developed jaundice/any intrauterine blood transfusion being required/severity of jaundice/need for phototherapy or exchange transfusion
  - Development of polyhydramnios/pre-eclampsia
  - Mode of delivery—vaginal or cesarean
  - Receiving antepartum or postpartum anti-D
  - Past history—any history of blood transfusion.

Q2. What will be your next investigations?

- *Determination of ICT titers:* If titers are < 1: 16 (critical level), 4 weekly titers should be done. (American College of Obstetricians and Gynecologists, 2012).
- *Determination of paternal genotype:*
  - If father is Rh negative, no further testing required
  - If father is Rh positive
  - If father is homozygous, 100% fetuses will be Rh positive and no need for fetal Rh testing
  - If father is heterozygous, 50% chance of fetuses being Rh negative indicates the testing of fetal Rh type. If fetus is Rh negative, no further testing required
- *Determination of fetal blood group and Rh status:* If fetus is Rh negative, no further testing required.

Q3. What is the primary aim while managing a Rh alloimmunized pregnancy?

- Earliest diagnosis of fetal anemia
- Rate of progression
- Plan of delivery if near term or 34 weeks
- If remote from termination, correction of fetal anemia.

Q4. Does positive ICT titers necessarily indicate affection of fetus?

No, despite maternal sensitization fetus may be unaffected.

- When the father is heterozygous, fetus may be Rh negative
- An amnestic response can be there in a pregnancy with Rh negative fetus due to previous sensitization.

Q5. What are the various methods to determine fetal blood group?

- Amniocentesis
- Free fetal DNA can be obtained from maternal circulation and identified, using highly sensitized fluorescence based polymerase chain reaction. (Accuracy—99-100%).

Q6. Outline the management of a mother whose ICT titers remain below the critical level?

- Patient should be followed up by serial ultrasound till term (ACOG, 2012)
- Pregnancy should be terminated not more than 40 weeks

- The pediatrician/neonatologist should be informed prior to delivery
- The cord blood should be collected for Rh typing, direct Coomb's test, hemoglobin and serum bilirubin.

Q7. Outline management of the mother whose titers are above the critical level?

Here in this case if two consecutive titers are > critical level, patient should be evaluated by Doppler velocimetry of the middle cerebral artery (MCA).

Q8. Elaborate briefly the role of ultrasound in the management of Rh alloimmunized pregnancy?

- Assessment of fetal growth
- Identify hydrops/fetal ascites/cardiomegaly/hepatosplenomegaly/pleural or pericardial effusion
- Detection of fetal anemia using middle cerebral, umbilical vein and ductus venosus Doppler studies
- Liquor abnormalities—poly/oligohydramnios
- Placental thickness
- Fetal anasarca.

Q9. What is the pathophysiology behind hydrops fetalis?

Exact mechanism not clear but proposed theories are:
- Hemolysis leading to severe anemia and cardiac failure
- Severe hypoxia secondary to anemia affecting capillary permeability leading to third space losses
- Portal hypertension secondary to extramedullary hematopoiesis leading to ascites
- Low colloid osmotic pressure due to liver dysfunction and associated hypoproteinemia
- These changes usually occur when fetal hemoglobin falls below 7 g%.

Q10. How do you diagnose hydrops fetalis?

- *On history:* There is usually previous perinatal losses or history of severely jaundiced babies requiring exchange transfusions
- *On examination:* Liquor may be clinically increased
- *On CTG:* sinusoidal pattern of fetal heart
- *On ultrasound:* Fetal ascites, hepatosplenomegaly, pericardial and pleural effusion, scalp and skin edema and placentomegaly
- *On maternal X-ray abdomen:* Not recommended, done in smaller centers—Buddha position

Q11. What is the role of MCA Doppler in management of Rh alloimmunized pregnancy?

- Serial measurement of peak systolic velocity (PSV) of middle cerebral artery (MCA) to detect fetal anemia has completely replaced amniocentesis.[11]
- MCA PSV has sensitivity of 100% for prediction of anemia in the fetus with false positive rate of 12%.[12]
- Mechanism: In fetal anemia blood is preferably shunted towards the brain to prevent any hypoxic damage leading to increased PSV of MCA.
- A value of >1.5 MOM (multiples of median) for that gestational age necessitates fetal blood sampling and need for in utero transfusion
- MCA velocity is generally done from 23 weeks onwards till 35 weeks POG at every 1-2 weekly interval. It should not be used beyond 35 weeks due to high false positive rates.

Table 1: Values of MCA PSV based on multiples of median (MoM) between 23–35 weeks POG

Gestational age (weeks)	Multiples of median for MCA PSV			
	1.0	1.29	1.50	1.55
23	35.44	45.72	53.16	54.93
24	35.48	45.77	53.22	55.00
25	35.81	46.20	53.72	55.51
26	36.45	47.03	54.68	56.50
27	37.43	50.01	56.15	60.09
28	38.77	50.01	58.15	62.75
29	40.49	52.23	60.73	62.75
30	42.61	54.97	63.91	66.04
31	45.16	58.26	67.74	70.00
32	48.17	62.13	72.25	74.66
33	51.65	66.62	77.47	80.05
34	55.63	71.76	83.44	86.22
35	60.13	77.56	90.19	93.20

Q12. What is the role of amniocentesis in management of Rh alloimmunized pregnancy?

- Detection of fetal anemia—in centers where facility for MCA PSV is not available
- Detection of lung maturity—prior to termination of pregnancy
- Detection of fetal genotype—in heterozygous fathers to detect 50% fetuses which will be Rh negative.

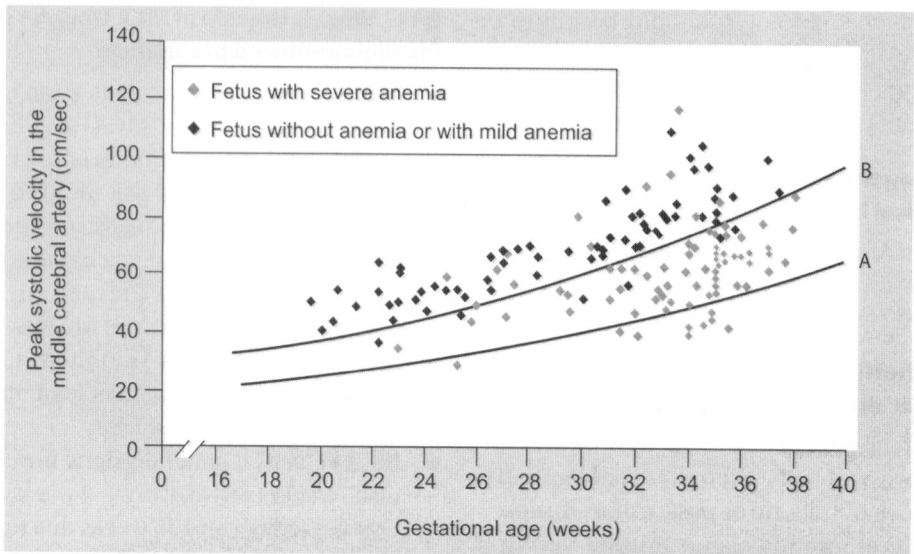

Fig. 1: PSV vs Gestational age chart showing a line A which indicates the median peak systolic velocity in normal pregnancies, and the line B showing 1.5 multiples of the median

Q13. How can you detect fetal anemia using amniocentesis?

- Liley (1961) used amniotic fluid spectral analysis to measure bilirubin concentration which is an indirect marker of hemolysis and thus predicts fetal anemia
- Using spectrophotometer, the change in optical density absorbance of amniotic fluid at 450 nm—referred to as ΔOD 450—is measured
- This ΔOD450 is plotted on a graph which is divided into several zones
- MCA PSV has completely replaced amniotic spectral analysis because of its greater sensitivity and accuracy. Amniocentesis is only done at centers where facility for MCA Doppler is not available or when pregnancy is beyond 35 weeks of gestation.
- The original Liley graph is valid from 27 to 42 weeks' gestation and contains three zones.
  - Zone 1
    - Indicates a Rh D-negative fetus or one with only mild disease
    - Pregnancy can be taken till term
    - Amniocentesis is repeated 3–4 weekly
  - Zone 2
    - Indicates moderately affected fetus with hemoglobin concentrations of 11.0–13.9 g/dL for values in lower zone 2 and those of 8.0–10.9 g/dL for upper zone 2
    - Monitor for signs of hydrops and repeat amniocentesis within 2 weeks
    - If value rises—manage as zone 3
    - If value remains same—deliver at 37 weeks.
  - Zone 3
    - Indicates severely affected fetus, with hemoglobin concentration <8.0 g/dL with a possibility of developing hydrops in next 7 days
    - If pregnancy is >34 weeks—deliver. Neonate may require exchange transfusion.
    - If pregnancy is <34 weeks—cordocentesis and intrauterine transfusion if hematocrit <30%. Give steroids at 32 weeks and repeat cordocentesis every 1–2 weeks to determine fetal Hct and need for transfusion and deliver at 34 weeks.

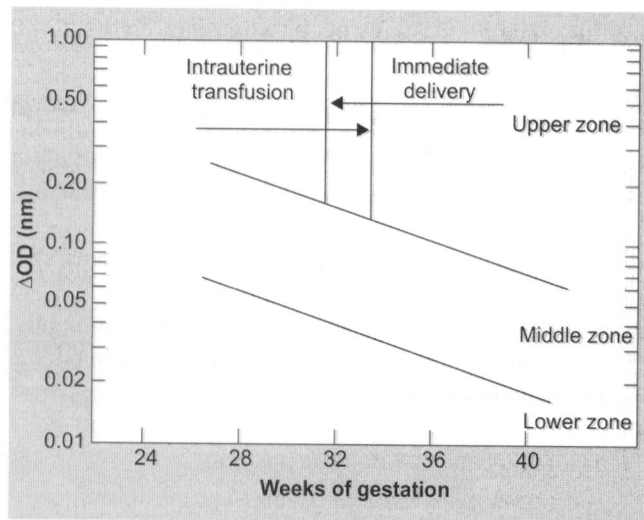

Fig. 2: Liley's graph—lower zone represents mildly or unaffected fetus, middle zone represents moderately affected fetus and upper zone indicates severe affection

Q14. What are the main indications for fetal blood sampling?

Cordocentesis allows precise measurement of fetal hemoglobin and hematocrit and the need for intrauterine blood transfusion.

The indications are:
- MCA PSV >1.5 MoM
- If OD 450 is in upper zone 2 or zone 3
- Rising trend of above two parameters
- Ultrasound features suggestive of fetal anemia
- Ultrasound suggestive of hydrops fetalis.

Q15. What are the indications for intrauterine transfusions?

The main indication for intrauterine transfusion is:
- Before 26 weeks gestation—hematocrit <25%
- After 26 weeks gestation—hematocrit <30%

  IUT can be started earliest at around 18-20 weeks. It is of three types:
1. Intravascular
2. Intraperitoneal
3. Combined.

Q16. Briefly enumerate important considerations prior and during the procedure of intrauterine transfusions?

- It should be performed in a tertiary care center with facilities for blood transfusion, neonatal ICU and fetal medicine specialist
- Informed consent should be taken and couple should be counselled regarding the procedure and possible risks involved
- Fresh O negative and CMV negative blood is cross matched against the mother
- It should be irradiated, leukocyte depleted and double packed to a Hct of 70-80%
- Strict asepsis should be maintained and the procedure should be carried out under antibiotic cover and tocolysis
- Confirm the fetal lie and attitude by ultrasound before starting the procedure
- Volume of blood needed for transfusion is:[13]

$$\frac{\text{(Desired hematocrit} - \text{actual hematocrit)}}{\text{Donor hematocrit}} \times \text{estimated fetoplacental blood volume}$$

- Usually 40-60 mL of blood is given in one sitting and this can be repeated every 1-2 weeks until 34 weeks.

Q17. What are the other alternative treatments for severely alloimmunized Rh negative pregnancy?

- Plasmapheresis
- Corticosteroids
- IVIg therapy
- Drugs like promethazine.

Q18. What factors decide termination of a Rh negative pregnancy?

Factors affecting termination include:
- Increased MCA PSV (>1.5 MoM)
- Previous history of still birth due to Rh alloimmunization
- ΔOD 450 in upper zone 2 or zone 3 on Liley's graph
- Hydropic fetus on ultrasound.

For mildly affected fetuses' delivery is conducted at 38 weeks.

For moderate—severely affected fetuses' intrauterine transfusions (if required) are given till 34 weeks and pregnancy is terminated at 34 weeks after giving steroid cover.

CASE SCENARIO

> A Rh negative G4 P3 L1 A0 with 20 weeks pregnancy comes with a past obstetric history of a first live born healthy child followed by the birth of a baby with jaundice who required phototherapy within 24 hours followed by an intrauterine fetal demise at 8 months of period of gestation. She did not receive anti-D at any time. Her anti-D titer is 1:16.

Q1. Describe the fetal and maternal effects of Rh alloimmunization?

Fetal

The various manifestations are as follows:
- *Immune hydrops (Erythroblastosis fetalis):* It is the most severe form of isoimmunization where excessive destruction of RBC's leads to severe anemia in fetus. This stimulates marked extramedullary hematopoiesis leading to hepatic and splenic dysfunction. As a result, there is cardiomegaly and marked fluid collection in third spaces. The hydropic fetus may be still born with signs of maceration.
- *Icterus gravis neonatorum:* It is a less severe manifestation wherein the baby develops jaundice within first 24 hours of birth. Red cell destruction leads to hyperbilirubinemia which in utero is cleared by placenta but as soon as the baby is born—the neonatal liver is unable to process such

high loads of bilirubin leading to jaundice. This may at times result even in kernicterus.
- *Congenital anemia of newborn:* It is the mildest form manifesting as mild to moderate pallor in the baby due to mild hemolysis. Jaundice is usually absent. This condition clears on itself by six weeks of life.

Maternal

The risk of following may be increased
- Pre-eclampsia
- Polyhydramnios
- Coagulopathy (If fetus is dead)
- Postpartum hemorrhage (secondary to coagulopathy, polyhydramnios and placentomegaly).

Q2. How will you manage this case?
- This is a case of severely sensitized Rh negative pregnancy
- Monitoring of mother for development of preeclampsia and polyhydramnios
- Biometry 2 weekly to monitor for fetal growth and hydropic changes
- MCA PSV every 2 weeks:
  – If <1.5 MoM with no USG changes in fetus—deliver the baby by 37–38 weeks
  – If >1.5 MoM
    ♦ Diagnose level of fetal anemia (fetal Hb and haematocrit)
    ♦ Intrauterine transfusion according to anemia, can be repeated every 10–14 days.
    ♦ USG monitoring to detect earliest features of hydrops
    ♦ Give steroid cover at 32 weeks and deliver by 34 weeks
    ♦ Transfusions can be continued till 35 weeks and delivery by 36–37 weeks if no features of hydrops on USG.
- Mode of delivery is decided upon gestational age and Bishops score.
- For preterm fetuses—cesarean section is a safe option
- For patients where Bishops is favorable and labor is induced, careful intrapartum monitoring is required.

Q3. Describe the neonatal management at birth?
- Neonatologist should be present at the time of delivery
- Neonatal intensive care unit should be readily available and prepared for exchange transfusion if required
- Rh negative, compatible blood should be available
- Cord blood samples are sent for estimation of blood group, DCT, Hct and bilirubin
- Cord to be kept longer to facilitate exchange transfusion if required
- Avoid squeezing the cord.

Q4. What are the indications for exchange transfusion?
- Cord hemoglobin <10 g% or Hct <30%
- Cord bil > 5 mg/dL
- Term infants with serum Bil >20 mg/dL
- Increase in newborns bilirubin @ >1mg/dL/hour even after phototherapy.

Q5. What are the other management options for the neonate?
- Phototherapy
- Intravenous immunoglobulin (IVIg)
- Erythropoietin
- Supplemental iron
- Drugs like phenobarbitone and metalloporphyrins.

Q6. What is the long-term prognosis of the baby?
- For unaffected babies—prognosis is good
- For affected babies the prognosis depends on development of hydrops or not. Though significant improvement has occurred following introduction of MCA PSV and intrauterine transfusions—despite that 30–40% fetuses develop irreversible hydropic changes and carry poor prognosis
- Affected babies have increased morbidity and mortality due to anemia and jaundice
- Long-term poor outcomes due to premature delivery include risk of developmental delays and cerebral palsy.

REFERENCES

1. Alloimmunization in pregnancy: Rhesus and other red cell antigens. In: Charles HR odeck, Anna P. Cockell; Turnbulls Obstetrics (3rd edition); Geoffrey Chamberlain, Philip Steer, 247-61.
2. Rh alloimmunization; Practical guide to high risk pregnancy and delivery (3rd edition); Fernando Arias, Daftary, Bhide. 358-71.
3. Prevention of Rh alloimmunization. SOGC Clinical Practice Guidelines No. 133, 2003.
4. Fung MK, Grossman BJ, Hillyer CD, Westhoff CM, (Eds). Technical manual. 18th edition. Bethesda (MD): American Association of Blood Banks; 2014.
5. Stasi R. Rozrolimupab, symphobodies against rhesus D, for the potential prevention of hemolytic disease of the newborn and the treatment of idiopathic thrombocytopenic purpura. Curr Opin Mol Ther. 2010;12:734-40.
6. Yver A, Homery MC, Fuseau E, et al. Pharmacokinetics and safety of roledumab: a novel human recombinant monoclonal

anti-RhD antibody with an optimized Fc for improved engagement of FcgammaRIII, in healthy volunteers. Vox Sang. 2012;103:213-22.
7. Morrow CP, Curtin JP. Tumors of the placental trophoblast. Tumors of the placental trophoblast. Synopsis of Gynecologic Oncology. 5th edition. New York (NY): Churchill Livingstone; 1998. p. 315-51.
8. Committee on Practice Bulletins-Obstetrics. Practice Bulletin No. 181: Prevention of RhD Alloimmunization. Obstet Gynecol. 2017;130(2):e57-e70.
9. Samson D, Mollison PL. Effect on primary Rh immunization of delayed administration of anti-Rh. Immunology. 1975;28: 349-57.
10. Gorman JG, Freda VJ. Rh immune globulin is indicated for Rh-negative mothers undergoing sterilization. Am J Obstet Gynecol. 1972;112:868-9.
11. Mari G, Deter RL, Carpenter RL, et al. Noninvasive diagnosis by Doppler ultrasonography of fetal anemia due to red cell alloimmunization. New Eng J Med. 2000;342:9-14.
12. Moise KJ. Hemolytic disease of fetus and newborn, Maternal Fetal Medicine: Principles and Practice (5th edition); Robert Creasy, Robert Resnik. 537-61.
13. Diseases of fetus and newborn; Williams obstetrics (23rd edn). 618-27.

CHAPTER 8

Pregnancy with Previous Cesarean Section

Bidisha Singha

"Once a cesarean always a cesarean" was a dictum of management of pregnancies with previous cesarean. Increased cesarean rate has been observed in both developing and developed countries, including India. Cesarean rates are much higher than the recommended level of 5–15%.[1] With emerging evidences, trial of labor after cesarean section (TOLAC) is an acceptable current practice.

CASE SCENARIO

G4P2L2A1 with nine months amenorrhea with false labor pain.

Mrs A, 30 years old, wife of Mr B, R/Paharganj, a housewife, came to gyne casualty on 22/8/17 with complaints of:
- Amenorrhea 9 months
- Pain in lower abdomen for 2 hours
- Her last menstrual period (LMP) was 22.11.16 so making her period of gestation (POG) 39 weeks on 22.8.17.

History of Presenting Complaint

- Patient is a booked case of our hospital
- She complained of pain lower abdomen for 2 hours, intermittent in nature, irregular in frequency, not associated with back pain
- No history of leaking or bleeding per vaginum
- Perceiving adequate fetal movements
- No history of backache, radiation of the pain, any aggravating or relieving factors
- No history of any abdominal trauma
- No history of abnormal bladder and bowel symptoms.

Course in the Hospital

- She was admitted to the labor room after her general physical, abdominal and internal examination
- Received an injection of analgesic and monitored for abdominal pain and fetal heart
- Relieved of symptoms after 3–4 hours
- After checking her fetal heart on a machine, most probably non-stress test (NST), she was shifted to maternity ward
- Blood sample was taken in the labor room.

Obstetric History

- *P1L1:* 6 years back full term lower segment cesarean section (LSCS) done in view of arrest of labor. Peripartum and postpartum period was un-eventful, baby healthy, breastfed, immunized till date.
- *P2L2:* 3 years back, vaginal birth after cesarean section (VBAC), baby healthy, rest un-eventful. Birth weight—3.0 kg.
- *A1:* 2 months gestation—spontaneous abortion. No history of dilatation and evacuation—2 years back.

Diagnosis

G4P2L2A1 at 39 weeks of gestation, previous cesarean section, term size with cephalic presentation with false labor pain.

Q1. What are the important points to be noted while taking history in a case of previous CS?

- Previous obstetric history
- Number of previous pregnancies
- Mode of delivery in the previous pregnancies
  In case of previous cesarean
  – Indication of CS
  – At what gestation
  – At what stage of labor
  – Was it done elective or emergency
  – Type of CS (history/records)

- Time since the last CS
- Any intrapartum complications
- Any history of blood transfusion
- Any postpartum complications (puerperal infection/wound infection)
- In case of wound sepsis, whether resuturing has been done or not
- Number of CS
- Prevoius records to be asked for and details are to be recorded
- Any history of any abortion, if yes whether dilatation and evacuation (D & E) was done or not
- Any previous vaginal delivery—prior to CS/VBAC (vaginal birth after CS).

Q2. What are the important specific points to be noted during examination?

General Examination
- Height—short stature may be associated with cephalopelvic disproportion (CPD)
- Pallor—to rule out anemia, prior to elective repeat cesarean section (ERCS)/labor
- Pulse—tachycardia is a sign of scar dehiscence.

Abdominal Examination
- Details of the scar, type (vertical/transverse), healing of the scar (primary intention/secondary intention/keloid)
- Fetal lie, presentation. Fetal weight
- Scar tenderness to be checked—engage patient in conversation, palpate the lower part of uterus just behind the pubic symphysis in between uterine contractions and watch whether the patient winces in pain during palpation.

Per Vaginal Examination
Pelvic assessment done at 36 weeks for pelvic adequacy and to rule out CPD.

Q3. What all investigations are important in this case and for what purpose?

Apart from routine blood and urine investigation, level II ultrasound sonography test (USG) in a case of previous CS
- Ultrasound for placental localization is important. In case of low lying placenta, morbid adherent placenta should be ruled out by USG Doppler and magnetic resonance imaging (MRI)

Risk of placenta previa in pregnancies following cesarean section[2]
- Previous 1 CS—1%
- Previous 2 CS—1.7%
- Previous 3 or more CS—2.8%

Incidence of placenta accreta in cases of placenta previa with previous cesarean section[2]
- Previous 1 CS—11–14%
- Previous 2 CS—23–40%
- Previous 5 or more—up to 60%

- Measurement of lower uterine segment thickness by USG antenatally can be used to predict the chances of uterine dehiscence or rupture in patient undergoing trial of labor after cesarean section (TOLAC). Recent meta-analysis suggested.[3]

Myometrial thickness cut-off of 2.1–4.0 mm—strong negative predictive value

Between 0.6 and 2.0 mm—strong positive predictive value for the occurrence of uterine defect.

Q4. What is the role of antenatal counseling in this patient?[4]
- Patient need to be counseled regarding the delivery options (VBAC/ERCS)
- Counseling to be documented in the records
- All risk and benefits of VBAC and ERCS explained
- Consideration of intended family size is important
- Final decision regarding the mode of birth should be finalized by 36 weeks and it should be agreed by patient and obstetrician team
- Plan of management to be recorded.

Q5. What suitable criteria are there for VBAC?
- Consent for VBAC
- Singleton pregnancy
- Cephalic presentation
- At 37 weeks or beyond
- Previous lower segment cesarean section
- With or without previous vaginal delivery.

Q6. What are the Contraindications of VBAC?
- Previous uterine rupture
- Previous classical cesarean section
- Absolute contraindications to vaginal birth (major placenta previa)
- Contracted pelvis/CPD
- Patient refusal for VBAC.

Q7. What are the risks and benefits of TOLAC and ERCS[5-10]

	Planned VBAC	ERCS at 39 weeks
Maternal outcome	• Success rate—72–75% • Few complications • Short hospital stay and recovery • Risk of uterine rupture —0.5% • The chances of future vaginal deliveries are increased • Increased rate of instrumental delivery • Risk of maternal death less	• 0.02% risk of uterine rupture • Longer recovery • Will require cesarean delivery for future pregnancies • Increased risk of placenta previa/accreta and adhesions • Reduces risk of pelvic organ prolapse and urinary incontinence • Sterilization can be done if not desirous of future pregnancies • Risk of maternal death is increased
Infant outcome	• 2–3% risk of transient respiratory morbidity • 0.08% risk of hypoxic ischaemic encephalopathy (HIE) • 0.1% risk of antepartum stillbirth > 39 weeks • 0.04% risk of delivery related perinatal death	• 4–5% risk of transient respiratory morbidity • <0.01% risk of HIE

Q8. What are the predictors of VBAC success or failure[11-16]

Increased chances of success	Decreased chances of success
Prior vaginal delivery (89%)	Maternal obesity
Prior VBAC (85–90%)	Short maternal stature
Spontaneous labor	Macrosomia
Favorable cervix	Increased maternal age (> 40 years)
Nonrecurring indication (malpresentations, placenta previa)	Induction of labor
Preterm delivery	Recurring indication (CPD), arrest in second stage
	Gestational age >41 weeks
	Increased interpregnancy weight gain

Q9. What the components for VBAC score?

VBAC score is a simple scoring system used at labor admission to predict a successful VBAC[17]

Five Features
- Bishop score on admission
- Indication of previous cesarean section
- Body mass index (BMI)
- Age
- Previous vaginal birth (both before or after cesarean section)

Higher the VBAC score, higher the success rate
Score >16—success rate of 85%
Score <10—success rate of 49%.

Q10. What are the different inducing agents that can be used?

- *Oxytocin:* Medical induction of labor with oxytocin may be associated with risk of uterine rupture and should be used carefully after appropriate counseling. Risk of uterine rupture is dose-dependent.
  - Start with 0.4 mu/mL and increase every 30 minutes
  - Maximum dose recommended is up to 20 milliunits/minute
  - Proper monitoring is essential and infusion pump to be used if available
  - Risk of rupture is 1.1% with oxytocin alone and 1.4% with oxytocin and prostaglandin together.[18]
- *Prostaglandin E2 or dinoprostone:* Medical induction with PGE2 is associated with increased risk of uterine rupture, so it should be used after appropriate selection of patient and counseling. Not more than one dose of PGE2 should be used
- *Prostaglandin E1 or misoprostol:* PGE1 is associated with high risk of uterine rupture and should not be used for induction in patients with previous cesarean section. In the recent WHO document comparing misoprostol with oxytocin, it was noted that misoprostol is associated with increased risk of rupture
- *Intracervical Foley Catheter:* Most accepted method of cervical ripening in a case of previous cesarean section.

Q11. What are the important points to be counseled while inducing or augmenting a patient with previous section?

- Induction of labor for maternal or fetal indication is an option in women undergoing TOLAC
- Two-to threefold increase risk of uterine rupture and 1.5 fold increased risk of cesarean delivery in induced or augmented cases compared to spontaneous labor

Risk of uterine rupture ranges between[19]
- 0.15–0.4% in spontaneous labor
- 0.54–1.4% in induced labor
- 0.9–1.9% in augmented labor.

Q12. What is the intrapartum management in a case of planned VBAC?

Patient is Considered as High Risk

Delivery to be conducted in a hospital setup with emergency cesarean and blood bank facility.

- Patients and relatives should be counseled, success and failure rates to be explained and informed consent is taken for all possible events
- Intravenous access
- Blood grouping and cross-matching to be done, blood availability to be ensured
- Maternal monitoring (vitals, any signs and symptoms of scar dehiscence or uterine rupture)
- Clear liquids are allowed orally
- Continuous electronic fetal heart rate monitoring should be done
- Epidural analgesia
- Partogram to be maintained
- Cut short the second stage of labor.

Q13. What are the predictors of uterine rupture?[20-24]

Increased rate of uterine rupture	Decreased rate of uterine rupture
Classical hysterotomy	Spontaneous labor
Two or more previous CS	Prior vaginal delivery
Single layer closure	Longer interpregnancy interval
Induction of labor	Preterm delivery
Use of prostaglandins	
Short interpregnancy interval (less than 12 months since last delivery)	
Infection at prior cesarean	

Q14. What are the signs and symptoms of uterine rupture and management?

Classic triad of complete uterine rupture—Pain/vaginal bleeding/fetal heart rate abnormalities. Present only in 10%.

Clinical Features

Presence of any of the features below, suggestive of uterine rupture
- Maternal tachycardia, hypotension or shock
- Abnormal **CTG** (most consistent finding)
- Severe abdominal pain
- Shoulder tip pain/chest pain
- Acute onset scar tenderness
- Abnormal vaginal bleeding
- Cessation of previously efficient uterine activity
- Loss of uterine contour
- Fetal parts easily palpable
- Absent fetal heart rate
- Loss of station of presenting part
- Hematuria.

* 90% of uterine rupture occur during labor with peak incidence at 4–5 cm of cervical dilatation, 18% during second stage and 8% detected postvaginal delivery.

Management

Resuscitation

Laparotomy followed by repair/hysterectomy/repair and sterilization

- *Repair:* Done in scar rupture cases, where margins are clean. Done after excision of fibrous tissue at the margins.
  - Desirous of future pregnancy
  - Repair is feasible
- *Cesarean hysterectomy*
  - Uncontrollable hemorrhage
  - Rupture involving broad ligament vessels
  - Morbidly adherent placenta
- *Repair and sterilization:* Done in clean scar rupture and not desirous of having further children.

Q15. What is scar dehiscence and scar rupture?

- *Scar dehiscence:* Disruption of a part of previous scar, fetal membranes are intact
- *Scar rupture:* Disruption of the entire length of the previous scar with separation of all layers of uterus including the serosa, rupture of fetal membranes.

Q16. How will you manage a case with history of previous rupture uterus?

- It is recommended that patient with previous history of rupture should undergo elective cesarean prior to onset of labor. Each case to be individualized and time of termination to be decided
- If previous scar rupture was confined to lower segment of uterus, rate of repeat scar rupture or dehiscence in labor is 6%. if the previous rupture involved the upper segment, repeat rupture rate is 32%.[25,26]

Q17. What is the plan of management in this case?

Patient had a prior vaginal delivery. After ruling out CPD, patient can have planned VBAC. One can wait for spontaneous labor till 41 weeks unless there is any contraindication.

Q18. What should be the plan if patient does not have spontaneous labor by 41 weeks?

- Induction of labor done only after clinical and cervical assessment[27]

- Risk of stillbirth at or after 39 weeks is 1.5- and 2-fold higher in women with previous cesarean compared with women without previous CS.

Q19. Is external cephalic version (ECV) in a case of previous cesarean with breech presentation, indicated?

External cephalic version is not contraindicated in a case of previous cesarean section with no other maternal or fetal risk.[28]

Q20. Can TOLAC be considered in a case of previous cesarean with twin gestation?

- TOLAC can be considered in a women with previous lower segment cesarean section[29]
- Patient with longitudinal lie with first cephalic baby with spontaneous labor has a better chance of success.

Q21. What are the preoperative requirements for elective repeat cesarean section?[4]

- Timing for ERCS—after 39 weeks of gestation
- Thromboprophylaxis in high risk cases, e.g. obese patients. Royal College of Obstetricians and Gynaecologist (RCOG) recommends it routinely as preoperative measure for ERCS
- Antenatal corticosteroids up to 39 + 6 weeks
- Pre-incision antibiotics to protect against wound infection, urinary tract infection and endometritis. Ideal antibiotics are cefuroxime and metronidazole
- In case of placenta previa with previous LSCS, multidisciplinary approach must be taken.

Q22. What is the management of previous cesarean for delivery of second trimester IUD?

- Prostaglandins (misoprostol) can be used for induction
- Studies published though small, shows that outcomes are similar when compared with unscarred uterus. Rate of uterine rupture is less than 1%[30-32]
- In cases of IUD after 28 weeks transcervical Foley catheter can be used.[33]

Q23. What are the different types of uterine incision and their associated risk of uterine rupture?[34]

- Lower segment transverse incision—commonly recommended, risk of rupture—0.2–1.5 %
- T-shaped—transverse lower uterine incision with vertical extension in upper segment. Risk of rupture 4–9%
- Lower segment vertical incision
  - Indications—placenta previa, large baby, shoulder presentation, conjoint twins
  - Can be considered if access to lower uterine segment is limited due to prematurity, obstructive lesion, presenting part high up. Risk of uterine rupture 1–7%
- Classical cesarean section—common indications-placenta accreta, densely adherent bladder, postmortem delivery, large leiomyoma in the lower segment. Risk of rupture is high 4–9%.

REFERENCES

1. WHO Statement on cesarean section rates, April 2015.
2. Guise JM, Eden K, Emeis C, et al. Vaginal Birth After Cesarean: New Insights. Evidence Reports/Technology Assessments, No. 191. Rockville, Maryland, USA: Agency for Healthcare Research and Quality; 2010.
3. Kok N, Wiersma IC, Opmeer BC, et al. Sonographic measurement of lower uterine segment thickness to predict uterine rupture during a trial of labor in women with previous Cesarean section: a meta-analysis. Ultrasound Obstet Gynecol. 2013;42:132-9.
4. Royal College of Obstetricians and Gynaecologist. Birth after previous Caeserean Birth. Green-top guideline No. 45, October 2015.
5. Landon MB, Hauth JC, Leveno KJ, et al.; National Institute of Child Health and Human Development Maternal–Fetal Medicine Units Network. Maternal and perinatal outcomes associated with a trial of labor after prior cesarean delivery. N Engl J Med. 2004;351:2581-9.76.
6. Smith GC, Pell JP, Dobbie R. Cesarean section and risk of unexplained stillbirth in subsequent pregnancy. Lancet. 2003;362:1779-84.
7. Go MD, Emeis C, Guise JM, et al. Fetal and neonatal morbidity and mortality following delivery after previous cesarean. Clin Perinatol. 2011;38:311-9.
8. Kamath BD, Todd JK, Glazner JE, et al. Neonatal outcomes after elective cesarean delivery. Obstet Gynecol. 2009;113:1231-8.
9. Richardson BS, Czikk MJ, daSilva O, et al. The impact of labor at term on measures of neonatal outcome. Am J Obstet Gynecol. 2005;192:219-26.
10. Zanardo V, Simbi AK, Franzoi M, et al. Neonatal respiratory morbidity risk and mode of delivery at term: influence of timing of elective cesarean delivery. Acta Paediatr. 2004;93:643-7.
11. Aaron B Caughey, Carl V Smith. Vaginal Birth After Cesarean Delivery. Overview, Preparation and Technique. Medscape. Dec 2015.
12. Zelop CM, Shipp TD, Cohen A, et al. Trial of labor after 40 weeks' gestation in women with prior cesarean. Obstet Gynecol. 2001;97:391-3. (Level II-2)
13. Chauhan SP, Magann EF, Carroll CS, et al. Mode of delivery for the morbidly obese with prior cesarean delivery: vaginal versus repeat cesarean section. Am J Obstet Gynecol. 2001;185:349-54. (Level II-2)

14. Srinivas SK, Stamilio DM, Sammel MD, et al. Vaginal birth after cesarean delivery: does maternal age affect safety and success? Paediatr Perinat Epidemiol. 2007;21:114-20. (Level II-2)
15. Goodall PT, Ahn JT, Chapa JB, et al. Obesity as a risk factor for failed trial of labor in patients with previous cesarean delivery. Am J Obstet Gynecol. 2005;192:1423-6. (Level II-3)
16. Zelop CM, Shipp TD, Repke JT, et al. Outcomes of trial of labor following previous cesarean delivery among women with fetuses weighing >4000 g. Am J Obstet Gynecol. 2001;185:903-5. (Level II-2).
17. Metz TD, Stoddard GJ, Henry E, et al. Simple, validated vaginal birth after cesarean delivery prediction model for use at the time of admission. Obstet Gynecol. 2013;122: 571-8.
18. SOCG guidelines for vaginal birth after previous cesarean birth. Feb 2005.
19. Ravasia DJ, Wood SL, Pollard JK. Uterine rupture during induced trial of labor among women with previous Cesarean delivery. Am J Obstet Gynecol. 2000;183:1176-9.
20. Shipp TD, Zelop CM, Repke JT, et al. Intrapartum uterine rupture and dehiscence in patients with prior lower uterine segment vertical and transverse incisions. Obstet gynecol. 1999; 94(5 Pt 1):735-40.
21. Macones GA, Peipert J, Nelson DB, et al. Maternal complications with vaginal birth after cesarean delivery: a multicentric study. Am J Obstet Gynecol. 2005;193(5): 1656-62.
22. Leung AS, Farmer RM, Leung EK, et al. Risk of factors associated with uterine rupture during trial of labour after cesarean delivery: a case control study. Am J Obstet Gynecol. 1993;168(5):1358-63.
23. Zelop CM, Shipp TD, Repke JT, et al. Effect of previous vaginal delivery on the risk of uterine rupture during a subsequent trial of labor. Am J Obstet Gynecol. 2000;183(5):1184-6.
24. Zelop CM, Shipp TD, Repke JT, et al. Uterine rupture during induced or augmented labor in gravid women with one prior cesarean delivery. Am J Obstet Gynecol. 1999;181(4): 882-6.
25. Ritchie EH. Pregnancy after rupture of the pregnant uterus. A report of 36 pregnancies and a study of cases reported since 1932. J Obstet Gynaecol Br Commonw. 1971;78:642-8. (Level III)
26. Reyes-Ceja L, Cabrera R, Insfran E, et al. Pregnancy following previous uterine rupture. Study of 19 patients. Obstet Gynecol. 1969;34:387-9. (Level III)
27. National Institute for Health and Clinical Excellence. Induction of labour. NICE clinical guideline 70. Manchester: NICE; 2008.
28. Flamm BL, Fried MW, Lonky NM, et al. External cephalic version after previous cesarean section. Am J Obstet Gynecol. 1991;165:370-2. (Level II-2)
29. Cahill A, Stamilio DM, Paré E, et al. Vaginal birth after cesarean (VBAC) attempt in twin pregnancies: is it safe? Am J Obstet Gynecol. 2005;193:1050-5.
30. Bhattacharjee N, Ganguly RP, Saha SP. Misoprostol for termination of mid-trimester post-Cesarean pregnancy. Aust N Z J Obstet Gynaecol. 2007;47:23-5. (Level II-2)
31. Marinoni E, Santoro M, Vitagliano MP, et al. Intravaginal gemeprost and second trimester pregnancy termination in the scarred uterus. Int J Gynaecol Obstet. 2007;97:35-9. (Level II-2)
32. Daponte A, Nzewenga G, Dimopoulos KD, et al. The use of vaginal misoprostol for second-trimester pregnancy termination in women with previous single cesarean section. Contraception. 2006;74:324-7. (Level III)
33. Hoffman MK, Sciscione A, Srinivasana M, et al. Uterine rupture in patients with a prior cesarean delivery: the impact of cervical ripening. Am J Perinatol. 2004;21:217-22. (Level II-2)
34. American College of Obstetricians and Gynaecologist. Vaginal birth after previous cesarean delivery. Practice bulletin No. 115, August 2010.

CHAPTER 9

Morbidly Adherent Placenta

Devender Verma

CASE SCENARIO

Mrs XX 26 years age wife of Mr XY resident of Delhi, a homemaker, came to gyne casualty with complaints of:
- 9 months pregnancy
- Pain lower abdomen for 3 hours and discharge PV for 3 hours.

Patient was apprehensive regarding a sonography report suggestive of abnormal placentation which can cause severe bleeding during delivery, as told to her by radiologist.

She was Gravida 3 Para 1 Live 1 and Abortion 1 and was carrying 37 weeks pregnancy [by last menstrual period (LMP)]. She was a booked case.

She had dull aching pain in lower abdomen and mucoid vaginal discharge for 3 hours. There was no episode of bleeding or leaking per vaginum (PV). She was perceiving fetal movements regularly.

- After admission she was given 2 injections following which she was relieved of her symptoms
- Her doctor told her about her condition that she would be delivered by cesarean section only, might require multiple blood and loose her uterus but first her ultrasonography (USG) would be repeated to reconfirm the diagnosis and extent of her problem
- 3 Years back, she had Emergency lower segment cesarean section at term pregnancy for fetal distress
- Baby was 2.8 kg at birth, exclusive breast fed for 6 months
- Antenatal and postnatal period was uneventful.

She had spontaneous abortion at 2 months of amenorrhea followed by evacuation in the hospital, 1 year back.

There was no other significant history.

Examination

- Patient was conscious, oriented and sitting comfortably in the bed
- Average built with gait normal, normal hairline, average orodental hygiene
- General condition good—height 155 cm
- Weight 65 kg
- Body mass index (BMI) was not calculated (as pre-pregnancy weight was not known)
- No pallor, icterus, cyanosis, clubbing or pedal edema observed
- Pulse rate 88/min, regular with no radiofemoral or radio-radial delay
- Blood pressure was 110/80 mm Hg in right arm in sitting position
- Respiratory rate—16/min
- Thyroid—normal.

Respiratory System

- Trachea centrally placed
- Normal vesicular sound heard all over the chest with bilateral air entry equal on both sides with no added sounds.

Cardiovascular System

S1 and S2 normal with no murmur.

Abdominal Examination

Inspection

- Abdomen was uniformly distended with all quadrants moving with respiration
- Linea nigra and striae gravidarum present, suprapubic transverse scar was seen
- Umbilicus was central and everted
- All hernial sites are free.

Palpation
- Fundal height—34 weeks
- Symphysio—fundal height (SFH)—34 cm
- Abdominal girth (AG)—32 inches.

Fundal Grip
A soft broad fetal pole was felt at fundus, suggestive of breech.

Lateral Grip
- Smooth and curved structure felt on the right lateral side of the abdomen, suggestive of back
- Multiple knobby parts felt on the left side, suggestive of limbs.

First Pelvic Grip
- A hard, globular and smooth structure felt on palpation, suggestive of head
- Head was freely mobile.

Second Pelvic Grip
- Head was not engaged and no scar tenderness felt Uterus relaxed, no contractions felt
- Liquor appears normal.

Auscultation
Fetal heart sound was heard at the right spinoumbilical line 134 beats/min, regular.

Perineal Examination
- External genitalia normal
- No bleeding and no leaking observed

Per Speculum Examination
- Os closed
- Cervix long
- No discharge, bleeding or leaking observed.

Diagnosis after Examination
G3 P1 L1 A1 with 37 weeks period of gestation with previous lower segment cesarean section (LSCS) with cephalic presentation and false labor pains with ? placenta previa adherent.

Q1. What will you do if this case is seen in casualty?
Patient and her relatives would be explained regarding the possibilities and consequences that she can have, i.e. placenta previa/accreta and its management and possible morbidities associated with it. She will be admitted in view of term pregnancy with previous LSCS with? abnormal placentation for workup, observation and fetal well-being.

Her antenatal records will be reviewed for the following: antenatal examinations, fetal growth, investigations and antenatal ultrasound. A repeat ultrasound will be advised for ascertaining the diagnosis of placenta previa.

Q2. What are features/findings you will note in USG report?
Number of fetus, fetal biometry, gestational age, anomalies, placental localization, features of morbid adherence (loss of hypoechoic layer between the placenta and myometrium) and liquor.

Q3. How will you define placental abnormalities (abnormal placentation) in such circumstances?
If the placenta is situated in lower segment within 2 cm from the internal os, it is called as placenta previa. In a case of anterior placenta previa with previous cesarean section, we must rule out morbidly adherent placenta.

Q4. What is adherent placenta?
When placenta (anchoring placental villi) is invading uterus beyond decidua basalis, it is called adherent placenta. Morbidly adherent placenta is a general term that includes placenta accreta, increta, and percreta depending on extent of invasion into the myometrium or beyond it (perforating uterine wall). This is commonly due to the complete or partial absence of the decidua basalis leading to defect in the Nitabuch membrane.
- *Accreta:* Adheres to myometrium
- *Increta:* Invades the myometrium
- *Percreta:* Perforates the myometrium and serosa.

Q5. Why should you worry about adherent placenta?
- Adherent placenta is commonly associated with placenta previa and hemorrhage during operative delivery due to nonseparation or partial separation of placenta
- It has high maternal & perinatal morbidity and mortality due to massive obstetrics hemorrhage (MOH) and emergency cesarean hysterectomy
- Maternal mortality reported is 10% in cases associated with placenta percreta[8]
- Involvement of the urinary bladder is associated with higher morbidity such as massive hemorrhage and bladder resection
- Maternal and fetal morbidity and mortality in such cases are associated with multiple blood and blood products transfusion, intensive care unit (ICU) and high dependent unit (HDU) admission
- Morbidly adherent placenta (38%) was one of the most commonly reported causes of hemorrhage leading to peripartum hysterectomy.[6]

Q6. What are the risk factors associated with morbidly adherent placenta?

The risk factors associated with morbidly adherent placenta are:
- Previous cesarean delivery (12%)
- Placenta previa (10%)
- Advanced maternal age
- High gravidity
- Multiparity
- Previous curettage.[9]

Q7. What is the incidence?

Incidence of placenta accreta continue to increase due to increased incidence of cesarean sections, placenta previa and/or increasing maternal age.[2] Placenta accreta occurs in approximately 1 of 2500 deliveries. Among women with placenta previa, the incidence is nearly 10%.[1]

Placenta percreta, represent 5–7% of all abnormal placentations and 75% of placenta percreta are associated with placenta previa.[7] A high degree of clinical suspicion is of utmost importance when the placenta is located over a previous uterine scar.

Q8. Can we clinically diagnose placenta previa or adherent placenta? Which cases should have high suspicion for adherent placenta?

- High suspicion is the key to management of adherent placenta
- One should have high suspicion in cases with previous cesarean sections or curettages due to scarring of uterine endometrium hence loss of decidua basalis
- Cases with previous uterine surgeries, e.g. myomectomy
- History of bleeding per vaginum beyond 20 weeks of pregnancy
- Cases with placenta previa
- In fact all cases of painless bleeding PV and malpresentations or high floating presenting part should be screened for abnormal placentation (placenta previa) and subsequently for adherence.

Q9. How do you diagnose adherent placenta?

There are different imaging modalities to diagnose adherent placenta.
- USG is the most common and sufficient mode to diagnose
- Doppler studies are required in suspected cases
- In cases where diagnosis is doubtful, magnetic resonance imaging (MRI) can be done.

Q10. What are the USG findings in adherent placenta?

USG is very useful and sensitive investigation for adherent placenta. Its sensitivity and specificity are as follows (Table 1):[3-5]

Table 1: Diagnostic performance of different ultrasound modalities

	Positive predictive value (%)	Sensitivity (%)	Specificity (%)
Ultrasonography (grayscale)	82	95	76
Color Doppler	76	92	68
3 D power Doppler	88	100	85

Ultrasound criteria for adherent placenta commonly used for diagnosis are as follows:

Grayscale
- Loss of the retroplacental sonolucent zone
- Irregular retroplacental sonolucent zone
- Thinning or disruption of the hyperechoic serosa–bladder interface
- Presence of focal exophytic masses invading the urinary bladder
- Abnormal placental lacunae.

Color Doppler (Fig. 1)
- Diffuse or focal lacunar flow
- Vascular lakes with turbulent flow (peak systolic velocity over 15 cm/s)
- Hypervascularity of serosa–bladder interface
- Markedly dilated vessels over peripheral subplacental zone.

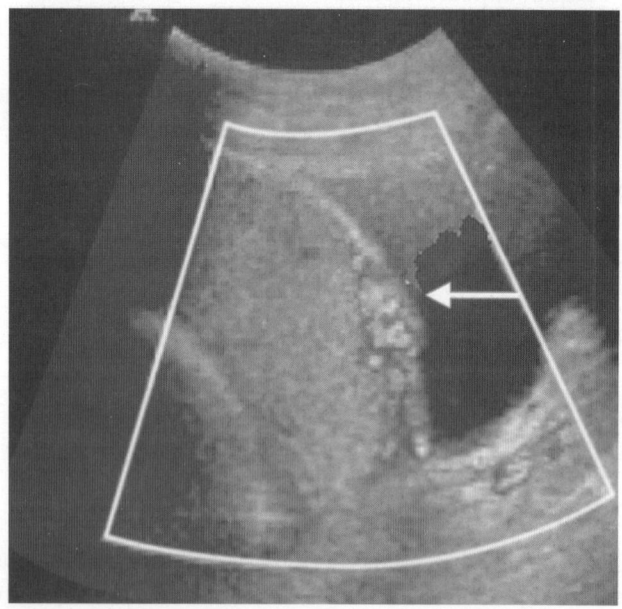

Fig. 1: Hypervascularity at bladder and lower segment junction with loss of intervening myometrium (marked with arrow) *(For color version, see plate 1)*

Three-dimensional power Doppler
- Numerous coherent vessels involving the whole uterine serosa–bladder junction (basal view)
- Hypervascularity (lateral view)

- Inseparable cotyledonal and intervillous circulations, chaotic branching, detour vessels (lateral view).

Q11. Is there any other investigation to diagnose or confirm?

MRI has significant role if USG findings are inconclusive. MRI is considered better at detecting the depth of infiltration in cases of placenta accreta. Literature has quoted sensitivity 93% versus 80% and specificity 71% versus 65% for ultrasound versus MRI. MRI has significant role when placenta is posterior and difficult to see on USG.

Q12. What are MRI findings in placenta accreta?

The main MRI features of placenta accreta include:
- Uterine bulge
- Heterogeneous signal intensity within the placenta
- Dark intraplacental bands on T2-weighted imaging.

Q13. How will you manage your case if USG shows adherent placenta with placenta previa?

All cases of major placenta previa and adherent placenta must be admitted in hospital where facility is available for:
- Massive blood transfusion
- Major surgeries (referral institutions)
- Critical care
    - Hemoglobin or anemic state should be corrected to keep in normal range (preferably > 10 g%)
    - Admission is advised ≥32 weeks or if any antepartum hemorrhage
    - Antenatal dexamethasone (6 mg, 4 doses 12 hours apart) should be given to mother for fetal lung maturity as preterm delivery is quite common in these cases
    - Patient and relatives should be apprised about prognosis as MOH, preterm delivery, cesarean section, laparotomy or cesarean hysterectomy is/are quite common in such cases. Written informed consents are mandatory
    - Adequate amount of blood and blood products should be arranged
    - Elective cesarean delivery is advised at 36–37 weeks in cases with obstetric indication like major placenta previa or cephalopelvic disproportion/contracted pelvis etc.
    - Placenta percreta may have associated hemoperitoneum and will require emergency laparotomy
    - All cases of morbidly adherent placenta should be operated by experienced obstetricians and anesthetists.

The seven elements considered to be reflective of good care are:
- Consultant obstetrician
- Consultant anesthetist
- Interventional radiologist
- Blood and blood products availability
- Multidisciplinary involvement in preoperative planning
- Discussion and consent includes possible interventions (such as hysterectomy, leaving the placenta in situ, and uterine embolization)
- Availability of critical care bed.

Q14. What is the role of classical CS in these patients?

Surgeons delivering the baby by cesarean section in the presence of a suspected placenta accreta should consider opening the uterus at a site distant from the placenta (classical cesarean), and delivering the baby without disturbing the placenta, in order to enable conservative management of the placenta or elective hysterectomy to be performed if the accrete is confirmed. Elective cesarean delivery and cesarean hysterectomy is the definite management of morbidity adherent placenta (Fig. 2).

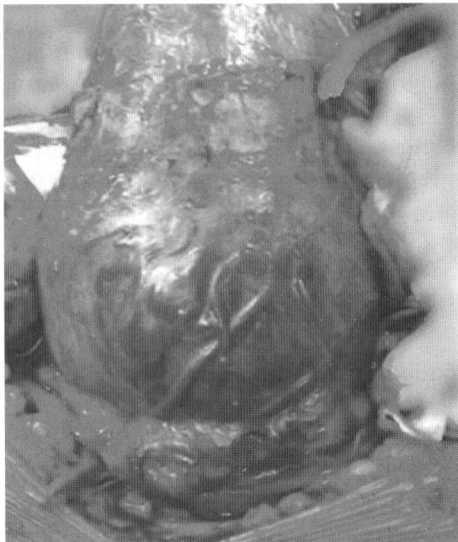

Fig. 2: Bulging lower segment of uterus with high vascularity
(For color version, see plate 1)

Q15. What radiological intervention can be done in such patients

- Interventional radiologist or cardiologist can embolise feeding vessels to the placenta, uterine or internal iliac arteries in conservative management of such cases
- If facilities allow, percreta with confirm diagnosis should be taken for cesarean, with full preparation of embolization, i.e balloon tipped intra-arterial catheters

can be placed in situ before proceeding for a cesarean section
- After baby's delivery with classical cesarean, patient should be shifted for embolization of feeding vessels of placenta, while placenta left in situ.

Q16. What follow-up do these patients require?
- If the placenta is managed conservatively (left in situ), patient do have shorter duration of surgery, less blood loss, few surgical morbidities but follow up can be hectic
- Serial USG is the mainstay of the follow-up
- No role of methotrexate and serial Beta HCG
- Severe and recurrent bouts of bleeding, sepsis, urinary tract infection, hematuria, pyelo-nephritis, and multiple blood transfusions are common complications encountered with follow-up
- Patient and relatives should be prognosticated regarding difficulties to deal with complications in follow-up.

Q17. What percentage of patients requires hysterectomy with uterine artery embolization (UAE) and how many resolve?
- Various studies, reporting series of conservative management, have found 10 to 15% patients require hysterectomy due to above mentioned complications
- Up to 75% resolution is reported
- Pregnancies, deliveries have been reported too
- Various menstrual abnormalities are seen in long term follow up, i.e. hypomenorrhea, amenorrhea (Asherman syndrome).

Q18. What is the role of elective hysterectomy in placenta accreta?
- Any patient with completed family should be planned for elective CS with expert personnel to perform the surgery
- Even if the family is not completed, massive hemorrhage warrants hysterectomy
- There is no role of conservative management when the woman is already bleeding. Surgeon should go ahead with hysterectomy without wasting time to save female's life.

Q19. What is the management of partially separated placenta?
- If the placenta partially separates, the separated portion(s) need to be delivered and any hemorrhage that occurs needs to be dealt immediately. Adherent portions can be left in place, but blood loss in such circumstances can be large and need massive transfusion protocols
- Internal iliac artery ligation, feeding vessel embolization can be considered if expertise and facility allow
- Small adherent part can be excised and uterus can be stitched as in routine hysterotomy.

Perioperative period for these mothers require intensive care/monitoring, antibiotics and regular counseling of relatives about prognosis (recording of prognosis is advised).

Chances of repeat placenta previa or adherent placenta is very high so patient should be advised to avoid next pregnancy and contraception should be advised and counseled.

REFERENCES

1. Miller DA, Chollet JA, Goodwin TM. Clinical risk factors for placenta previa-placenta accreta. Am J Obstet Gynecol. 1997;177(1):210.
2. Wu S, Kocherginsky M, Hibbard JU. Abnormal placentation: twenty-year analysis. Am J Obstet Gynecol. 2005;192(5):1458.
3. Dwyer BK, Belogolovkin V, Tran L, et al. Prenatal diagnosis of placenta accreta: sonography or magnetic resonance imaging? J Ultrasound Med. 2008;27:1275-81.
4. Masselli G, Brunelli R, Casciani E, et al. Magnetic resonance imaging in the evaluation of placental adhesive disorders: correlation with color Doppler ultrasound. Eur Radiol. 2008;18:1292-9.
5. Cali G, Giambanco L, Puccio G, et al. Morbidly adherent placenta: evaluation of ultrasound diagnostic criteria and differentiation of placenta accrete from percreta. Ultrasound Obstet Gynecol. 2013;41:406-12.
6. Knight M on behalf of UKOSS. Peripartum hysterectomy in the UK: management and outcomes of the associated haemorrhage. BJOG. 2007;114:1380-7.
7. Morken NH, Henriksen H. Placenta percreta—two cases and review of the literature. Eur J Obstet Gynecol Reprod Biol. 2001;100:112-5.
8. Bennett MJ, Sen RC. 'Conservative' management of placenta praevia percreta: report of two cases and discussion of current management options. Aust N Z J Obstet Gynaecol. 2003;43:249-51.
9. Gielchinsky Y, Rojansky N, Fasouliotis SJ, et al. Placenta Accreta—Summary of 10 Years: A Survey of 310 Cases. Placenta. 2002;23(2-3):210-4.

10
CHAPTER

Preterm Labor

Poonam Sachdeva, Niharika Dhiman, Sneha Sharma

CASE SCENARIO

*G2P1L1 at 30 weeks period of gestation with preterm labor pains 26 years old, Mrs F, wife of Mr M, resident of Paharganj, a housewife, belonging to low socioeconomic status came to Gyne casualty on 10/3/17 with complaints of
- Amenorrhea 7 months
- Pain lower abdomen for 5 hours. Discharge for 3 hours
- Her LMP was 12/8/16 so making her period of gestation (POG) 30 weeks.

History of Presenting Complaints

She was an unbooked antenatal case presented to the gyne casualty with complaints of pain in lower abdomen for last 5 hours. Pain was sudden in onset, dull in nature, coming at every half hourly interval, associated with tightening of abdomen and mucoid vaginal discharge. Pain is not increasing in intensity, there are no aggravating or relieving factors. She is perceiving normal fetal movements. There is no associated history of leaking per vaginum or burning micturition, blood in urine or pain while passing urine. There is no history of any bowel complaints/trauma over the abdomen/fall. No history of recent coitus.

Course in the Hospital

- She was admitted to the labor room after her abdominal and internal examination.
- She received few injections in her buttocks and monitored for abdominal pain and fetal heart.
- Blood sample was taken in the labor room.
- History of present pregnancy—Spontaneous conception—Planned pregnancy.

First Trimester

- Pregnancy was confirmed, at home by urine pregnancy test when she was overdue by 7 days.
- She had no history of any bleeding or discharge P/V, pain lower abdomen, fever with rashes, bladder and bowel symptoms, self medication or radiation exposure.
- Folic acid was started once her pregnancy test came positive after she consulted some doctor.

Second Trimester

- Amenorrhea continued.
- Quickening felt at around four and a half months. Iron and calcium started. Folic acid continued.
- Two doses of tetanus toxoid were received.
- Blood and urine tests were done and patient was told, all normal.
- Level ll ultrasound was done in 5th month of pregnancy and was normal.
- Patient had quickening at around four and a half month.
- No history of breathlessness, easy fatigability, swelling over the feet, abnormal weight gain, leaking or bleeding P/V, recurrent urinary infection or increased blood sugars was there.
- Her blood pressure was normal on all antenatal visits. She now presented with the above-mentioned complaints to the gyne casualty.

Obstetrics History (O/H)

- Married since 3 years
- Non-consanguinous marriage G2P1L1.

G1: It was a spontaneous conception. There is history of delivery of baby at the beginning of 8th month when she was hospitalized in view of pain in abdomen, she delivered a preterm baby weighing 1.5 kg after two days of admission, baby was kept in ICU for 20 days and was discharged at a weight of 1.8 kg.

No history of any contraception except occasional barrier contraception.

Menstrual History (M/H)
Unremarkable.

Diagnosis on History
G2P1L1 with 30 weeks POG with preterm labor pains.

Examination
- Patient is conscious, oriented and sitting comfortably in the bed
- Average built with gait normal, normal hairline, poor oro-dental hygiene
- General condition good
- Height 155 cm
- Weight 45 kg
- BMI not done as prepregnancy weight is not known
- No pallor/icterus/cyanosis/clubbing/pedal edema
- Pulse rate—88/min, regular with no radio-femoral or radio-radial delay
- Blood pressure—110/80 mm Hg in right arm in sitting position
- Respiratory rate—16/min
- Thyroid—normal
- No lymphadenopathy.

Respiratory System
Unremarkable.

Cardiovascular System
Unremarkable.

Abdominal Examination

Inspection
- Abdomen is uniformly distended with all quadrants moving with respiration
- Linea nigra and striae gravidarum present, no other scar marks are seen
- Umbilicus is central and flat
- All hernial sites are free.

Palpation
- Fundal height—30 weeks
- Symphysio-fundal height (SFH)—29 cm
- Abdominal girth—28 inches
- Uterus relaxed with occasional contraction—2 in every 10 mins.

Fundal Grip
A soft broad ballotable structure felt at fundus, suggestive of breech.

Lateral Grip
- Smooth and curved structure felt on the right lateral side of the abdomen, suggestive of back
- Multiple knobby parts felt on the left side, suggestive of limbs.

Pelvic Grips
- A hard, globular and smooth structure felt on palpation, suggestive of head
- Head was freely mobile, not engaged, preterm feel.

Auscultation
Fetal heart sound was heard at the right spino-umblical line 134 beats/min, regular.

Perineal Examination
- External genitalia normal
- No bleeding, leaking or abnormal discharge observed.

Per Speculum Examination
- Os open
- Cervix length <2.5 cm
- No discharge, bleeding or leaking observed.

Diagnosis after Examination
G2P1L1 at 30 weeks POG with cephalic presentation with preterm labor.

Q1. In a patient with preterm labor, what are the important points to be noted on examination?
- Patient is conscious, oriented and lying comfortably in bed.
- Average built and nutrition (Thin built and poor nutrition are more prone).

- Pulse, BP, temperature.
- Pallor, pedal edema, icterus, thyromegaly and lymphadenopathy.
- Any focus for infection should be looked for, i.e. oral cavity, respiratory infection or urinary infection.

Q2. What is the management of this case?

A. This Patient Should be Admitted to Labor Ward
- Adequate rest.
- Reassurance, counseling and written consent regarding risk of preterm delivery should be done.
- Vitals charting (pulse and temperature) charting, monitoring of uterine contractions and fetal heart.
- Patient should be started on tocolysis—Steroid cover should be started promptly.

B. Investigations
- Hemoglobin, TLC, DLC
- Routine antenatal investigations
- C-reactive protein (CRP)—(>3–4 mg/dL indicate infection)
- High vaginal swab for microscopy and culture sensitivity
- Vaginal fluid for pH and fetal fibronectin levels
- Cardiotocography for fetal heart rate pattern
- Ultrasonography: For fetal biometry, gross congenital anomalies, amount of liquor, location and grade of placenta
- Transvaginal sonography—cervical length, internal os status and cervical index.[1]

C. Management
These patients should be managed conservatively till fetal lung maturity is attained or she completes 35+6 weeks of pregnancy. Termination of pregnancy is indicated only if any of the following features are present:
- Chorioamnionitis
- Nonreassuring nonstress test or repeated severe variable decelerations
- USG suggestive of severe FGR or severe placental insufficiency
- Associated complicating factors like, eclampsia or preeclampsia with severe features, abruption.

1. *Steroids:*
   Dose:
   - Injection betamethasone two doses of 12 mg each at an interval of 24 hours or
   - Injection dexamethasone four doses of 6 mg each at an interval of 12 hours
   - Delivery should be delayed by 12 hours after the last dose of steroid although optimal benefit begins 24 hours after therapy and lasts for a week. The benefit of a repeat course is doubtful and not recommended at present.[2,3,6]

2. *Tocolytic agents:* Only to be given to buy time for steroid cover
   Contraindications to tocolytic therapy.
   - Advanced labor (cervix >4 cm dilated)
   - Features of chorioamnionitis
   - Severe preeclampsia and eclampsia
   - Abruptio placentae and placenta previa with hemodynamic instabilities
   - Fetal distress
   - Hyperthyroidism
   - Severe anemia
   - Nifedepine: It is considered as the first line tocolytic agent.
     - Dose: 20–30 mg orally stat followed by same dose after 30 min if contractions persist. Maintain at 10–20 mg 6 hourly for 48–72 hours. Maximum dose is 160 mg in 24 hours.
     - Side effect: Maternal hypotension, tachycardia, headache, dizziness and facial flushing.
     - Contraindications: Maternal cardiac disease, maternal hypotension (<90/50 mm Hg). It should be used cautiously in patients with renal compromise.
     - Its use with magnesium sulfate should be avoided.
     - Maternal tachycardia >120 bpm, BP <100/60 mm Hg, pulse oximetry <95% or presence of fever are reasons for discontinuation of therapy.[4]
     - In cases where nifedipine is contraindicated, the oxytocin receptor antagonist can be used.
   - Oxytocin antagonist-Atosiban: It is an oxytocin antagonist, recommended as a first line agent in the management of preterm labor though its cost may be a limiting factor for its use in developing countries.[2,8]
     - Dose: 6.75 mg IV stat over one minute followed by an infusion of 18 mg/hr for 3 hours and then 6 mg/hr for up to 45 hours. Total duration of treatment should not exceed 48 hours and the total dose not to be more than 330 mg.
     - Side effects: Palpitations, tachycardia, chest pain, dyspnea, hypotension, nausea, vomiting and headache (Evidence level Ia).[8]

3. *Antibiotics:* Prophylactic antibiotics has got role only in PPROM as oral Erythromycin 250 mg four times day for maximum of 10 days or until the woman is in established labor, whichever is earlier. For patients not tolerating erythromycin, oral penicillin can be given.[10]

4. Treatment of associated infections.

Q3. How should the patient be managed during labor?

- Adequate bed rest to prevent premature rupture of membrane.
- Delivery by LSCS not preferred as there is no significant difference in the frequency of periventricular or intraventricular hemorrhage.
- Use of sedatives and oxytocics should be avoided.
- Monitoring of mother (vitals) and fetus (intermittent auscultation or CTG).
- Repeated digital examination should be avoided to prevent risk of infection.
- Epidural analgesia can be given in second stage of labor.
- Episiotomy is recommended especially in primigravida to minimize head compression.
- Prophylactic forceps should not be used.[12-14]

Q4. What is the role of TVS in management of preterm labor?

Transvaginal scan (TVS) is used as diagnostic test to determine likelihood of delivery within next 48 hours. If cervical length is more than 25 mm then her chances of preterm labor are less and can be managed on outpatient bases after ruling out other causes of preterm. If cervical length is less than 25 mm then consider the woman as diagnosed preterm labor and offer treatment as mentioned.[9]

Cervical index (CI)—a ratio of cervical length and width.

Q5. What is the role of fetal fibronectin in preterm labor?

Fetal fibronectin as per RCOG guidelines is considered as a diagnostic test to determine likelihood of birth within 48 hours for women more than 30+0 weeks if TVS is indicated but is not available or not acceptable. Result of fibronectin should be viewed as following:

- If fetal fibronectin is negative (50 ng/mL or less), she should be explained that she is unlikely to be in preterm labor. Benefits and risks of going home can be discussed with her as compared to conservative management at hospital and advised to come back with recurrence of symptoms.
- If fetal fibronectin testing is positive (>50 ng/mL),[5] she is considered to be in preterm labor and managed accordingly.
- TVS for cervical length and fibronectin should not be combined to diagnose preterm labour as per RCOG guidelines.[5]

Q6. What is the role of magnesium sulfate in neuroprotection of the baby?

There is a definite role of Injection magnesium sulfate for neuroprotection of the baby from 24+0 to 33+6 weeks as per NICE Guidelines.

Dosage

4 g IV bolus of Inj magnesium sulfate over 15 minutes followed by an IV infusion of 1 g per hour until the birth or for 24 hours (whichever is sooner).[20]

Q7. What is the role of prophylactic vaginal progesterone and prophylactic cervical cerclage in preterm labor?

As per NICE guidelines there is a definitive role of giving prophylactic progesterone to women with no history of spontaneous preterm birth or mid trimester loss in whom TVS has revealed cervical length less than 25 mm.[11]

Prophylactic cervical cerclage should be considered in women between 16+0 and 24+0 weeks with cervical length less than 25 mm who have had:

- History of P-PROM in previous pregnancy or
- History of cervical trauma

Q8. What should be the timing of cord clamping for preterm babies.

If the mother and the baby are stable then one can wait till 30 seconds but no longer than 3 minutes for cord clamping.

Q9. What is the acceptable mode of birth of preterm baby?

Vaginal delivery is considered with continuous fatal monitoring during labor, preterm breech between 26 + 0 and 36 + 6 weeks should be delivered by a cesarean section.[12]

Q10. Difficulties during cesarean section in case of preterm baby.

Poor formation of lower uterine segment.

Q11. Complications of preterm baby.[15]

- Hypothermia
- Asphyxia
- Respiratory distress syndrome
- Neonatal septicemia
- Jaundice
- Dehydration
- Retinopathy.

Q12. Maternal risk factors for preterm labor.[16,17]

Social Factors

- Low socioeconomic status
- Extremes of age

- Smoking
- Low maternal weight
- Psychological stress

Uterine Factors
- Overdistension of uterus (multiple pregnancy, polyhydramnios)
- Congenital anomaly of uterus (bicornuate, septate uterus)
- Cervical incompetence

Maternal Diseases
- Preeclampsia
- Antepartum hemorrhage
- Diabetes in pregnancy
- Renal diseases
- Asymptomatic bacteriuria
- Infections
- Previous history of preterm delivery, spontaneous abortions
- Idiopathic.

Q13. Instrumental delivery in preterm labor.
- Vacuum delivery is avoided in infants <34 weeks of gestation due to the percieved risk of IVH.[12-14]
- Forceps is the only option for delivery of premature fetuses because of the risk of cephalohematoma and intracranial hemorrhage with vacuum extraction.[13]

Q14. Use of vitamin K.

No difference was found in the incidence of other neurodevelopmental abnormalities at pediatric follow-up at 18 to 24 months or seven years of age between children born to mothers given vitamin K and children not so exposed.

Q15. Use of steroids for lung maturity in preterm labor.

A single course of corticosteroids is recommended for pregnant women between 24 0/7 weeks and 33 6/7 weeks of gestation, and may be considered for pregnant women starting at 23 0/7 weeks of gestation who are at risk of preterm delivery within 7 days.[16-18]

Although betamethasone and dexamethasone differ only by a single methyl group, betamethasone has a longer half-life because of its decreased clearance and larger volume of distribution. There are no differences in perinatal death or alterations in biophysical activity, but there was a decreased incidence of intraventricular hemorrhage with dexamethasone treatment.[19] Alternatively, an observational study reported less-frequent adverse neurological outcome at 18–22 months after betamethasone exposure.[20] These inconsistent and limited data are not considered sufficient to recommend one corticosteroid regimen over the other.

CASE SCENARIO

G4P1L0A2 with 18 weeks POG with short cervical length.

Mrs X 28 years old G4P1L0A2 at 18 weeks pregnancy presented to the ANC OPD as an unbooked patient with complaints of pain in lower abdomen on and off. It is dull in nature, coming at half hourly interval, associated with tightening of the abdomen; there is no relieving or aggravating factor.

Trimester History

First Trimester
- Spontaneous conception, planned pregnancy, pregnancy was confirmed by local practitioner by urine pregnancy test when she was five days overdue. She was started on tab folic acid till 4 months of pregnancy.
- She had no history of any nausea or vomiting, BP/V, fever with rash, drug intake or radiation exposure.
- No history of bladder or bowel complaints.

Second Trimester
- Quickening was felt around four and a half months.
- Iron and calcium was started. Folic acid stopped after four months.
- Received two doses of Inj TT 0.5 mL IM 6 weeks apart.
- All blood investigations done and were reported as normal.
- Level II ultrasound was done and was normal.

Obstetric History (O/H)
- Married since 7 years
- Non-consanguinous marriage.

G4P1L0A2
- A1 was 7 years back, induced abortion at 3 months, followed by dilatation and curettage in a private hospital.
- A2 was 2 years back, spontaneous abortion at 20 weeks POG.
- G2—was a supervised pregnancy, spontaneous preterm vaginal delivery (PTVD) at 28 weeks, delivered at home,

3 years back—Baby was female, 1.2 kg birth weight. Baby expired after 6 days due to respiratory distress.
- G4—present pregnancy.

Q1. What are the important points should be asked in history?

- History of previous recurrent abortions especially second trimester (spontaneous or induced) or previous history of preterm labor.
- Short intervals between two pregnancies (less than 12 months) more prone to preterm labor.
- History of hypertension, diabetes, renal disease, heart disease, asthma, thyroid disease or severe periodontal disease or any other chronic illness can predispose to preterm labor.
- Past surgical history:
  - History of cervical conization (or any history of cervical encerclage to be elicited in multigravida).
  - History of alcohol or drug abuse or smoking is associated with higher incidence of preterm labor.
  - Any history of domestic violence especially trauma due to physical abuse is also associated with preterm birth.
  - History of prolonged standing, fatigue due to physical work and high stress job (these are strong predictors of preterm labor).

Q2. What is the probable cause of bad obstetric history in your case?

The probable cause can be cervical incompetence.

Q3. What are the causes of cervical incompetence?

- Congenital: With or without presence of other uterine anomaly
- Acquired:
  - History of D and C, D and E
  - Cervical amputation, conization
  - History of premature bearing down in previous pregnancy.

Q4. What are the circumstances when cervical encirclage be used to prevent preterm birth?

- Prophylactic encirclage in women who have history of recurrent midtrimester losses and who are diagnosed with cervical insufficiency
- Women identified during sonographic examination to have short cervix
- Third indication is rescue encirclage when cervical incompetence is recognized in women with preterm labor.

Q5. How will you diagnose cervical incompetence?

- History of repeated midtrimester pregnancy losses
- Easy passage of Hegar's cervical dilator no 8 during non-pregnant state
- During pregnancy:
  - On per speculum examination—dilatation of the cervix with herniation of membranes can be seen
  - Diagnosis by USG—transvaginal USG is preferred over transabdominal and serial ultrasonography is helpful
  - Length of the cervix becomes less than 25 mm
  - Funneling of the internal os.

Q6. How is cervical shortening seen in transvaginal ultrasound?

The progression of changes in the cervix during the course of parturition has been visualized with the help of transvaginal sonography. The temporal sequence of cervical changes and described the change as T, Y, V and U. As the cervix effaces, the relationship of the cervical canal to the lower uterine segment changes from a **T** to the notched **Y**. With further effacement, the **Y** becomes a **V** and ultimately a **U**.

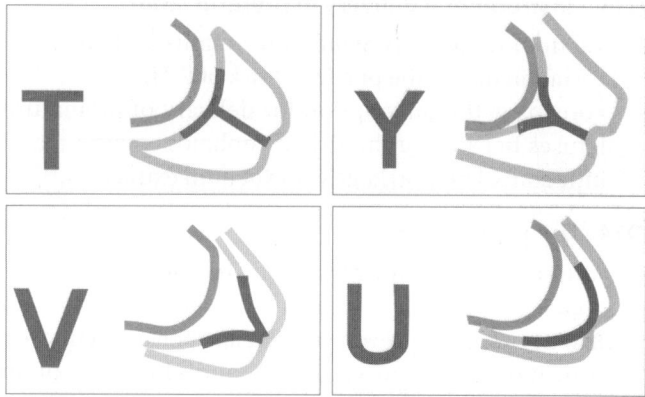

Q7. Management of cervical incompetence?

Cervical encirclage operation either McDonald's procedure or Shirodkar's method.

McDonalds procedure: Nonabsorbable suture like mersilene tape or silk is passed from posterior to anterior like purse string suture all around the cervix as high as possible taking successive deep bites. Two ends of suture are tied anteriorly. Success rate is same as Shirodkar's operation and there is less blood loss, chance of cervical scar is less.

Shirodkar's method: Small transverse incision is made at the cervicovaginal junction below the base of the bladder, bladder is pushed up, small vertical incision is made on the posterior wall of the cervix at cervicovaginal junction. A nonabsorbable suture is passed from anterior to posterior aspect submucosally using Shirodkar's needle. Two ends of the suture are tied posteriorly and the anterior and posterior incisions are closed with interrupted catgut.

Q8. What are the complications of cerclage operation?

Complications of circlage are
- Premature rupture of membranes
- Onset of uterine contractions
- Later fibrosis leading to cervical dystocia
- Hemorrhage
- Sepsis.

Q9. Postoperative care following cervical encirclage?

- Bed rest
- Tocolytic agents started preoperatively
- Avoid constipation
- Avoidance of sexual intercourse.

Q10. When will you remove the circlage sutures?

Usually at 37 weeks or at the onset of labor pains whichever is earlier. At the time of discharge patient must be counseled that she must attend hospital immediately in case of abdominal pains and the stitch must be removed otherwise it might lead to tear and laceration of the cervix leading to excessive bleeding.

REFERENCES

1. Ross MG. Preterm labor emedicine. Obstetrics and Gynaecology. 2010;1-9.
2. Anotayanoth S, Subhedar NV, Garner P, et al. Betamimetics for inhibiting preterm labor. Cochrane Database Syst Rev 2004; issue 3: CD004352.
3. Fernando Aries. Preterm labor. In: Practical Guide to High Risk Pregnancy and Delivery. 3rd edn; 217-23.
4. Aries F. Premature rupture of membranes. In: Practical Guide to High Risk Pregnancy and Delivery, 3rd edn.
5. Faron G, Boulvain M, Irion O, et al. Prediction of preterm delivery by fetal fibronectin: a meta analysis. Obstet Gynecol. 1998;92:153-8.
6. Crowley Patricia. Antenatal corticosteroids prior to preterm delivery.In: Recent Advances in Obstetrics and Gynecology; Churchill Livingstone; 20:81-96.
7. Elimian A, Verma U, Camnterino J, et al. Effectiveness of antenatal steroids in obstetrics subgroups. Obstet Gynecol. 1999;93:174-9.
8. http://www.rcog.org.ulc/guidelines/tocolytic.htlm.
9. Edwin C, Arulkumaran S. Recent advances in management of preterm labor. Journal of Obstet Gynecol India. 2005;2(55): 118-24.
10. Romero R, Gomez R, et al. The role of infection in preterm labor and delivery. Paediatric and Perinatal epidemiology 2001;15(Suppl 2):41-56.
11. nice.org.uk/guidance/ng 25 published November 2015.
12. American College of Obstetricians and Gynaecologists. Operative vaginal delivery: use of forceps and vacuum extractors for operative vaginal delivery. ACOG practice bulletin no.17, June 2000.
13. Vacca A. The trouble with vacuum extraction. Curr Obstet Gynaecol. 1999;9:41-5.
14. Society of obstetricians and Gynaecologists of Canada. SOGC Clinical practice guideline no. 148, August 2004: guidelines for vaginal birth. J Obstet Gynaecol Can. 2004;26:747-53.
15. Cochrane pregnancy and childhood group.
16. Periviable birth. Obstetric Care Consensus No. 4. American College of Obstetricians and Gynecologists. Obstet Gynecol. 2016;127:e157-69.
17. Management of preterm labor. Practice Bulletin No. 171. American College of Obstetricians and Gynecologists. Obstet Gynecol. 2016;128:e155-64.
18. Antenatal corticosteroids revisited: repeat courses. NIH Consens Statement. 2000;17:1-18.
19. Brownfoot FC, Gagliardi DI, Bain E, et al. CA. Different corticosteroids and regimens for accelerating fetal lung maturation for women at risk of preterm birth. Cochrane Database of Systematic Reviews 2013, Issue 8. Art. No.: CD006764. DOI: 10.1002/14651858.CD006764.pub3.
20. Lee BH, Stoll BJ, McDonald SA, et al. Neuro-developmental outc xposed prenatally to dexamethasone versus betamethasone. National Institute of Child Health and Human Development Neonatal Research Network. Pediatrics. 2008;121:289-96.

11
CHAPTER

Preterm Premature Rupture of Membranes

Shakun Tyagi, Vandana Sehrawat

CASE SCENARIO

Primigravida with seven and a half months amenorrhea with preterm premature rupture of membranes (PPROM) a 22 years old, Mrs S, wife of Mr R, resident of Delhi, a teacher by profession. Booked patient at a private clinic. Primigravida.
Last menstrual period (LMP): 31/12/16
Estimated date of delivery (EDD): 09/10/17
Therefore making her period of gestation (POG) 32 weeks and 2 days on 00/0/2017.
She reported to gyne emergency on 14/8/17 with presenting complaints of:
- Amenorrhea for seven and half months
- Leaking per vaginum for 2 days.

History of Present Illness

- Patient was booked with an obstetrician at a private clinic and was continuing with her pregnancy uneventfully till two days back when she complained of watery discharge per vaginum. The discharge was copious, non-mucoid and increased on coughing. Patient required use of a sanitary pad.
- There was no episode of bleeding or pain abdomen following leaking per vaginum.
- There was no history of foul smelling liquor.
- She was perceiving normal fetal movements.
- No history of backache radiating to thighs or pain lower abdomen.
- No history of any abnormal bladder and bowel symptoms
- No history of any abdominal trauma.

Course in the Hospital

She was admitted to the labor ward after her abdominal and internal examination. She was explained that there was risk of infections to both her and the baby but as the baby was premature it was advisable to wait before delivery.

An intravenous access was secured and patient's blood sample was drawn and sent for some investigations. She was periodically given some injections through the intravenous catheter. She was observed in the labor ward for about 6 hours and then transferred to maternity ward. Here she was advised to apply a sterile pad. Her temperature, pulse and fetal heart were observed regularly and her abdominal ultrasound was also done. There is no history of fever, burning micturition or discharge per vaginum preceding or following the episode of leaking per vaginum. In the ward the patient was advised foot end elevation of the bed that she is practicing.

History of Present Pregnancy

Spontaneous conception, planned pregnancy.

1st Trimester

- Pregnancy was confirmed, at home by urine pregnancy test when she was overdue by 7 days.
- She had no history of any bleeding or discharge per vaginum, pain in lower abdomen, fever with rashes, bladder and bowel symptoms, self-medication or radiation exposure.
- Folic acid was started once her pregnancy test came positive after she consulted some doctor.
- She reported mild symptoms of morning sickness but no treatment was required for that.

2nd Trimester

- The lady booked with the local obstetrician and was prescribed iron and calcium.
- Quickening felt at around four and a half months.
- She received two doses of tetanus toxoid one month apart.

- Her various blood and urine tests were normal.
- Level II ultrasound was done in 5th month of pregnancy and was normal.
- No history of raised BP recording, breathlessness, easy fatigability, swelling over the feet, abnormal weight gain, or recurrent urinary infection. Glucose challenge test (GCT) was performed at 24 weeks and was normal.

3rd Trimester
- Pregnancy continued uneventfully.
- She continued her iron, calcium and folic acid once daily.
- In early third trimester she visited the clinic twice and got ultrasound done for the baby's wellbeing on her own.

Obstetrics History (O/H)
- Married since 4 years
- Nonconsanguinous marriage
- Primigravida.

Menstrual History
Menarche-attained at 13 years.
LMP—15/01/2017
EDD—22/10/2017
- Previous cycles were regular, 4–5 days of bleeding with 28–30 days cycle with normal flow.
- No history of dysmenorrhea, menorrhagia
- No history of pills intake for contraception or missed periods prior to conception
- Contraceptive history—barrier method.

Medical History
- No history of hypertension, diabetes mellitus, tuberculosis, asthma or any seizure disorder in the past.
- No history of any prolonged medical illness.
- No history of blood transfusions.

Surgical History
No history of any surgical intervention.

Family History
- Mother of the patient is hypertensive since one year and her Blood Pressure (BP) is controlled on some antihypertensive medication.
- No history of hypertension in father and diabetes mellitus (DM) in her parents.
- No history of TB in family.

Personal History
She is a housewife with normal bowel and bladder pattern with normal sleep pattern. No history of any mood disorders. Vegetarian, Non-smoker, non-alcoholic and no other addictions.

Socioeconomic History
- She lives in a nuclear family of 2 members. Husband has passed high school.
- Her house is a pucca house with MCD water supply with modern sanitation and electricity facilities.
- She belongs to a lower middle class as per modified Kuppuswamy scale.

Dietary History
- She is a vegetarian by choice.
- Patient takes approximately 2200 kcal as per the 24 hours recall method.
- Her protein intake is approximately 50–60 g. Her diet is almost balanced and adequate in terms of proteins and calories.

Diagnosis on History
Primigravida with 32 weeks and 2 days POG with PPROM.

Examination
- Patient is conscious, oriented and sitting comfortably in the bed.
  - Average built with gait normal, normal hairline, average orodental hygiene
- General condition good:
  - Height 155 cms
  - Weight 65 kg
- Pulse rate—88/min, regular normal rhythm with no radiofemoral or radioradial delay
- Blood pressure—110/80 mm Hg in right arm in sitting position
- Respiratory rate—16/min
- Temperature 37.4°C
- No pallor
- No icterus
- No cyanosis
- Thyroid—normal
- No lymphadenopathy

- Breast lump (B/L)—breast show no retracted or cracked nipple
- No clubbing
- No pedal or presacral edema.

Respiratory System
- Trachea centrally placed
- Normal vesicular sound heard all over the chest with bilateral air entry equal on both sides with no added sounds.

Cardiovascular System
S1 and S2 normal with no abnormal sound.

Abdominal Examination

Inspection
- Abdomen is uniformly distended with all quadrants moving with respiration. No scar marks.
- Linea nigra and stria gravidorum present, no other scar marks are seen
- Umbilicus is central and everted
- All hernial sites are free.

Palpation
- No organomegaly
- Fundal height—30 weeks
- Symphysiofundal height (SFH)—29 cm
- Abdominal girth—32 cm.

Fundal Grip
A soft broad balotable structure felt at fundus, suggestive of breech.

Lateral Grip
- Smooth and curved structure felt on the right lateral side of the abdomen, suggestive of back
- Multiple knobby parts felt on the left side, suggestive of limbs.

Pelvic Grips

Superficial Pelvic Grip
A hard, globular and smooth structure felt on palpation, suggestive of head. Head was free. Head feels corresponding to 32 weeks. Liquor appears to be reduced. Estimated baby weight 1.8 kg. Uterus relaxed. Non-tense non-tender.

Auscultation
Fetal heart sound was heard at the right spino umbilical line—134 beats/min, regular.

Perineal Examination
- External genitalia normal
- Vulva moist.

Per Speculum Examination
- Os closed
- Cervix long
- Clear watery discharge present on the speculum on valsalva and coughing, no bleeding or foul smelling discharge present.

Per Vaginal Examination
Not done.

Diagnosis After Examination
G3P1L1A1 with 32 weeks plus 2 days POG corresponding to dates, cephalic presentation with PROM with no symptoms and signs of choriomnionitis.

Q1. How will you confirm your diagnosis of PPROM?

- History suggestive of leaking: Copious watery discharge which is nonsticky and initially non-foul smelling.
- Per speculum examination: Pooling of liquor over the speculum is confirmatory
- Following bedside tests may be done in case of any doubt:
  - pH test of vaginal fluid: normal, pH of vagina is 3.8 to 4, it increases to 6 in case of PPROM
  - Ferning: Drying of amniotic fluid on slide results in crystallization of salts and a ferning pattern when viewed under light microscope
  - Reduced liquor on ultrasound can be suggestive of leaking
  - Ultrasound guided intra-amniotic instillation of indigo carmine dye
  - Actim PROM vs AmniSure: AmniSure better when diagnosis in doubt[1]
  - Actim PROM detects insulin-like growth factor binding protein (IGFBP) and AmniSure detects placental alpha microglobulin-1 (PAMG-1) protein marker.

Q2. How will you manage PPROM?

I will prognosticate the patient and the relatives regarding the risks of chorioamnionitis and prematurity, and take high risk consent. After hospitalization, I will rule out any chorioamnionitis, abruptio placentae or fetal compromise.

I will confirm that routine antenatal investigations have been performed and are within normal limit. I will prescribe antibiotics and steroids and monitor the mother and the fetus:

- Sterile pad
- Rest in left lateral
- Daily fetal movement record (DFMR)
- Temperature, pulse and respiration (TPR) charting 4 hourly. BP charting 12 hourly
- Continue hematinics and calcium
- Watch for any sign and symptoms of chorioamnionitis, abruptio placentae and fetal compromise
- Perform complete blood counts and high vaginal swab gram stain and culture and sensitivity tests at least once a week
- Continue antenatal monitoring of the mother and the baby
- Avoid per vaginal examination.

Q3. How will you monitor for complications of PPROM?

With the help of history, examination and investigations aim for early detection of chorioamnionitis, abruptio placentae and fetal compromise:

Chorioamnionitis

- *History of*
  - Foul smelling discharge
  - Fever
  - Pain abdomen
- *Examination*
  - Temperature >100.4° F and pulse rate monitoring every four hourly
  - Tenderness over abdomen
  - Foul smelling discharge per vaginal
- *Investigations*
  - Leukocytosis: Complete blood counts should be performed at least once a week and more frequently if there is a rising trend or any clinical features of chorioamnionitis.
  - High vaginal swab should be performed once a week or as clinically appropriate
  - Erythrocyte sedimentation rate (ESR) and C-reactive protein (CRP) are non-specific for chorioamnionitis.

Abruption

- History of bleeding per vaginum and pain abdomen.
- Abdomen tense and tender on examination, fundal height more than period of gestation.
- USG examination may show evidence of retroplacental clot, non-reassuring fetal heart rate on cardiotocography (CTG).

Fetal monitoring

- Daily fetal movement record
- Patient should be explained to report any abnormality of fetal movement earliest.
- Nonstress test (NST) should be done, on alternate day to detect umbilical cord compression. Fetal tachycardia is the earliest sign of fetal infection
- Fetal growth should be monitored if the PPROM takes place remote from delivery.

Q4. Should corticosteroids be administered before 34 weeks period of gestation?

Corticosteroids are not recommended before viability. Corticosteroid should be given between 24–34 weeks if the risk of delivery within 7 days.

Q5. What is the role of magnesium sulfate?

Magnesium sulfate for fetal neuroprotection is not recommended before viability.

It is administered in cases of PPROM before 32 0/6 weeks of gestation in women who are at risk of imminent delivery.

Q6. What is the preferred prophylactic Antibiotic regimen for PPROM?

Injection Ampicillin 500 mg 6 hourly IV after test dose for 48 hours followed by Tab Erythromycin for 250 mg four times a day and Tab Amoxicillin 250 mg 8 hourly for 7 days.

Q7. What is the role of domiciliary management?

Domiciliary treatment after viability has not been recommended because:

a. Primary infection may present suddenly.
b. Risk of cord compression.

Therefore, hospitalization and dose surveillance is recommended after viability. Before viability patient may be advised domiciliary management under close self monitoring of temperature.

Q8. What is the role of tocolysis?

Tocolysis should be given only to facilitate in-utero transfer or for the action of corticosteroids to take place.

Q9. What are indications for delivery in PPROM?

- Clinical or lab evidence of chorioamnionitis
- Fetal compromise, non-reassuring fetal heart rate status or fetal demise
- Significant placental abruption
- Classically induction of labor has been performed at gestational age > 34 weeks. But according to the latest Cochrane review,[2] there was no clinically important difference in the incidence of neonatal sepsis between women who delivered immediately and those who were managed expectantly in PPROM prior to 37 weeks' gestation. Induction of labor before 37 weeks of gestation was associated with an increase in the incidence of complications of prematurity like neonatal respiratory distress syndrome (RDS), need for ventilation, neonatal mortality, admission to neonatal intensive care as well as endometritis and cesarean section.

Q10. What is the preferred mode of Delivery?

Lower segment cesarean section (LSCS) is performed for any obstetric indication. Most of the patients go into spontaneous labor. For induction of labor oxytocin infusion is preferred over dinoprostone gel in view of higher chances of infection with dinoprostone gel instillation in PPROM.

Q11. How will you manage a case of Chorioamnionitis?

Clinical chorioamnionitis is associated with increased maternal and fetal morbidity and mortality. Patient and the relative need to be counseled regarding the status. Delivery should be instituted along with broad spectrum antibiotics like combination of Ampicillin, Gentamicin and Metronidazole. In the absence of any contraindication to vaginal delivery induction of labor with Oxytocin infusion should be performed. Antibiotics should be continued post partum also with close monitoring for puerperal sepsis.

Q12. What are important postpartum complications with PPROM?

Puerperal sepsis (mild, moderate, severe) is the most important complication and patient should be administered broad spectrum antibiotics for 48 hours to prevent postpartum sepsis.

Q13. What are the indication of cervical cerclage in next pregnancy?

Patient should be watched for risk factors and singleton pregnancy with prior spontaneous preterm birth (<34 weeks) with cervical length <2 cm) with gestational age <24 weeks should be considered for cerclage.

Q14. How will management differ in presence of human immunodeficiency virus (HIV) and herpes simplex virus (HSV)?

With antiretroviral therapy (Tinifovir, Lamivudine, Efaverenz) regime being given universally, the management remains same as in non-HIV patient with close surveillance, as for any infection.

For HSV, cesarean is performed if active lesions are present at time of delivery. In addition Tab. Acyclovir 200mg three times a day has to be given.

Q15. What are the possible causes of PPROM?

- Genital tract infection, UTI (urinary tract infection)
- Low socioeconomic status
- Poor nutrition
- Genital tract anomalies
- Intrauterine invasive procedures—amniocentesis, cordocentesis
- Fetal factors—polyhydramnios, twin pregnancy, transvers lie, intrauterine detal death (IUFD).

CASE SCENARIO

G2P1L0 with five and a half months amenorrhea with PPROM
- G2P1L0
- LMP: 12/01/2017
- EDD: 17/10/2017
- POG: 24 weeks

Reported to gyne emergency on 29/6/17 with presenting complaints of:
- Amenorrhea for five and half months
- Leaking per vaginum for 2 days.

Diagnosis After Examination

G2P1L0 with 24 weeks POG corresponding to dates, with PPROM wih single live fetus with no symptoms and signs of chorioamnionitis.

Q1. How will you manage a case of midtrimester PPROM?

The most important issue in case of midtrimester PPROM is to balance the potential neonatal benefits of prolongation of the pregnancy and the risk of chorioamnionitis, intra-amniotic infection and its consequences for the mother and neonate. The management encompasses close monitoring for symptoms, signs and investigations for chorioamnionitis, and antibiotics (Erythromycin and Amoxycillin or according to reports of High Vaginal Swab: Culture and Sensitivity

Report); timing of corticosteroids for pulmonary maturity should be decided based on the survival rates of preterm neonates of the institution. Maximum effect of steroids on pulmonary maturity is achieved within one week of administration of corticosteroids.

- Pulse and temperature monitoring 4 hourly
- Monitoring for abdominal tenderness and foul smelling discharge per vaginum
- Daily NST
- Total leukocyte count on alternate day
- Patient's CRP levels and amniotic fluid IL-6 and procalcitonine levels tested as means of early detection of intra-amniotic infection.

Q2. How will you prognosticate this patient with PPROM at 24 weeks and what are the complications of PPROM?

Midtrimester PPROM (before 28 weeks POG) is associated increased rate of chorioamnionitis in the patient and high rate of neonatal morbidity and mortality.[3]

- 40–50% patients give birth within 1st week
- 70–80% give birth 2–5 weeks after membrane rupture
- 10–20% develop pulmonary hypoplasia, whereas, its rarely lethal as alveolar growth have already taken place at 24 weeks.

Neonatal complications are listed below:[4]

- Prematurity and respiratory distress syndrome
- Fetal deformities—potter like facies (low set ears, epicanthal folds)
- Limb contractures
- Pulmonary hypoplasia chronic lung disease
- Periventricular leukomalacia
- Intraventricular hemorrhage.

Q3. What is the role of amnioinfusion in cases of mid trimester PPROM ?

Long-term oligohydramnios is responsible for complications of pulmonary hypoplasia and position deformities. It has been suggested that amnioinfusion might reduce these complications. However, literature is lacking on this aspect. Results of an ongoing multicentric randomized controlled trial (PPROMEXIL - III trial) are awaited.[5]

Q4. In the absence of features of chorioamnionitis and any maternal or fetal complication, what is the right time for delivery in cases of PPROM?

Induction should be planned to balance the risk of prematurity with fetomaternal complications due to PPROM. The delivery is planned at 34 weeks of pregnancy. However, a recent Cochrane review suggested delivery at 37 week might reduce complications related to prematurity in these women but will increase duration of stay in hospital.

Q5. How will you manage a case of chorioamnionitis?

Delivery under broad spectrum antibiotic cover is primary aim. Patient and the relative need to be counseled regarding associated maternal and fetal morbidity and mortality. Preferably vaginal delivery should be considered unless there is an obstetric indication of cesarean section. Close watch for puerperal sepsis and neonatal sepsis is essential in post partum period.

Q6. What is the role of progesterone in PPROM?

Recent trials are not showing any benefit to the patient in terms of continuation of pregnancy although prior it was suggested that it has some role.[6]

REFERENCES

1. Palacio M, Kuhnert M, Berger R, et al. Meta-analysis of studies on biochemical marker tests for the diagnosis of premature rupture of membranes: comparison of performance indexes. BMC Pregnancy and Childbirth. 2014;14:183.
2. Bond DM, Middleton P, Levett KM. Planned early birth versus expectant management for women with preterm prelabor rupture of membranes prior to 37 weeks' gestation for improving pregnancy outcome. Cochrane Database Syst Rev. 2017 Mar 3;3:CD004735. doi:10.1002/14651858.CD004735.pub4.
3. Tchirikov M, Schlabritz-Loutsevitch N, Maher J, et al. Mid-trimester preterm premature rupture of membranes (PPROM): etiology, diagnosis, classification, international recommendations of treatment options and outcome. Perinat Med. 2017 Jul 15. pii:/j/jpme.ahead-of-print/jpm-2017-0027/jpm-2017-0027.xml. doi:10.1515/jpm-2017-0027. [Epub ahead of print]
4. Crowley AE, Grivell RM, Dodd JM. Sealing procedures for preterm prelabor rupture of membranes. Cochrane Database Syst Rev. 2016 Jul 7;7:CD010218. doi: 10.1002/14651858.CD010218.pub2.
5. van Teeffelen AS, van der Ham DP, Willekes C, et al. Midtrimester preterm prelabor rupture of membranes (PPROM): expectant management or amnioinfusion for improving perinatal outcomes (PPROMEXIL - III trial). BMC Pregnancy Childbirth. 2014 Apr 4;14:128. doi: 10.1186/1471-2393-14-128.
6. Briery CM, Veillon EW, Klauser CK, et al. Women with PPROM do not benefit from weekly progesterone. Am J Obstet Gynecol. 2011;204:54.e1-54.e5.[PUBMED]

CHAPTER 12

Pregnancy with Fetal Congenital Anomaly

Gazala Shahnaz, Asmita Muthal Rathore

Congenital anomalies can be defined as presence of structural or functional anomalies, which are present at the time of birth.[1] The prevalence is around 2-3% in newborn. Congenital malformations have become important causes of perinatal mortality in developing countries like India, with improved control of infections and nutritional deficiency diseases.[2] In India, prevalence is 6-7%, most common being congenital heart disease (8-10 per 1000 live birth) followed by congenital deafness (5.6-10 per 1000 live birth) and neural tube defect (4-11.4 per 1000 live birth).[3] It is responsible for 8-15% of perinatal deaths and around 13-16% of neonatal deaths.[2] It also contributes significantly to preterm birth, childhood and adult morbidity. This chapter will discuss the clinical evaluation and management principles of common congenital anomalies in fetus.

CASE SCENARIO

A 28 years old Mrs X, G3P1L1A1 with 28 weeks period of gestation (POG) present with complain of some abnormalities in fetal heart on ultrasound report. She had no other complaints. Ultrasound (USG) report, which was done at 7 months, suggestive of single live intrauterine fetus corresponding to 28 + 3 weeks with congenital heart disease (tricuspid valve with septal leaflet toward apex and moderate tricuspid regurgitation). Fetal echo was done at 30 weeks, confirmed dysplastic tricuspid valve and moderate to severe pulmonary stenosis (Ebstein anomaly). She is married for last 6 years, consanguineous marriage with previous one full term normal vaginal delivery of healthy fetus and a missed abortion at 3 months amenorrhea. This pregnancy is spontaneous conception, confirmed at 8 weeks POG by urine pregnancy test, late booked at 4 months POG, no history of folic acid intake in first trimester. First trimester was uneventful, no history of (H/O) fever, drug and radiation exposure, no biochemical screen was done. Second and third trimesters were also uneventful, patient took iron-calcium supplementation and received 2 doses of tetanus toxoid. Her routine blood and urine investigation including oral glucose tolerance test were normal.

Her routine general and systemic examinations were normal.

On obstetric examination: Fundal height is less than period of gestation, other findings corresponds to singleton pregnancy with cephalic presentation.

Diagnosis: 28 years old, G3P1L1A1 with 30 weeks POG with congenital heart disease (? Ebstein anomaly) in fetus with fetal growth restriction.

Q1. What are the relevant points in history of this patient?

History of Present Pregnancy

- Maternal age, consanguinity, mode of conception
- Multiple gestation, periconceptional intake of folic acid, number of antenatal visit
- History of fever especially in first trimester, drug exposure (retinoic acid, ethanol, anticonvulsants, lithium) and maternal smoking
- Any abnormal test reports—biochemical screen and/or USG.

Past Obstetric History

Previous baby with chromosomal abnormalities, birth defects, miscarriages, early neonatal death.

Past Medical History

Congenital heart disease in mother, diabetes mellitus, systemic lupus erythematous or any other condition which points toward chromosomal anomalies.

Family History

A detailed family history up to 3-generation should be obtained and look for neonate born with congenital anomalies and early deaths in family.

Q2. What points will you look for in examination?

Maternal

Look for undiagnosed congenital heart disease.

Obstetric Examination

There may be no significant changes but may present with fetal growth restriction/oligohydramnios/polyhydramnios.

Q3. What is the etiology of fetal congenital malformation?

- Unknown — 40–60%
- Genetic/chromosomal — 10–15%
- Environmental — 10%
- Intrauterine infection
- Drug exposure
- Radiation exposure
- Deficiency of iodine
- Non-intake of folic acid in periconceptional period.

Q4. What are the different types of congenital heart disease, which are commonly diagnosed prenatally?

According to the National Heart, Lung and Blood Institute, the most common types of congenital heart defects which can be diagnosed prenatally are:

Anomalous pulmonary venous return	Ebstein's anomaly	Tricuspid valve atresia
Atrial septal defect (ASD)	Hypoplastic left heart syndrome	Truncus arteriosus
Atrioventricular septal defect (AVSD)	Pulmonary valve atresia/stenosis	Ventricular septal defect (VSD)
Aortic valve stenosis	Patent ductus arteriosus (PDA)	Fetal arrhythmias
Coarctation of the aorta	Tetralogy of Fallot	Cardiac tumors
Double outlet right ventricle	Transposition of the great arteries or vessels	Cardiomyopathies

Q5. How will you manage this case?

- Patient should be referred to a tertiary ultrasound unit and genetic counseling should be provided to optimize diagnosis.
  - Detail USG by experienced sonologist to rule out other associated malformations and fetal echo by pediatric cardiologist to diagnose type of lesion and functional status should be done.
  - Genetic counseling after diagnosis:
    - Prognosis—poor if associated with other anomaly [may be undetected on USG], part of genetic syndrome,
    - Risk of recurrence
    - Course of ebsteins anomaly—prognosis, need for surgery
    - Place of delivery
- Invasive prenatal and parental blood testing may also be offered to confirm the diagnosis.
- Multidisciplinary care: Referral to the pediatric cardiologist should be considered.

  Subsequent management will include:
  - Follow up: Ultrasound examination and echocardiography should be repeated at regular interval to evaluate status of the ebstein and its consequences (congestive heart failure a and hydrops), to detect other anomalies not previously identified and FGR.
  - Delivery should be planned at tertiary center with availability of pediatric cardiologist and cardiac surgeon. Vaginal delivery unless there are obstetric indications for another mode of delivery.
  - A detained evaluation of newborn is essential for diagnosis and counseling on the etiology, prognosis, and recurrence risk for future pregnancies.
- Parents should be encouraged for performance of autopsy in cases of termination of pregnancy, stillbirth, or neonatal death, to provide maximum information.

Q6. What are the limitations of anomaly scan?

Ultrasound at 18 to 20 weeks of POG is usually performed to diagnose most of major fetal anomalies. However, there sensitivity varies from overall 15–80% with sensitivity of approximately 40%[4,5] for detecting fetal anomalies.[5] The sensitivity of USG varies with diagnosis of fetal anomalies whether major or minor, the background risk of anomalies, the expertise of the operators, and the completeness of anomaly confirmation report. The detection rate is higher for central nervous system and urinary tract anomalies than for cardiovascular system.[6] Obesity also lowers detection rates of fetal anomalies during prenatal ultrasonography.[7] USG performed at tertiary care centers have a higher detection rate for fetal anomalies.[8] The RADIUS study also highlights the importance of a USG in tertiary unit for detection of major anomalies in fetus.

Some of congenital heart lesions may be missed at the time of routine anomaly scan (18–20 weeks) and ideal time for cardiac scanning is around 22–24 weeks. Other anomalies like Hydrocephalus, CDH, etc. may also evolve later.

Q7. What is the role of invasive diagnostic testing in this case?

Invasive testing should be generally done in all pregnancies with fetal structural congenital anomalies. It is a method to assess the fetal karyotype, via chorionic villus sampling or amniocentesis, or fetal blood sampling (cordocentesis). It will be indicated especially when the estimated risk of aneuploidy is greater and there is presence of other structural anomalies, as most cases of Ebstein anomaly are sporadic. Chromosomal abnormalities were reported but rare mainly Trisomy 21 and rearrangements of chromosome 11q in association with renal malformation and Pierre Robin sequence.

Q8. How will you prognosticate this woman?

The Ebstein anomaly when diagnosed prenatally has a high perinatal mortality (87.5%).[9] Short-term survival depends on degree of fetal heart failure or hydrops, degree of pulmonary hypoplasia and left ventricular dysfunction. The poor prognosis in fetal stage of Ebstein anomaly depends on—cardiothoracic index >0.55, relative foramen ovale—atrial septal <0.3, the obstruction to the outflow tract, a degree of valve displacement >2.5, absence of reverse flow in the duct arteriosus, ratio of right ventricle-left ventricle >2.

Fetus with mild form of Ebstein anomaly require no specific treatment and the infants generally do well, moderate-to-severe Ebstein anomalies baby will need prostaglandin (PGE), an intravenous medication that keeps the patent ductus arteriosus open. The patent ductus arteriosus (PDA) will allow blood flow to the lungs. For more severe cases surgery in the newborn period may be necessary.

Long-term prognosis after surgery for Ebstein's anomaly depends on the severity of the defect. The child will need lifelong follow up.

CASE SCENARIO

A 28 years old Mrs X, G2P1L1 at 24 weeks period of gestation came with concern of abnormal USG report. She had no other complaints. She is married since last 3 years, non-consanguineous marriage with previous one full term normal vaginal delivery of healthy baby. This pregnancy is spontaneous conception, booked at 4-month period of gestation (POG), no history of folic acid intake in first trimester. First trimester was uneventful, no history of fever, drug and radiation exposure. No biochemical screen and aneuploidy screening were done. Second and third trimesters were also uneventful. Patient took iron calcium supplementation and received 2 doses of tetanus toxoid. USG done at 6 months, showed single live fetus with 24 weeks POG with bilateral prominent cerebral ventricle. Her routine blood and urine investigation including oral glucose tolerance test were normal. She had no history of any medical disorder in herself or family.

Q1. What are the relevant points in history and examination in case of ventriculomegaly (VM)?

History of Present Pregnancy

Parental age and consanguinity, parity, smoking, diabetes, epilepsy, hypertension, fever with rashes, medication (retinoic acid), X-rays and occupational exposure.

Past Obstetric History

Previous pregnancies with malformations and stillbirths.

Family History

X-linked hydrocephalous (HCP) spectrum have variable presentation within same families, with some present with VM antenatally and are severely affected, while others may have no macrocephaly and long survival.

Q2. How do you diagnose ventriculomegaly (VM) on USG?

Any enlargement in axial diameter >10 mm across the atrium of lateral ventricle is called ventriculomegaly. It is usually constant at 7.6 ± 0.6 mm (mean ± SD) from 14th to 38th weeks of gestation.

If the difference is greater than 2 mm between the right and left sides, VM is considered asymmetric. Separation of the choroid plexus from the medial wall of the lateral ventricle (if >3 or 4 mm) is also used to diagnose VM, even with borderline parameters.[10]

The X-linked HCP spectrum may develop VM in late gestation or even after birth. The patients at risk for X-linked HCP spectrum should be therefore informed that a normal mid trimester US does not rule out this condition.[11]

Fetal MRI—should be offered as adjunct to detect occult CNS abnormalities (present in up to 40–50%).

Q3. What are the common causes of congenital ventriculomegaly?

- *Obstruction to cerebrospinal fluid flow:* Aqueduct stenosis/X-linked hydrocephalus spectrum.
- *Congenital failure of brain growth:* Agenesis of corpus callosum, Dandy-Walker malformation, lissencephaly, cerebellar hypoplasia.
- *Reduced absorption of cerebrospinal fluid:* Congenital absence of arachnoid villi

- *Intrauterine infections*: Maternal prenatal infection (toxoplasmosis, syphilis, CMV, rubella)
- Intrauterine hemorrhage
- Extracranial abnormalities (30%)
- Multiple anomalies (25%)
- Chromosomal aberration (11%)
- Idiopathic.

Q4. How will you manage if fetal cerebral ventriculomegaly is diagnosed antenataly?

Women presenting with fetal ventriculomegaly will need detail evaluation according to period of gestation:
- Detailed anatomic survey and fetal echocardiography
- Genetic counseling and amniocentesis for karyotyping or infection studies
- Consider MRI brain to look for additional brain anomalies
- Consultation with maternal fetal medicine, neonatology, pediatric neurology
- Discuss pregnancy options such as termination of pregnancy and in-utero fetal surgery
- Serial USG to monitor progression of VM.

> Patient has been admitted for evaluation and management. Routine investigation was normal. TORCH profile done which turn out to be cytomegalovirus (CMV), IgM and IgG positive with low avidity. Repeat USG done to confirm, symptoms of bilateral ventriculomegaly (12 mm). Amniocentesis done and amniotic fluid send for karyotyping and infection. CMV was isolated in amniotic fluid by PCR and karyotype was normal. On fetal MRI, no other associated lesion seen. Serial follow up scan done at 4 weeks interval, lateral ventricle diameter reduced to 10–11 mm in 28 weeks scan.

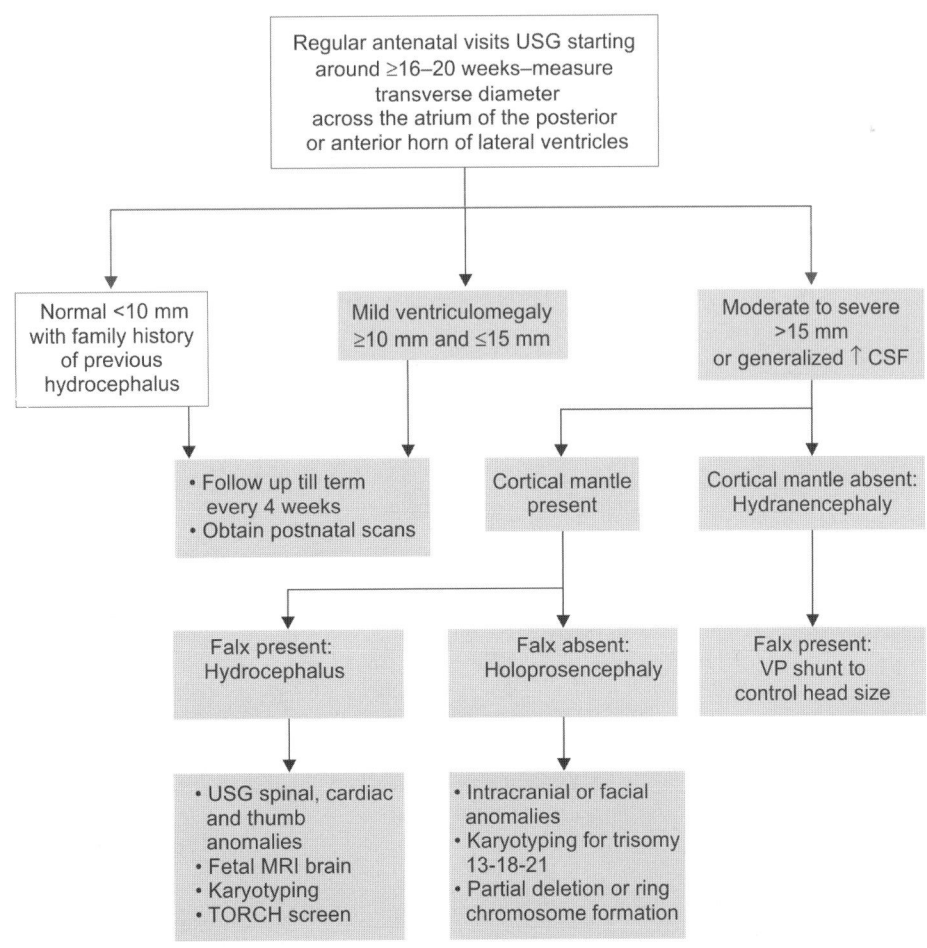

Flowchart 1: Evaluation of fetal cerebral ventriculomegaly

Q5. How will diagnose cytomegalovirus infection in pregnancy?

Patient with CMV infection are usually asymptomatic or may present with fever but diagnosis by clinical symptoms alone is rare. Presence of maternal seroconversion and low avidity test are required to confirm the diagnosis of a primary infection.

Amniotic fluid culture or PCR is recommended for detection of CMV, in situations where maternal primary or undefined CMV infection is detected especially in the first half of pregnancy or in cases where fetal abnormalities are suggestive of infection. A comprehensive ultrasound examination is therefore being required for determining the extent of fetal insult. The principal ultrasound findings suggestive of congenital CMV infection are placentomegaly, intrauterine growth restriction, microcephaly, ventriculomegaly, periventricular calcifications, isolated serous effusions, and echogenic bowel. However, only 15% CMV infected fetuses will display ultrasound abnormalities.[12]

Q6. How will you manage CMV infection in pregnancy?

Primary maternal CMV infection possess only 30-40% risk of vertical transmission, and among those only 10-20% of the fetuses will have evidence of clinical infection at birth.

However, because of the poor prognosis associated with fetal CMV infection, diagnosed early in pregnancy, elective termination should be discussed as an option.

Women who wish to continue the pregnancy may be offered medical therapy with hyperimmunoglobulin, however, it is still be regarded as investigational.[13] Therapy with antiviral agents such as ganciclovir, foscarnet, and cidofovir is not recommended during pregnancy. Given the limited success of vaccine prevention of CMV, attention has been directed at patient education as a means of preventing the acquisition of infection.

The flowchart for diagnosis and management of CMV infection in pregnancy is given in Flowchart 2.

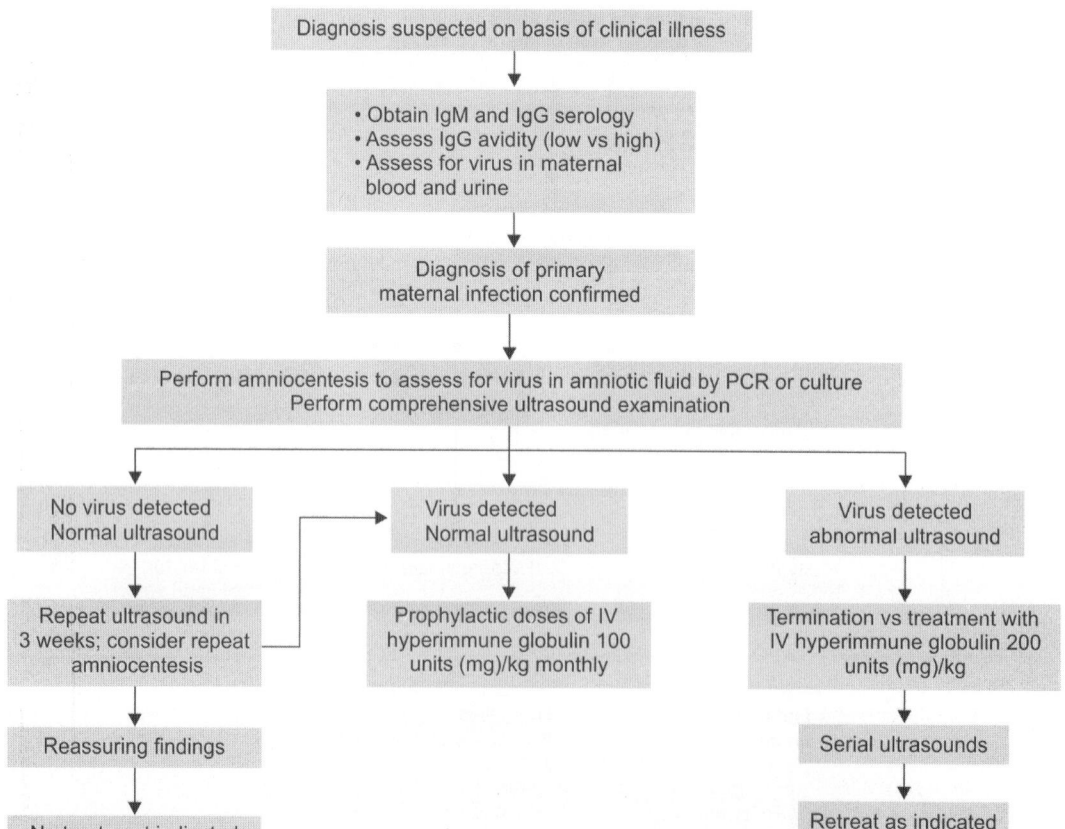

Flowchart 2: Algorithm for the diagnosis and management of congenital CMV infection

Q7. What is the clinical significance of isolated borderline ventriculomegaly?

Isolated VM is a diagnosis of exclusion, termed only if there is no other associated malformations or aneuploidy markers are also negative at the time of the initial presentation. It can be a benign finding, but can also be associated with some chromosomal abnormalities, congenital infection, cerebral vascular accidents or hemorrhage, and other fetal cerebral and extracerebral abnormalities. A careful examination of the fetal anatomy should be carried out using fetal MRI, where available. Invasive testing for chromosomal analysis should be offered. Maternal serum CMV and toxoplasma studies should be considered if suspected.

Isolated VM have normal perinatal and neurodevelopment outcomes in 85% of fetuses.[14] Around 62% case of mild isolated VM resolve before 24 weeks gestation, 11% present with neurodevelopmental delay in postnatal period. The most important prognostic factors are presence of occult abnormalities, which remain undetected at the time of the first diagnosis (about 13% of cases) and progression of the ventricular dilatation (about 16% of cases).

Q8. What treatment options are available for VM?

Termination of pregnancy: It is option for severe VM or those with associated structural malformations such as spina bifida as carries poor prognosis.

Witholding therapy: If the diagnosis is made too late for termination and severe malformations

or

Fetal surgery: In isolated progressive VM, ventriculoamniotic shunt (the placement of a tube between the fetal ventricular system and the amniotic cavity to reduce pressure and to improve brain development) is an option. Although in-utero treatment with ventriculoamniotic shunts has not led to improved perinatal outcomes.[15]

Q9. How would you deliver a fetus with ventriculomegaly?

Delivery to be planned in tertiary care center with access to NICU and pediatric surgery and delayed until fetal lung maturity achieved.

Cephalocentesis should be avoided, unless baby is nonviable.

The pediatric team should be informed before delivery, and a definitive plan and arrangements should be made from both the obstetric and neonatal team.

Cesarean section is only for obstetrical indications or if there is cephalopelvic disproportion. A trial of labor is given in most infants with VM and vertex presentation, as most of them usually do not have macrocrania.

Q10. What is the prognosis of ventriculomegaly?

The prognosis for fetal VM varies from poor to very good. The most important prognostic factors are the specific cause of VM, association to other abnormalities and the progression of ventricular dilation.

Bilateral VM is associated with a poorer prognosis compared to unilateral cases. Isolated unilateral borderline VM carries a favorable prognosis.

Q11. The role of cephalocentesis in hydrocephalous?

It is destructive procedure performed by passing 14–18 G needle transabdominally or transvaginal under ultrasound guidance and removing sufficient cerebrospinal fluid to allow overlapping of cranial sutures. It reduces the cranial size and allow vaginal delivery.

Cephalocentesis is associated with a high perinatal mortality (more than 90%) and it should be reserved for babies with questionable viability to allow vaginal delivery after informed consent of parents.

Q12. Risk of recurrence of VM?

Congenital VM is mostly multifactorial and have a recurrence risk of 4% except for X-linked HCP (recurrence risk 50% of males) and Dandy-Walker anomaly (autosomal recessive) 25% risk of transmission.

Q13. Management of neonatal hydrocephalus?

- Evaluation by neonatology, pediatric neurology and/or neurosurgeon.
- Repeat head USG and/or MRI to reassess in-utero findings.
- Serial head measurement in case of progressive ventriculomegaly.
- Consider chromosomal studies, if neonate appear dysmorphic or other anomalies are diagnosed in neonatal period and these are not performed prenatally
- Surgical treatment in case of severe VM or rapidly progressive post-hemorrhagic hydrocephalus
- Follow up till 1 year of age.

CASE SCENARIO

G5P2L2A2 with 28 weeks period of gestation (POG) was referred in view of multiple congenital anomalies in fetus with gestation hypertension. She was booked in private hospital in seelampur at 28 weeks POG, USG was done there, suggestive of SLIUF of 28 weeks with bilateral hydronephrosis and distended bladder and oligohydramnios. Admitted in our hospital for further evaluation and management. Repeat scan was done to confirm findings. USG KUB of mother was normal. Counselling was done regarding poor prognosis of fetus. Follow-up scan were done at 2 weeks interval, showed fetal growth restriction and anhydroamnios. Her blood and urine investigation were normal. Her blood pressure was controlled with oral antihypertensive. She went in preterm labor at 34 + 5 weeks, fetal heart rate decreased during uterine contraction and she delivered a dead male fetus (fresh stillborn with potter facies, small bell-shaped chest, distended abdomen with bilateral palpable kidney and distended bladder with inability to cathaterize urinary bladder with smallest size feeding tube) of birth weight 1kg. Postpartum period was uneventful.

Q1. What was the fetal pathology in this case?

Lower urinary tract obstruction (LUTO) was probably main pathology which prevent normal fetal micturition and causing the bladder and subsequently kidney to distend. Pressure on the developing nephrons causes renal dysplasia and poor function and eventually long standing anhydroamnios, resulting in lethal pulmonary hypoplasia.

Q2. What are the diagnostic features of LUTO on USG?

Lower urinary tract obstruction (LUTO) present with:
- Megacystis (markedly enlarged bladder)
- Thickened bladder wall (>3 mm)
- Dilated posterior urethra (keyhole sign)
- Bilateral hydronephrosis or cortical cysts indicating renal dysplasia
- Oligohydramnios.

Q3. What are the other renal anomalies, which can be diagnosed antenatally?

Congenital anomalies of the urinary tract which can be diagnosed antenatally are:
- *Renal parenchymal disease:* Multicystic dysplastic kidney disease, polycystic kidney disease, renal agenesis, hyperechogenic kidney, solitary cyst.
- *Abnormalities of migration and fusion*: Ectopic kidney and horse-shoe kidney.
- *Abnormalities of urinary collecting system:* Duplicated system, dilated ureter and hydronephrosis, ureterocele.
- *Abnormalitie of bladder and urethra:* Posterior urethral valve obstruction, urethral atresia, bladder exostrophy.

Q4. What are the condition associated with LUTO?
- Oligohydramnios
- Urinary ascites with ruptured bladder, perinephrourinoma with ruptured kidneys
- Echogenic atrophic kidneys
- Pulmonary hypoplasia
- Other genitourinary anomalies, present in approximately 40%
- Aneuploidy
- Potter sequence malformation with long-standing oligohydramnios
- Other neurologic anomalies.

Q5. How will you evaluate a case of fetal LUTO in antenatal period?

Initial evaluation of the fetus with suspected LUTO should include:
- Detailed anatomic survey and fetal echocardiography to rule out associated anomalies
- Serial scan for assessment of amniotic fluid index, fetal growth and development of pulmonary hypoplasia
- Genetic counseling and amniocentesis for karyotyping (10 % of LUTO cases are associated with trisomy's 13, 18, or 21).
- Consultation with maternal fetal medicine, neonatology, pediatric nephrology
- TORCH titer if other findings indicate possible intrauterine infection
- A minimum of three sequential vesicocentesis 48–72 hours apart, should be performed to assess fetal urine function
- Isolated cases of LUTO with normal amniotic fluid volume denotes a milder form of disease, and does not require fetal intervention
- Consider in-utero fetal therapy in isolated LUTO cases with oligohydramnios and favorable prognostic indicators. Consider termination if anhydroamnios is suspected
- In non-isolated cases of LUTO and/or with genetic abnormality consider elective termination of pregnancy
- Fetal nonstress or biophysical profile testing twice weekly, beginning at 32–34 weeks
- Delivery in tertiary care facility, vesicocentesis may be warranted in LUTO to decompress the fetal bladder to prevent abdominal dystocia with vaginal delivery and improve respiratory compliance in the neonate
- Cesarean delivery is reserved for obstetric indication, may be necessary to prevent abdominal dystocia from massively enlarged kidney.

Q6. What is the role of fetal therapy in this case?

Fetal therapy in LUTO is predominantly aimed at restoration of amniotic fluid volume for prevention of pulmonary hypoplasia, and urinary decompression for attenuation of on-going renal damage. Treatment options for this subset of fetuses includes:

- *Vesicoamniotic shunting (most commonly used):* A percutaneous procedure performed under ultrasound guidance, using local anesthesia. Double pigtail catheter is placed with the distal end in the fetal bladder, and proximal end within the amniotic cavity. Amnioinfusion may be required. The outcomes associated with vesicoamniotic shunting are not clear.
- *Valve ablation via cystoscopy:* Percutaneous fetal cystoscopy is useful for diagnostic as well as therapeutic purposes. It is an emerging treatment option for only posterior urethral valve obstruction, the valves can be treated using hydroablation, guide-wire or laser fulguration.
- *Vesicostomy:* Fetal vesicostomy, via open fetal surgery, is yet another treatment option for LUTO. However, this technique does not improve the bladder function.

These interventions are experimental, and large-scale studies are needed to assess its utility and safety.

Q7. What is fetal therapy? What are the other indications of fetal surgery?

It is a therapeutic intervention for correcting or treating a fetal anomaly or condition. The fetal anomaly should be correctly diagnosed and its severity should be assessed before starting fetal therapy. Other serious malformations should be excluded. The benefits of treatment should outweigh the risks if anomaly is left untreated and the risks of the procedure itself. The pulmonary maturity should be ascertained prior to delivery, and adequate follow-up care should be provided after the intervention.

Surgical (Invasive) Fetal Therapy

Fetal Image-guided Procedure

- *Hemolytic disease of the fetus:* Intrauterine transfusions, direct intravascular transfusions through umbilical vein puncture or a combination of intraperitoneal and intravascular transfusions.
- *Isolated hydrocephalus:* Ventriculoamniotic shunt.
- *Uni- or bilateral pleural effusions:* Placement of pleuro-amniotic shunt (double-pigtail catheter).

Fetal Endoscopic Surgeries

- *Acardiac twin:* Bipolar diathermy or radiofrequency ablation of umbilical cord.
- *Twin-to-twin transfusion syndrome:* Obliteration (laser) of communicating vessels between two twins, in monochorionic gestation.
- *Congenital diaphragmatic hernia:* Balloon occlusion of trachea.

Exit (Ex-utero Intrapartum Treatment) Procedure

- Removal of balloon after treatment of diaphragmatic hernia
- Surgical intervention for congenital high airway obstruction.

Open Fetal Surgeries

- Congenital cystic adenomatous malformation
- Sacrococcygeal teratoma.

Q8. Describe the role of medical therapy in prenatal treatment?

Preventive

- *Neural tube defect:* Folic acid beginning at least 1 month prior to conception through 3 months of pregnancy 0.4 mg/day PO, and 4 mg/day for women with a previously affected child.
- *Congenital adrenal hyperplasia:* Dexamethasone is started at 7–9 week in dose of 0.25 mg PO qid and stopped when it is confirmed as male or unaffected female fetus. Treatment is continued until term only in affected fetuses.
- *Lung maturity induction:* Maternal Betamethasone 12 mg IM 12 hourly for two doses or dexamethasone 6 mg IM 12 hourly for four doses is recommended for fetuses of less than 34 weeks of gestation who are at risk of preterm delivery.
- *Fetus with maternal SLE:* Dexamethasone 4 mg per day to prevent congenital heart block in fetus.
- *Methylmalonic acidemia:* Prenatal cyanocobalamin orally to the mother at titrated dose to achieve high maternal plasma B_{12} levels and normal maternal urinary methylmalonic acid excretion.
- *Multiple carboxylase deficiency:* Maternal biotin supplementation.

Therapeutic

- *Fetal cardiac arrhythmia:* Digoxin and/or amiodarone
- *Fetal thyrotoxicosis:* Propylthiouracil 300 mg/day orally initially and subsequently titrated according to effect or methimazole.
- *Fetal hypothyroidism:* Intra-amniotic L-thyroxine 500 µg every 2 weeks, initiated at 34 weeks gestation.

Q9. Prognosis of LUTO in fetus?

Fetal mortality is 30–40%, prognosis depends on sonographic appearance of kidney, fetal urine concentration and amniotic fluid volume. Good prognosis (10% mortality) with normal kidneys and normal fetal urine. Worst prognosis (95% mortality) with severe oligohydramnios or anhydroamnios, neonatal mortality results from pulmonary hypoplasia or renal failure or both.

Long term—increased risk to develop hypertension, vesicoureteric reflux, frequent urinary tract infections and end-stage renal failure requiring dialysis or transplant.

Q10. This patient delivered a stillborn baby. How will you evaluate further?

All stillborn fetuses especially with anomalies should undergo autopsy.

The main objectives of the fetal autopsy are to determine gestational age, document growth and development, detect congenital abnormalities, make clinical diagnosis and treatment, and determine the cause of death and possible recurrence risk. Autopsy findings are useful even when no clear clinical diagnosis is available or when there is a fetal malformation.

Steps of Fetal Autopsy

- *Biometry:* The size and weight of the body, the crown–heel and crown–rump lengths, occipitofrontal circumference, inter-canthal distances, chest circumferences, abdominal circumference and foot lengths. Other specialized measurements can be obtained and compared with published norm (width and length of fontanelles, nasal height, philtrum length, mouth width, ear length, inter-nipple distance, lengths of limbs).
- *Photographs:* A frontal, lateral, and dorsal pictures of the fetus with a close of the cleaned face, any unusual findings, and of both maternal and fetal placental surfaces, are a strict minimum.
- *External examination*: This examination is of great importance especially when the autopsy is declined. It should be performed by experienced clinicians (perinatal/pediatric pathologist or clinical genetics or by a pediatrician).
- *Infantogram*: X-ray of fetus anteroposterior and lateral view.
- *Internal examination and routine microscopic sections:* All major organs must be weighed and compared with expected values. Organ maturity and structure should be assessed by macroscopic (e.g. cerebral gyration) and/or histologic (e.g. lungs and kidneys) evaluation.
- *Additional sampling:* The need for additional sampling is guided by the results of previous investigations, along with the type of anomalies identified in the fetus.
- *Placenta:* The placental examination is useful for identifying infection, investigating stillbirth, and conditions where maternal disease plays a major role in pregnancy outcome. Includes gross examination of the placenta followed by a routine methodology (culture, cytogenetics, RNA) and it should ideally be performed on a fresh tissue.

Q11. If parents are not willing for a full autopsy, what are alternatives?

The alternatives option must be offered after explaining the limitation to couples who deferred full autopsy. These are:

- *Limited autopsy:* It include examination of specific body cavities, or full body imaging techniques. Biometric measurements, clinical photographs, external examination, and radiographs are generally acceptable to most parents. That may answer specific questions or concern. Obtaining samples of blood, body fluids, skin, and placenta is important to allow specific ancillary testing.
- *MRI of fetus:* It may be offered to parents who decline for an autopsy.[16] However, MRI does not supply tissue samples, and important information may be missed, and it is of uncertain value when there is an advanced degree of maceration or autolysis.[17] MRI also provides suboptimal resolution in assessing certain malformations such as skeletal dysplasia.
- *New options:* Postmortem needle biopsy, laparoscopic autopsy, and small incision access are other alternatives.

Conclusion

Congenital anomalies are important causes of fetal and neonatal morbidity and mortality even in developing countries. Although 50% of all congenital anomalies cannot be linked to a specific cause, there may be presence of some known genetic, environmental risk factors. Preconception and periconception screening can be useful to identify those at risk of passing a disorder onto their children. Preconception and periconception preventive health measures can help to decrease the frequency of certain congenital anomalies through either by removal of risk factors or the reinforcement of protective factors with the advances in imaging and invasive technique, early diagnosis is also possible. Management should be multidisciplinary and comprehensive neonatal screening after birth is essential. Parents should be informed about various treatment option. Fetal autopsy to performed whenever possible.

REFERENCES

1. World Health Organization. Section on congenital anomalies. [Cited on 2012 Oct]. Available from: http://www.who.int/mediacentre/factsheets/fs370/en/
2. Bhat BV, Ravikumara M. Perinatal mortality in India—Need for introspection. Ind J Matern Child Health. 1996;7:31.
3. March of Dimes report. 2006, congenital anomalies (birth defects); national health portal.
4. Grandjean H, Larroque D, Levi S. Sensitivity of routine ultrasound screening of pregnancies in the Eurofetus database. The Eurofetus Team. Ann N Y Aced Sci. 1998; 847:118–24.
5. Levi S. Ultrasound in prenatal diagnosis: polemics around routine ultrasound screening for second trimester fetal malformations. Prenat Diagn. 2002; 22:285-95. (Level III)
6. Grandjean H, Larroque D, Levi S. The performance of routine ultrasonographic screening of pregnancies in the Eurofetus Study. Am J Obstet Gynecol. 1999; 181:446-54. (Level II)
7. Obesity in pregnancy. Practice Bulletin No. 156. American College of Obstetricians and Gynecologists. ObstetGynecol. 2015;126:112-26. (level III)
8. Crane JP, LeFevre MsL, Winborn RC, et al. A randomized trial of prenatal ultrasonographic screening: impact on the detection, management, and outcome of anomalous fetuses. The RADIUS Study Group. Am J Obstet Gynecol. 1994; 171:392–9. (Level I)
9. Luis-Miranda RS, Arias-Monroy LG, Alcantar-Mendoza MA, et al. Fetal diagnosis and prognosis of Ebstein's anomaly. Ginecol Obstet Mex. 2013;81(5):221-30.
10. Filly RA, Goldstein RB, Callen PW. Fetal ventricle: importance in routine obstetric sonography. Radiology. 1991;181:1-7.
11. Stumpel S, Fryns JP. Congenital hydrocephalus: nosology and guidelines for clinical approach and genetic counselling. Eur J Pediatr. 1998;157:355-62.
12. Guerra B, Simonazzi G, Puccetti C, et al. Ultrasound prediction of symptomatic congenital cytomegalovirus infection. Am J Obstet Gynecol. 2008;198:380.e1-7.
13. Carlson A, Norwitz ER, Stiller RJ. Cytomegalovirus infection in pregnancy: should all women be screened? Rev obstet gynec. 2010;3(4):172-9.
14. Laskin MD, Kingdom J, Toi A, et al. Perinatal and neuro-developmental outcome with isolated fetal ventriculomegaly: a systematic review. J Matern Fetal Neonatal Med. 2005;18(5):289-98.
15. Bruner JP, Davis G, Tulipan N. Intrauterine shunt for obstructive hydrocephalus-still not ready. Fetal Diagn Ther. 2006;21:532-9.
16. Alderstein MP. Perinatal mortality: clinical value of postmortem magnetic resonance imagining compared with autopsy in routine obstetric practice. BJOG. 2003;110: 378-82.
17. Huisman T. Magnetic resonance imaging: an alternative to autopsy in neonatal death. Semin Neonatol. 2004; 9:347-53.

13

Recurrent Pregnancy Loss

Deepali Dhingra, Anjali Tempe, Komal Rastogi

CASE SCENARIO

Mrs X, a 24 years old wife of Mr Y, a 28 years old, residence of Sunder Nagar, came to gyne OPD with history of three spontaneous miscarriages at 6–8 weeks.

Q1. What are the important points in the history to be asked?

When she comes to gyne OPD for the advice on next pregnancy, the couple should be asked the following points in the history:
- Weeks at which miscarriage occurred
- How was the pregnancies confirmed?
- Whether any ultrasound was done or not?
- Whether cardiac activity was present or not?
- Any history of curettage
- Whether the couple had a consanguineous marriage?
- Any history of any prior term or preterm pregnancy
- Any history of raised blood pressure records
- Any history of diabetes mellitus or thyroid disorder
- Any history of any surgical procedure on the cervix
- Any family history of congenital abnormalities, recurrent miscarriage, or pregnancy complications
- Any history of smoking or alcohol intake.

Q2. What important points to look for in examination?
- Vitals: Blood pressure, pulse, temperature, weight, BMI
- General physical examination: Any evidence of thyroid swelling, galactorrhea, pallor, icterus, cyanosis or pedal edema.
- Systemic examination
- Per speculum and per vaginal examination is to be done.

Q3. What is the definition of recurrent pregnancy loss (RPL)?

RPL is also known as recurrent miscarriage or habitual abortion. It is defined historically as three consecutive pregnancy losses prior to 20 weeks. However, as per American Society of Reproductive Medicine (ASRM) Practise Committee statement 2008, presence of two consecutive miscarriages can be labeled as RPL.

The risk of subsequent miscarriage is 30% after 2 losses and 33% after 3 losses and there is no reliable data of finding a cause of RPL with 2 versus 3 losses, the current evidence indicate starting work-up after two miscarriages.[1]

Q4. How common is RPL?
- It affects 1 % of population.[2]
- Prevalence ranges between 0.6% and 2.3% among couples.[2]
- In nearly 50% of patients with RPL, the underlying cause remains unknown.[3]

Q5. What are the risk factors for RPL?
- Prior history of miscarriage is found to be the strongest predictor
- Maternal age above 40 years
- Genetic risk
- Life style factors: Obesity, smoking and alcohol intake.

Q6. What are the causes of RPL?

In about 50 % of cases, no cause is identified. Other accepted aetiologies are as follows:[4]
- Idiopathic   : 50%
- Genetic   : 2–5%
- Autoimmune : 20%
- Anatomic   : 10–15%
- Infections : 0.5–5%
- Endocrine   : 17–20%

Q7. What are various genetic causes?

Parental Chromosomal Rearrangements

In a population 2–5% of RPL occurs because of balanced parental translocations. Phenotypically carriers (parents)

are normal but pregnancies from these carriers are chromosomally incompetent resulting in increased risk of miscarriages. Most common are balanced translocations, which can be reciprocal or robertsonian.
- In reciprocal translocations, the parts of chromosome break and re-attaches at other place reciprocally.
- In robertsonian translocations, the two acrocentric chromosomes fuse near the centromere region with loss of the short arms.
- In both of the above translocations genetic material is exchanged but content remained equal, so they are phenotypically normal.
- If a parent carries balanced translocation, the pregnancies arising may inherit an extra or missing piece of chromosomal material.
- The child may be normal, may be a carrier of balanced translocation, the pregnancy ends in miscarriage or a baby is born with multiple congenital malformations due to unbalanced chromosomal rearrangements.

Embryonic Chromosomal Abnormalities

These occur due to abnormalities in the egg, sperm or both. Most common are aneuploidies (trisomies or monosomies). Strong association occurs with maternal age. These abnormalities usually result in sporadic miscarriages.

Q8. How to rule out genetic abnormalities? What to do if one of the parents carries a balanced translocation?

All couples with history of RPL should have:
- Peripheral blood karyotype of parents
- Karyotyping of products of conception should be done from third conceptus onwards, if not previously done.

It most often reveals aneuploidies which is usually not a cause of RPL. If unbalanced chromosomal component is found in conceptus, couple is then offered parental karyotyping to detect balanced translocations.[5]

Presence of balanced translocations in one of the parent warrants genetic counseling. Current management options include:
- In-vitro fertilization (IVF) with pre-implantation genetic diagnosis.
- Antenatal genetic testing including amniocentesis or chorionic villus sampling, if parents do not want an option of IVF or the cost issue arises or already conceived.

Q9. What is antiphospholipid antibody syndrome (APS) and how it is detected?

Antiphospholipid antibodies (aPL) are the autoantibodies directed against membrane phospholipids. Thrombosis caused by aPLs in utero placental circulation remains most common hypothesis for adverse pregnancy outcome. Three types of antibodies are identified, anticardiolipin (aCL), lupus anticoagulant (LAC), and anti-β_2 glycoprotein I antibodies. Presence of these antibodies has been linked to *antiphospholipid syndrome* (APS), i.e. first trimester RPL, adverse pregnancy outcome and vascular thrombosis. About 15% of RPL is contributed by APS. APS is diagnosed when at least one clinical and one laboratory criteria are met.

Table 1: Antiphospholipid antibody syndrome criteria[6]

Criteria	Attributes
Clinical	*Vascular thrombosis*: One or more episodes of vascular thrombosis of arteries, veins or small vessels, confirmed by Doppler studies or histopathology
	Obstetrical: 3 or more consecutive miscarriages before 10 weeks 1 or more deaths of a morphologically normal fetus at or after the 10 weeks gestation 1 or more premature births of a morphologically normal neonate before 34 weeks gestation due to severe preeclampsia or severe placental insufficiency
Laboratory	Lupus anticoagulant (LA) present in plasma on ≥2 occasions at least 12 weeks apart Anticardiolipin (aCL) antibody of IgG / IgM isotype in serum in medium or high titer (i.e. >40 GPL or MPL) on ≥ 2 occasions at least 12 weeks apart by ELISA measurement Anti-β2 glycoprotein-1 antibody of IgG / IgM isotype in serum (in titer > the 99th percentile) on ≥ 2 occasions at least 12 weeks apart

Q10. What is the management of APS?

The first line management options are low-dose aspirin and heparin. Both unfractionated and low molecular weight heparin (LMWH) can be used, latter is preferred as it avoids less heparin induced thrombocytopenia and osteoporosis. Currently there is no role of prednisolone and intravenous immunoglobulin for management of APS.

Q11. Elaborate endocrine causes associated with RPL.

- Poorly controlled diabetes mellitus
- Hypothyroidism and presence of thyroid autoantibodies
- Luteal phase defect with decreasing progesterone levels
- Polycystic ovary syndrome and hypersecretion of LH
- Prolactin disorders

Q12. How to manage various endocrine causes implicated for RPL?

Table 2: Endocrine causes of RPL

Disorder	Management
Hypothyroidism/ autoantibodies	Thyroid replacement therapy. Careful monitoring of thyroid function in preconceptional and early pregnancy period
Diabetes mellitus	Achieve euglycemia before conception. Maintain good metabolic control
Polycystic ovary syndrome (PCOS)	Hyperinsulinemia seems to be the cause of RPL.[7] Normalization of weight, addition of metformin may help in reducing risk of RPL.
Luteal phase defect	No definitive diagnostic criteria. Progesterone started during luteal phase, i.e. two days after ovulation and continuing till end of first trimester remains most widely practised management option. Current guidelines do not support use of progesterone to support early pregnancy in a case of RPL.

CASE SCENARIO

A 29 years old G4A3 with 6 weeks pregnancy presented to antenatal OPD with history of three miscarriages. All three miscarriages occurred between 16–18 weeks. There is no significant medical, gynecological and surgical history.

Q1. What is most likely cause of RPL in this patient? What important points to be asked in history to confirm the cause? How to manage this case now?

- This is most likely a case of cervical incompetence leading to pregnancy losses.
- There is no history of pain, bleeding preceding the expulsion.
- Typical history of painless cervical dilation and spontaneous rupture of membranes is present.
- Any prior history of surgical procedures on cervix should be asked.

This patient needs cerclage to prevent pregnancy loss:
- Ultrasound monitoring is started 2–3 weeks prior to period of gestations at which prior losses occurred.
- Cervical cerclage is offered prophylactically to women when there is presence of three or more previous second trimester losses.[5,8]
- If the cervical length in current pregnancy is less than 25 mm, cervical cerclage is indicated only if history of painless second trimester loss is present.
- Cerclage only on basis of cervical length without history of pregnancy loss is not recommended.

So, this patient is offered prophylactic cerclage. Cerclage placement is done two weeks prior to period of gestation at which prior losses occurred, i.e. at around 14 weeks of gestation.[8]

Prerequisites
- Ultrasound scan for viability
- Exclude significant malformations
- If possible combine with first trimester screening for aneuploidies
- Urinalysis for routine and culture
- Vaginal culture is needed before cerclage placement and should be treated if positive.

Q2. What are different types of cerclage techniques?

There are two main types of transvaginal cerclages technique:
1. McDonald cerclage
2. Shirodkar cerclage

- *In McDonald's approach* the cervical stitch is placed as close as possible to the junction of cervix with vagina, without dissection of tissue planes.
- *In Shirodkar's technique* the stitch is placed above the junction of cervix with vagina with dissection of bladder and rectum.
- No technique is better over another but simplicity of McDonald approach favors its use.
- Any non-absorbable suture, e.g. silk or prolene can be used.
- If not contraindicated, regional anesthesia is preferred over general anesthesia.
- Most commonly used is 17 hydroxy-progesterone 500 mg IM given before cerclage placement and may be continued weekly up to 34 weeks depending upon risk factors for preterm birth.[9]
- There is insufficient evidence to support or discourage the use of antibiotics as an adjunct to preterm labor prevention. Large RCTs are needed to define the role of antibiotics and the exact regime to prevent preterm birth.
- Tocolytic is not routinely recommended proximate to cerclage placement. A 2012 Cochrane review concluded no tocolysis during cerclage placement.
- Emergency cerclage placement is considered when cervix is already dilated to >1–2 cm, with no uterine contractions and with or without membranes bulging through external os.[8]
- There should be no evidence of chorioamnionitis before cerclage placement.

- Progesterone use along with cerclage has not been supported by literature as isolated data is limited but it has been used historically to prevent preterm birth, so the rationale to use progesterone along with cervical cerclage placement is justified.

Q3. What are other anatomic causes of recurrent pregnancy loss and how are they diagnosed?

a. Uterine anomalies
   The prevalence of uterine anomalies ranges from 1.8% and 37.6[10] in RPL.
   Congenital uterine malformation usually presents as:
   - Second trimester recurrent pregnancy losses
   - Preterm labor
   - Abnormal presentation
   - Increased risk of cesarean delivery.

b. Uterine septum is the most common congenital anomaly associated with RPL.
   - Poor endometrial vasculature leading to abnormal placentation appears to be the cause resulting in RPL.
   - Intrauterine adhesions and intramural fibroids > 5 cm may also cause RPL.
   - The diagnosis of uterine anomalies includes hysterosalpingography (HSG), transvaginal sonography and hysteroscopy.
   - Correction of septum improves pregnancy outcome by 70%.[10]
   - Correction of intrauterine synechiae, polyps, fibroids and other anomalies appears to be controversial as well randomized controlled trials are lacking.

Q4. Discuss the role of progesterone in an otherwise unexplained recurrent pregnancy loss.

Although there is no evidence to support routine use of progesterone to prevent early and mid-trimester miscarriages, there is some convincing proof in patients having recurrent miscarriages.[11] Large RCT are needed to support routine use of progesterone in RPL.

One such RCT is progesterone use in women with recurrent miscarriages (PROMISE) trial,[12] which concluded that progesterone use in first trimester in patients with otherwise unexplained RPL does not result in significant improvement of pregnancy outcome. Recent ASRM committee opinion did not support progesterone use in non-artificial reproductive techniques (ART) pregnancies.[13]

Q5. What is role of infections in RPL?

Organisms implicated in causing abortion include: *Chlamydia*, *Mycoplasma*, *Ureaplasma*, Herpes, Cytomegalovirus and *Toxoplasma*. But, genital infections mostly cause sporadic pregnancy loss. There is no convincing proof that infections cause repeated pregnancy loss. So, routine TORCH screening or genital infections screening is not required in RPL.

Q6. Do you think inherited thrombophilia testing is justified in cases of RPL?

Screening for mutations for inherited thrombophilia i.e. factor V Leiden, prothrombin gene mutations, protein C, protein S and antithrombin deficiencies is justified only when there is personal or first degree family history of thromboembolism.

Q7. What is the role of aspirin/low molecular weight heparin (LMWH) in unexplained RPL?

There are limited numbers of studies supporting the role of aspirin and/or LMWH in unexplained RPL. At present there are no recommendations to support the use of aspirin and/or LMWH for unexplained recurrent pregnancy loss.[14]

Q8. What is TLC in context to recurrent pregnancy loss?

TLC stands for *tender loving care*. Even after investigating, 50–70% of cases of RPL will remain idiopathic. So, TLC was defined as psychological support with weekly medical and instructions to avoid heavy work and travel. It is known to increase the live birth rates among these women compared to routine ANC care.

Table 3: Etiology of RPL, diagnosis and management

Cause of RPL	Diagnosis	Management
Genetic	Karyotype of parents, if karyotype of products of conception (POC) still not performed	In utero fertilization (IVF) with preimplantation diagnosis, amniocentesis, or chorionic villus sampling (CVS)
Endocrine	Thyroid stimulating hormone (TSH)/diabetes mellitus/prolactin/polycystic ovary syndrome (PCOS)	Progesterone/thyroxine/metformin
Antiphospholipid antibodies (APLA) syndrome	Lupus anticoagulant/beta 2 microglobulin/anti-cardiolipin antibody	Aspirin / low molecular weight heparin
Anatomic evaluation	Hysterosalpingography (HSG)/ transvaginal scan (TVS)	Appropriate correction
Lifestyle	Alcohol, tobacco consumption/obesity	Eliminate consumption Weight loss advocated if obese

Q9. If a patient with history of three spontaneous miscarriages in first trimester with all the possible etiologies ruled out, presents with 6 weeks of pregnancy, how are you going to manage?

First trimester	- Start folic acid if not started
- Start progesterone (intramuscular/vaginal) till 12 weeks
- Antenatal investigations
- Complete blood count, T3/T4/TSH, HbA1c, fasting blood sugar, urine routine and microscopy (RM), hepatitis B surface antigen (HBsAg), veneral disease research laboratory (VDRL), human immunodificiency virus (HIV)
- Avoid heavy activity, vigorous sexual intercourse, travel and X-ray exposure
- Ultrasound for cardiac activity
- First trimester screening [free beta human chorionic gonadotrophin (HCG), pregnancy-associated plasma protein A (PAPPA)]
- USG for nuchal transluncy 11-13 weeks
- Psychological support
- Start aspirin empirically
Second trimester	- Start iron tablets at 16-20 weeks
- Ultrasound monitoring of cervical length from 16 weeks onwards or two weeks prior to period of gestation (POG) of previous losses
- Offer prophylactic cerclage after three losses, if no cause is identified and history favors cervical weakness or cervical length borderline
- Level II ultrasound at 18-20 weeks
- Progesterone continued if risk factors of prior preterm birth are present
- 2 hr OGTT(75 mg)
- Complete blood count (CBC), urine RM , T3/T4/TSH
- Triple marker screening
Third trimester	- Continue progesterone till 34 weeks if risk factors for preterm births persists
- Iron/calcium/folic acid (FA) continued
- Ultrasonography with biophysical profile at 32-34 weeks
- Umbilical artery Doppler if intrauterine growth restriction is suspected
- Remove cerclage at 36-37 weeks
- Stop aspirin at 34 weeks
- Stop heparin at term once labor begins
- Daily fetal movement count
- Weekly visits

REFERENCES

1. Management of Recurrent Early Pregnancy Loss. Washington, DC: The American College of Obstetricians and Gynecologists; 2001. The American College of Obstetricians and Gynecologists. (ACOG Practice Bulletin No. 24).
2. Stirrat GM. Recurrent miscarriage. Lancet 1990;336:673–5
3. Toth B et al. Reccurrent miscarriage: current concepts in diagnosis and treatment. Journal of Reproductive Immunology 2010:85;25-32.
4. Ford HB, Schust DJ. Recurrent pregnancy loss: etiology, diagnosis, and therapy. Rev Obstet Gynecol. 2009;2(2):76–83.
5. Regan L, Backos M, Rai R. The Investigation and Treatment of Couples with Recurrent First-trimester and Second-trimester Miscarriage. RCOG Green-top Guideline No. 17. April 2010. http://www.rcog. org.uk/files/rcog-corp/GTG17recurrentmiscarriage.pdf (accessed 1 April 2011).
6. Miyakis S, Lockshin MD, Atsumi T, et al. "International consensus statement on an update of the classification criteria for definite antiphospholipid syndrome (APS)," Journal of Thrombosis and Haemostasis, vol. 4, no. 2, pp. 295–306, 2006.
7. Craig LB, Ke RW, Kutteh WH. Increased prevalence of insulin resistance in women with a history of recurrent pregnancy loss. Fertil Steril 2002;78:487–90.
8. Brown R, Gagnon R, Delisle MF, et al; Maternal Fetal Medicine Committee, Society of Obstetricians and Gynaecologists of Canada. Cervical insufficiency and cervical cerclage. J Obstet Gynaecol Can. 2013;35(12):1115-27.
9. Norwitz ER, Caughey AB. Progesterone Supplementation and the Prevention of preterm birth. Reviews in Obstetrics and Gynecology. 2011;4(2):60-72.
10. Grimbizis GF, Camus M, Tarlatzis BC, et al. Devroey P. Clinical implications of uterine malformations and hysteroscopic treatment results. Hum Reprod Update 2001;7:161-74.
11. Haas DM, Ramsey PS. Progestogen for preventing miscarriage. Cochrane Database of Systematic Reviews 2013, Issue 10. Art. No.: CD003511. DOI: 10.1002/14651858.CD003511.pub3
12. Coomarasamy A, Williams H, Truchanowicz E, et al. A randomized trial of progesterone in women with recurrent miscarriages. N Engl J Med. 2015;373:2141-8.
13. Practice Committee of the American Society for Reproductive Medicine Current clinical irrelevance of luteal phase deficiency: a committee opinion American Society for Reproductive Medicine. Birmingham, Alabama Fertility and Sterility® 2015.
14. De Jong PG, Kaandorp S, Di Nisio M, Goddijn M, et al. Aspirin and/or heparin for women with unexplained recurrent miscarriage with or without inherited thrombophilia. Cochrane Database of Systematic Reviews 2014, Issue 7.

CHAPTER 14

Pregnancy in Extremes of Ages

Komal Rastogi, Niharika Dhiman, Nupur Ahuja, Pushpa Mishra

TEENAGE PREGNANCY

Teenage or adolescent pregnancy is the pregnancy occurring in teenagers from puberty to 19 years of age. Births to adolescent mothers represent 10% of births worldwide and contribute to 23% of maternal morbidity and mortality.[1] In India early age of marriage is the leading cause for a higher incidence of teenage pregnancy. Adolescent fertility rate contributes 17% to the total fertility rate in India and about 14% of births in women aged below 20 are unplanned.[2]

CASE SCENARIO

Miss X, 16 years old girl, comes to antenatal OPD at 12 weeks of period of gestation.

Q1. What are the risk factors for teenage pregnancy?

- Early marriage
- Exposure to domestic or sexual violence
- Drug addiction like alcohol, smoking and substance abuse
- Lower socioeconomic status
- Low level of schooling
- Social isolation
- Lack of sexual and reproductive health information
- Stress and depression
- Single parent homes
- Limited job opportunities.

Q2. What is the significant history to be asked in this patient and what are the important points in examination?

- *History of smoking or substance abuse:* Adolescents who are pregnant have higher rates of smoking and substance abuse. Any such history should be elicited and every effort should be made to reduce the effects of smoking and substance abuse on pregnancy
- *History of past physical abuse and violence in pregnancy:* Violence in adolescent pregnancy is quite common and is associated with adverse perinatal outcomes such as preterm birth, low birth weight, fetal death and postpartum depression
- *Presence of any depressive symptoms:* Adolescent mothers are twice as likely to experience depression as compared to adult mothers,[3] the rate varies from 16–44%. Untreated maternal depression is associated with preterm delivery and SGA infants. There is also increased risk of postpartum depression in adolescent mothers. Therefore, adolescent mothers should be routinely screened for mood disorders and treated accordingly
- *Socioeconomic history:* Poverty, poor socioeconomic status and lower educational attainment are risk factors for adolescent pregnancy.

On Examination

- Apart from usual general and systemic examination these patients should be examined for any evidence of physical abuse, i.e. bruises, cuts, old scars, etc.
- Signs of anemia and preeclampsia, i.e. pallor, blood pressure, edema, fetal growth restriction, etc. should be seen repeatedly
- Speculum examination: At first visit to look for vaginal infections
- Per vaginal examination: Done at term to rule out cephalopelvic disproportion which is more common in these patients.

Q3. What investigations will you order in a case of teenage pregnancy?

- Blood group, hemoglobin
- Human immunodeficiency virus (HIV) antigen 1 and 2, Australia antigen, venereal disease research laboratory (VDRL)

- Oral glucose tolerance test (75 g)
- Urine routine and microscopy
- A first trimester ultrasound is recommended for dating if girl comes early to prevent preterm birth and its consequences. An ultrasound between 18–20 weeks of gestation should be performed to rule out congenital anomalies because of increased rates of congenital anomalies in this age group. These include central nervous system anomalies (microcephaly, anencephaly, spina bifida), musculoskeletal anomalies (cleft lip, cleft palate, syndactyly, polydactyly) and gastrointestinal anomalies (gastroschisis, omphalcoele)[4,5]
- An ultrasound should be done at 32–34 weeks of gestation to assess fetal well-being as these patients are at risk of developing fetal growth restriction due to poor nutritional status, substance abuse and lack of antenatal care.

Q4. How will you manage this case?

- After getting an ultrasound for dating the pregnancy, we will offer her medical termination of pregnancy
- Counsellors should be made available to help her in making a decision and provide support
- Adolescents are at greater risk for sexually transmitted infections (STIs) because they have unprotected intercourse, have multiple partners and are biologically more vulnerable to sexually acquired infections and face multiple obstacles to utilization of health care
- Medications to prevent sexually transmitted infections should also be given to the patient. Contraception, especially barrier, should be explained and advised.

Q5. How will you manage if pregnancy has progressed beyond 20 weeks of gestation?

- Adolescents are high-risk pregnancies and should be given multidisciplinary care by a team of obstetricians, pediatricians, psychiatrists and counsellors
- Social worker, family and social organizations should also be involved in the care of pregnant adolescents and future options like giving the baby for adoption should be discussed with the girl and her family
- She should be followed up regularly in antenatal clinic and all investigations discussed above should be done
- Anemia is a very common complication in pregnant adolescents, with a reported prevalence of 50% to 66%.[6] This is mainly due to inadequate replacement or nutrition. She should be given regular iron and folic acid and calcium tablets and should be advised to have diet, adequate in calorie (2000–2500) and protein (60–75 g/day)
- Adolescents are at greater risk for STIs and in pregnancy STIs have been associated with preterm delivery, chorioamnionitis, and postpartum infections. Testing for sexually transmitted infection and bacterial vaginosis should be performed on presentation and again in the third trimester and treatment should be given. Testing for sexually transmitted infection should also be performed during the postpartum and when needed symptomatically[7]
- As these patients are at risk of developing fetal growth restriction, serial ultrasound should be done for fetal growth. Fetal monitoring should be performed by fetal kick count, non-stress test and biophysical profile
- These patients should be routinely screened for alcohol use, substance use, and violence and mood of disorders in each trimester
- Adolescents have lower cesarean delivery rate and improved vaginal delivery rates than their adult counterparts but those aged 15 years and younger are more likely to experience cesarean births for the indication of presumed cephalopelvic mismatch. Peripartum care in hospital should be multidisciplinary, involving support for breastfeeding and lactation, social care and the involvement of children's aid services should be provided after delivery of the baby
- Contraception must be offered during puerperium to decrease the high rates of repeat pregnancy in this population and to reduce risk of RTIs too.

Q6. What are the complications associated with teenage pregnancy?

Maternal Complications

- Anemia
- Abortion
- Preeclampsia
- Psychological problems like depression, suicidal tendencies due to inadequate family support and unplanned pregnancy
- Postpartum depression
- Preterm labor
- Lower genital tract infections
- Difficult delivery in small pelvis.

Fetal Complications

- Prematurity
- Low birth weight due to prematurity, smoking and substance abuse
- Behavior problems
- Infections
- Exposure to domestic violence
- Lack of immunization
- Developmental delays.

Q7. A 15 years old girl comes to you with alleged history of sexual assault. How will you manage?

- The police has to be informed as per the law, in case the survivor does not want to pursue a police case, a medicolegal case (MLC) must be made and she must be informed that she has right to refuse to file first information report (FIR). An informed refusal must be documented in such cases
- An informed consent should be taken for examination, sample collection for clinical and forensic examination, treatment and police intimation and any informed refusal for examination and evidence collection must be documented
- A consent form must be signed by the person herself if she is above 12 years of age. Consent must be taken from guardian/parent if the survivor is under the age of 12 years
- Psychosocial care: All survivors should be provided the first line support. The health professional must provide this support or ensure that there is someone trained at the facility to provide this
- The history taking and examination should be carried out in complete privacy in the special room set up in the hospital. All relevant medical/surgical history should be taken and examination should be done including the examination for injuries, local examination of genital parts and other orifices and sample collection for central/state forensic science laboratory
- If a woman reports within 96 hours (4 days) of assault, all evidence including swabs must be collected based on the nature of assault that has occurred. However, the likelihood of finding evidence after 72 hours is greatly reduced
- If clinical signs are suggestive of sexually transmitted disease (STD) on examination, collect relevant swabs and start postexposure prophylaxis (PEP). For pregnant women, amoxycillin/azithromycin with metronidazole is preferred
- Draw a blood sample for hepatitis B surface antigen (HBsAg) and administer 0.06 mL/kg HB immunoglobulin immediately (anytime up to 72 hours of sexual act)
- Postexposure prophylaxis for HIV should be given if a survivor reports within 72 hours of the assault
- Emergency contraception
  - Two tablets of levonorgestrol 0.75 mg within 72 hours or 2 tablets of COCs i.e MALA D—2 tablets stat repeated after 12 hours within 72 hours
  - Pregnancy assessment must be done on follow up and the survivor must be advised to get tested for pregnancy in case she misses her next period.
- All injuries should be cleaned with antiseptic or soap and water and if the survivor is not already immunized with tetanus toxoid, 0.5 mL of TT intramuscularly (IM) should be administered
- Follow up: The survivor should be called for re-examination after 2 days to note the development of bruises and other injuries; thereafter at 3 and 6 weeks.
  - Repeat test for gonorrhea if possible
  - Test for pregnancy
  - Repeat test after 6 weeks for VDRL
  - Assess for psychological sequel and re-iterate need for psychological support
- In case a rape survivor comes with pregnancy at later period of gestation—a medicolegal case should be made, counseling should be done and antenatal care given for safer delivery. Provision for child adoption should be given to the survivor after delivery.

PREGNANCY IN ELDERLY PRIMIGRAVIDA

Pregnancy and child birth are normal physiological processes and outcomes of most pregnancies are good, but pregnancy in woman with advanced age is considered high risk. Women who become pregnant for the first time after the age of 35 are termed as elderly primigravida. Age 35 was first designated as the threshold for being labeled as "elderly" while pregnant during a National Institutes of Health (NIH) conference in 1978. Progressively, this has become more common in our contemporary society and traditionally such pregnancy is regarded as high risk.

CASE SCENARIO

> Mrs X, age 38 years, married for 8 months presents to you with history of amenorrhea of 9 weeks. How will you manage this patient?

Q1. What is the incidence of elderly primigravida?

In Western countries, the proportion of maternities in women aged 35 years or over has increased from 8% in 1985–87 to 20% in 2006–2008 and in women aged 40 years and older has trebled in this time from 1.2–3.6%.[7]

Q2. What is the role of preconceptional counseling in these patients?

Preconceptional counseling is very important in this age group and many women willingly seek it. This is very important for women with pre-existing medical problems in which case pregnancy can be planned after stabilizing the medical condition.

Q3. What special investigations will you offer her apart from routine investigations?

The elderly primigravida is generally believed to have decreased fertility and increased risk for adverse pregnancy outcomes. Reduced fertility with increasing maternal age is evidenced by decline in ovarian oocyte reserve and quality with increasing number of ovulatory cycles. Poor oocyte quality is associated with an increased risk for aneuploidy, chromosomal abnormalities, and spontaneous abortions in this group of women.

First Trimester Screening

Certain genetic risks are more common in pregnancies of older pregnant people. One risk is that the embryo will have Down syndrome, which has the following distribution:

Age	Rate of embryo having Down syndrome at 10 weeks	Rate of having a baby with Down syndrome at term
25	1 in 1,064	1 in 1,340
30	1 in 686	1 in 939
35	1 in 240	1 in 353
40	1 in 53	1 in 85
45	1 in 19	1 in 35

- Combined screening (nuchal translucency measurements, serum markers [PAPP-A and beta-hCG], and maternal age) is effective for testing for Down syndrome. For women younger than 35, combined screening in the first trimester has a detection rate similar to that of quadruple screening in the second trimester. For women 35 years and older, combined screening has a detection rate of 90% but it has a higher screen-positive rate (16–22%).[8]
- However, screening will not identify all affected fetuses. Diagnostic testing has the ability to detect all autosomal trisomies and reliably detect sex chromosome aneuploidies, large deletions and duplications of chromosomes, and mosaicism.
- Women 35 years and older are typically considered to be at highest risk of having a child with Down syndrome. Screening methods for these women include chorionic villus sampling (CVS) in first trimester or genetic counseling and amniocentesis in second trimester.[8]
- The decision to offer screening or invasive testing should not be based on age alone but should take into account patient preferences.
- There has been a growing body of evidence regarding the high negative predictive value of noninvasive prenatal testing (NIPT) using cell-free DNA (cfDNA) and its potential to reduce iatrogenic fetal loss. Several countries have already started to recommend the use of NIPT using cfDNA for contingent screening in women who are at a higher risk of a fetus with trisomy 21, including women of advanced maternal age but cost is the limiting factor.[9]

First Trimester CVS Versus Second Trimester Amniocentesis[10]

- Counselors should discuss the risk for miscarriage attributable to both procedures: the risk from amniocentesis at 15–18 weeks' gestation is approximately 0.25–0.50% (1/400–1/200), and the miscarriage risk from CVS is approximately 0.5–1.0% (1/200–1/100).
- Current data indicate that the overall risk for transverse limb deficiency from CVS is 0.03–0.10% (1/3,000–1/1,000) and no increase in risk for limb deficiency after amniocentesis at 15–18 weeks' gestation.
- The risk and severity of limb deficiency appear to be associated with the timing of CVS: the risk at <10 weeks' gestation (0.20%) is higher than the risk from CVS done at greater than or equal to 10 weeks' gestation (0.07%). Most defects associated with CVS at greater than or equal to 10 weeks' gestation have been limited to the digits.
- Timing of procedures
  - The timing of obtaining results from either CVS or amniocentesis is relevant because of the increased risks for maternal morbidity and mortality associated with terminating pregnancy during the second trimester compared with the first trimester.
  - Second trimester ultrasound markers have low sensitivity and specificity for detecting Down syndrome, especially in a low-risk population.
  - The highest detection rate is acquired with ultrasound markers combined with gross anomalies. Although the detection rate with combination of markers is high in a high-risk population (50–75%), false-positive rates are also high (22% for a 100% Down syndrome detection rate). Relying only on ultrasonography to identify Down syndrome is not recommended.

Q4. What are the risks likely to be encountered in these women?

- Preexisting maternal medical conditions including—
  - Hypertension,
  - Obesity and
  - Diabetes increase with advancing maternal
- Pregnancy-related maternal complications such as
  - Preeclampsia
  - Gestational diabetes.

These medical comorbidities can all influence fetal health and are likely to compound the effect of age on the risk of pregnancy in an older mother. However, after controlling for these comorbidities, advanced maternal age is still found to be independently associated with an increase in antenatal and intrapartum stillbirth. It is also associated with an increase in neonatal mortality.

Compared to younger women, the types of complications that women over 35 years are at increased risk of during pregnancy include:

During pregnancy
- Spontaneous abortions (9% at age 22 years, 20% at age 35 years, 40% at age 40 years)[11]
- Gestational diabetes (2.85% at age 35–40 years, 4.56% at age >40 year)[12]
- Hypertension with pregnancy
- Multiple pregnancy (due to greater use of ART)
- Placenta Praevia (0.26% at age 18–36 years, 0.56% at age 35–40 years, 0.97% at age >40 year)[11]
- Abruptio Placentae.
- Higher incidence of fibroid with pregnancy.

During Labor
- Malpresentations
- Uterine inertia and prolonged labor
- Rigid perineum so instrumental deliveries
- Post-term pregnancy
- Induction of labor
- Increased cesarean section rate.

Aging impairs myometrial function, with several large population studies reporting increased rates of cesarean section for dystocia and instrumental delivery in older mothers who have gone through both spontaneous and induced labor.

Fetal Complications
- Intrauterine growth restriction (IUGR)
- Preterm labor (6% at age 18–34 years, 6.63% at age 35–40 years, 8.17% at age >40 years).

Fetal anomalies (2.5%)
- IUD (3.75% below 35 years, 6.41% between 35–39 years, 8.65 at 40 years and older).[8]

There is no evidence to support routine assessment of fetal growth or umbilical artery and uterine artery Doppler in older mothers to identify those who definitively have FGR.

Q5. When should delivery be planned in these women?

What do the guidelines say?

RCOG does not make specific recommendations, but they do state that "Women ≥40 years of age having a similar stillbirth risk at 39 weeks of gestation to women in their mid-20s at 41 weeks of gestation, at which stage the consensus is that induction of labor should be offered to prevent late stillbirth."[7]

The current Up-To-Date recommendation for women aged 40 and older is to give birth at 39 weeks.

REFERENCES

1. United Nations Pouplation Fund. UNPFA annual report 2007. Available at http://www.unfpa.org/publications/unpfa-annual-report-2007. Accessed on May 30, 2015.
2. Strategy Handbook. Rashtriya Kishor Swasthya Karyakram. Adolescent Health Division Ministry of Health and Family Welfare Government of India. January 2014 [Internet]. [cited 2014 September 8]. Available from: https://www.dropbox.com/s/0oj4p422y7st4ku/RKSK%20Strategy%20Handbook.pdf.
3. Barnet B, Liu J, Devoe M. Double jeopardy: depressive symptoms and rapid subsequent pregnancy in adolescent mothers. Arch Pediatr Adolesc Med. 2008;162:246-52.
4. Chen XK, Wen SW, Fleming N, et al. Teenage pregnancy and adverse birth outcomes: a large population-based retrospective cohort study. Int J Epidemiol. 2007;36:368-73.
5. Shrim A, Ates S, Mallozzi A, et al. Is young maternal age really a risk factor for adverse pregnancy outcome in a Canadian tertiary referral hospital? J Pediatr Adolesc Gynecol. 2011;24:218-22.
6. Fleming N, O'Driscoll T, Becker G, et al. Adolescent pregnancy guidelines. J Obstet Gynaecol Can. 2015;37(8):740-56.
7. Induction of Labour at Term in Older Mothers. RCOG. Scientific Impact Paper No. 34, February 2013.
8. ACOG Releases Guidelines on Screening for Fetal Chromosomal Abnormalities. Am Fam Physician. 2007;76(5):712-6.
9. Soothill PW. Non-invasive Prenatal Testing for Chromosomal Abnormalities using Maternal Plasma DNA. Scientific Impact Paper No 15, March 2014.
10. Chorionic Villus Sampling and Amniocentesis: Recommendations for Prenatal Counseling. CDC 2005.
11. Andersen AM, Wohlfahrt J. Maternal age and fetal loss: population based register linkage study. BMJ. 2000; 320(7251): 1708-12
12. Jolly M, Sebire N, Harris J, Robinson S, Regan L. "The risks associated with pregnancy in women aged 35 years or older." Hum Reprod. 2000;15(11):2433-7.

15
CHAPTER

Postdated Pregnancy

Neelam Yadav, Preeti Singh

The World Health Organization has defined post-term pregnancy as pregnancy that has extended to or beyond 42 weeks (294 days) of gestation.[1] According to American terminology, pregnancy that has extended beyond the due dates is called postdated pregnancy. Prolonged gestation occur in 5–10% of pregnancies.[2] Pregnancies extending beyond expected date of delivery, i.e. 40 weeks holds a great concern for both patient and obstetrician. The incidence of post-term pregnancies may vary by population, due to differences in regional management practices for pregnancies that go beyond the estimated date of delivery. The reason why this subject holds a great importance in obstetrics as prolonged pregnancy leads to increased perinatal morbidity and mortality. The risk of perinatal death is 1:7000 at 36 weeks compared 1:350 at 42 weeks.[3] Boyed et al. found the incidence of post-term pregnancy is 7.5% when diagnosis is based upon menstrual history, 2.6% when based on early ultrasound, 1.1% when diagnosis based on concurrent menstrual history and ultrasound examination.[4]

CASE SCENARIO

A 22 years old primigravida came to gyne casualty as she has completed 40 weeks today (she has been told that her expected date of delivery is today), she has no complain. How will you approach the case?

A 22 year old primigravida came to gyne casualty as she has approached the EDD (Expected date of delivery), she is very anxious what will happen next as she has reached her due date.

History

We should enquire whether she has any complain like labor pain, leaking per vaginum, bleeding per vaginum or decreased fetal movement.

History of Present Pregnancy

Detailed trimester-wise history should be taken to come across any risk factor which will effect the continuation of pregnancy to both mother and fetus like history of chronic hypertension, gestational hypertension, preeclampsia, gestational diabetes mellitus, overt diabetes, isoimmunized pregnancy, any e/o fetal growth restriction or macrosomia.

Menstrual History

Date of first day of last menstrual period (LMP) should be asked, whether the lady is sure about the date, whether previous menstrual cycles are regular, no history of preceding contraceptive intake if all these criteria are met then gestational age which is calculated by LMP is taken as reliable. EDD is calculated by adding 9 months and 7 days to the date of LMP.

Obstetric History

Primi MF X 2 years, whether pregnancy was spontaneous or conceived after treatment.

Past History

Any history of chronic medical and surgical illness like history of hypertension, diabetes, tuberculosis, seizure disorder, heart disease.

Family History

Any history of medical and surgical disorder, any history of postdated pregnancy in mother side.

Dietary History

Taken by 24 hours recall method, since obesity is a risk factor for postdatism the diet should be reviewed for extra fat and carbohydrate.

Socioeconomic History

Social class will be assigned according to modified Kuppuswamy classification, as it was seen that postdated pregnancy is more common in higher socioeconomic class with sedentary lifestyle.

Examination

- General physical examination to be done as per the routine protocol
- *Palpation:* Any e/o organomegaly like hepatosplenomegaly, height of uterus, measurement of symphysio-fundal height, abdominal girth to decide whether you are dealing with term pregnancy, preterm pregnancy, intrauterine growth restriction (IUGR), macrosomia
- *Obstetric grip:* Fundal grip, lateral or umbilical grip, Pawlick grip—presenting part is being felt if it is head one should look whether head has term or preterm baby feel—preterm fetus has soft skull bones with wide fontanelle compared to term fetus. Deep pelvic grip-To see whether presenting part is freely mobile or engaged as it is seen that in term pregnancy the presenting part has generally crossed the pelvic inlet, amount of liquor should also be commented upon—as the gestation advances amount of liquor decreases. Estimated fetal weight should be documented as there are chances of macrosomia in posterm pregnancy
- *Pelvic examination:* Assign a bishop score. In preterm fetus—Bishops score is generally unfavorable, head has generally soft feel and station is high up. In term fetus and post-term pregnancy—bishop score generally improves, head is engaged and has hard skull bones.

Q1. How to establish accurate dating?

Accurate assessment of gestational age is the first and foremost part of the management of postdated pregnancy. It is done by the following methods:

- *Clinical dating:* By LMP, if previous menstrual cycle are regular, normal in duration and amount of flow, no history of oral contraceptive intake for preceding 3 cycles, expected date of delivery is calculated by adding 9 months and 7 days to the first day of last menstrual period. Around 30% of patient do not fulfill this criteria and thus making the dating by LMP unreliable. It is a matter of surprise that only 1% women deliver on the day of EDD.[2] In case of prolonged or short cycles, if the interval of cycles is longer, the extra days are to be added and if the interval is shorter, the lesser days are to be subtracted to get the exact EDD; for example, a women having LMP 01/01/2017 with cycles of 21 days EDD will be calculated by subtracting 7 days from calculated EDD, i.e. 01/10/17.
- *Dating by ultrasound:* First trimester ultrasound should be offered to women ideally between 11 and 14 weeks, as it is more accurate in estimating gestational age than LMP. If there is difference of greater than 5 days in estimating the gestational age using LMP and first trimester USG then gestational age is to be determined by first trimester USG (Level I-A). If there is a difference of greater than 10 days between gestational age calculated using the last menstrual period and second trimester ultrasound, the estimated date of delivery should be determined by the second trimester ultrasound (Level I-A). When there has been both a first and second trimester ultrasound are available, gestational age should be determined by the earliest ultrasound done preferably between 11 and 14 weeks (Level I-A)
- *Urine pregnancy test:* Done after first missed period adding 36 weeks to the date when urine pregnancy test was first came out positive will give EDD
- *Date of quickening:* Adding 22 weeks in primigravida and 24 weeks in multipara to the date of quickening gives the rough estimate of EDD
- *Dates on which fetal heart tones first audible:* By Doppler ultrasound device 10 weeks, adding 30 weeks to this date and by obstetrical stethoscope—20 weeks adding 20 weeks to this date
- Antenatal record of bimanual examination in first trimester and fundal height palpation in second trimester corroborate with dates.

Q2. How will you assign the dates as excellent, good, poor dates?

- *Excellent dates:* Patient with adequate clinical information plus ultrasound of first trimester between 11 and 14 weeks corresponding with gestational age with LMP. Patient with inadequate or incomplete clinical information but with two ultrasound exams between 16 and 24 weeks showing linear fetal growth and similar EDD.
- *Good dates:* Patient with adequate clinical information and one confirming ultrasound examination obtained after 24 weeks of gestation. Patient with inadequate clinical information with two or more ultrasound exams showing adequate growth and similar EDD.
- *Poor dates:* Any clinical situation different from those listed above.

Q3. What are risk factors associated with postmaturity?

- Error in calculation of gestational age (most common cause of postmaturity is miscalculation of EDD)
- Nulliparity is a significant risk factor for postmaturity.[5]
- Obesity-BMI >25 is significantly associated with prolonged pregnancy[5]
- Abnormalities in biochemical and physiological mechanism responsible for initiation of labor—congenital anomaly in baby like anencephaly, adrenal hypoplasia, X-linked placental sulfatase deficiency (disruption of fetal pitutary adrenal axis, maternal placental sulphatase deficiency)
- History of post-term pregnancy in previous pregnancy (recurrence rate of 19.1%)[6]
- Genetic predisposition.[7]

Q4. What investigation will you do in the above case scenario?

Investigations

Confirmation of fetal maturity—Ultrasonography—best is first trimester ultrasound which can predict the maturity by just an error of ±5 days and a second trimester ultrasound which can detect the gestation by just an error of ±10 days.

Assesment of Fetal Well-being

- Done by twice weekly biophysical profile and nonstress test (NST)
- Recent recommendation is to do NST and amniotic fluid volume labeled as modified biophysical profile—to be done twice weekly.

Q5. What counseling should be done in the above case?

Women should be counseled regarding both expectant management and induction of labor explaining the advantages and disadvantages of both the methods. If she opts for expectant management fetal surveillance twice a week with modified biophysical profile (NST+ AFI) should be done. Membrane sweeping and stretching should be done if women is willing for expectant management. Women should be counseled that the rate of vaginal delivery is more when labor was spontaneous in onset as compared to increased chances of cesarean sections in cases when labor was induced. It was seen that 7–14% of women went into spontaneous labor between 40 and 41 weeks of gestation.[8]

Q6. How will you do antepartum fetal surveillance if one opt for expectant management?

- *Fetal kick count:* After having her meal women is asked to lie in left lateral position and to observe carefully the fetal movement for at least 1 hour this is multiplied by 4 to get exact fetal movements over 12 hours
- *Nonstress test:* Biophysical profile—Nonstress test, fetal gross body movement, fetal muscles tone, fetal breathing movement, amniotic fluid. Each parameter is given a max score of 2 and min of 0. BPP score of 8–10 indicates no fetal hypoxia, 4–6 is suspicious of asphyxia, score of 0–2 strongly suspect asphyxia
- *Modified biophysical profile (NST+AFI):* Twice a week is simple than complete biophysical profile and thus currently most commonly used for fetal surveillance (Level I-A).

Delivery is recommended if there is fetal compromise or oligohydramnios.

Q7. What is the opinion of evidence-based medicine regarding fetal surveillance?

The American College of Obstetrician and Gynecologists have a Level C recommendation for initiation of fetal surveillance between 41 and 42 weeks because of evidence that perinatal morbidity and mortality increase as gestational age advances and that a twice weekly assessment of amniotic fluid and an NST (Modified biophysical profile) should be adequate.[9] The Royal College of Obstetricians and Gynecologists recommends increased antenatal surveillance consisting of a twice weekly NST and an ultrasound estimation of maximum amniotic pool depth from 42 weeks in women who decline labor induction.[10] The Society of Obstetricians and Gynaecologists of Canada (SOGC) includes antenatal fetal surveillance between 41 and 42 weeks by NST and AFI (Level I-A).

Q8. Is there any role membrane sweeping beyond 38 weeks of gestation and nipple stimulation?

Sweeping (or stripping) of fetal membrane off the lower uterine segment during vaginal examination by inserting finger in cervical os between fetal membranes and lower uterine segment and rotating it through 360°. Sweeping results in the release of endogenous prostaglandin thereby resulting in cervical softening and augmenting uterine contraction by releasing oxytocin.[11] Cochrane review has shown that routine sweeping beyond 38 weeks onward reduces the number of pregnancy going beyond 41 weeks. The adverse effect includes maternal discomfort, vaginal bleeding and irregular uterine contractions. Therefore, women should be offered the option of membrane sweeping between 38 and 41 weeks following a discussion of risk and benefit of the procedure (Level I-A). There is not enough evidence to evaluate the role of breast and nipple stimulation in the prevention of post-term pregnancies.

CASE SCENARIO

A 24 years old G2P1L1 with 41+1 week of gestation came for routine antenatal checkup, she has no labor pain how will you proceed further?

History

Patient should be asked for any specific complain like labor pains, leaking per vaginum or bleeding per vaginum, decreased fetal movement, any comorbidity necessitating early pregnancy termination.

Detailed Menstrual History

LMP first day of last menstrual period, previous menstrual cycle regular at least previous 3, no h/o preceding oral contraceptive intake for last few weeks, EDD is calculated by adding 9 calendar months and 7 days to LMP. This detailed menstrual history gives us idea of reliability of gestational age calculated by LMP.

Obstetric History

G2P1L1, she has 3 years old male child delivered vaginally, labor was induced in view of postdatism has no intrapartum complications, baby is well immunized, presently alive and healthy. The history is significant as we have seen that post-term pregnancy has recurrence rate of 19.1%.

Trimester History

Any important relevant history in any trimester of pregnancy which will influence pregnancy outcome in current and future pregnancy.

Examination

General physical examination, systemic examination, P/A-feel of head whether it is term or preterm, head is free floating or fixed in pelvis, P/V examination to asses bishops score—generally becomes favorable as gestation advances, very unfavorable bishops score may be one of the indicator that we are dealing with preterm pregnancy although exceptions are there.

Investigation

First Trimester

USG—one of the important tool in calculating the period of gestation

Second Trimester

USG—detailed anomaly description, if the patient is not sure of date then it can be used for calculating period of gestation.

Q1. What are the maternal risk associated with postdatism?
- *Dystocia:* Prolonged labor, shoulder dystocia
- Increased risk of pelvic trauma, instrumental delivery and cesarean section
- Increased risk of postpartum hemorrhage and endometritis.

Q2. What are the fetal risk associated with postdatism?

Stillbirth

Rate of stillbirth increased from 0.35/1000 ongoing at 37 week to 2.12/1000 women still pregnant at 43 weeks.[12] The recent database has demonstrated increasing risk of stillbirth with advancing gestational age.

Two-fold Increased Risk of Macrosomia

Perinatal complications: Post-term pregnancies were associated with increased risk of neonatal convulsion, meconium aspiration syndrome and 5 min APGAR score of less than 4, 3 meconium aspiration, asphyxia before, during and after delivery, cord complications, fractures, peripheral nerve injury, pneumonia, septicemia, etc

Q3. What is management protocol of prolonged pregnancy?

See Flowchart 1.

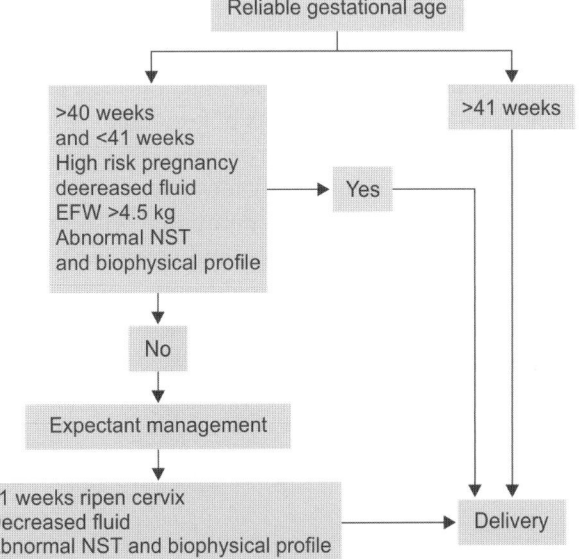

Flowchart 1: Algorithm shows management of prolonged pregnancy

Q4. What is the evidence-based management of post-dated pregnancy?

Induction versus expectant management—perinatal and neonatal mortality increases in pregnancy continued beyond 41 weeks. Therefore, women who have reached or exceed beyond 41 weeks should be delivered.

A review of the literature on post-term pregnancy published by Hannah et al. included meta-analysis of 11 randomized or quasi randomized trials in which a policy of routine induction at 41 weeks was compared with expectant management with serial fetal surveillance. A total of 5057 women were included in these trials. Results showed that inducing labor at 41 weeks resulted in a significantly lower cesarean section rate (OR 0.85; 95% CI 0.74–0.97), lower rate of fetal distress (OR 0.81; 95% CI 0.68–0.97), lower rate of meconium staining of amniotic fluid (OR 0.79; 95% CI 0.69–0.90), lower rate of macrosomia (usually defined as birth weight >4000 g) (OR 0.80; 95% CI 0.69–0.92) and lower rate of fetal or neonatal death (excluding lethal congenital anomalies)than expectant management (OR 0.23; 95% CI 0.06–0.90). The reduction in perinatal death was largely due to a reduction in fetal death (OR 0.14; 95% CI 0.02–0.98).

The authors conclude that the induction of labor groups are less likely to undergo delivery by cesarean, to have an operative vaginal delivery, or to have fetal distress, macrosomic babies, or babies who die during the perinatal period. She states that women who reach 41 weeks should be appropriately counseled about the higher risks to themselves and to their babies if they pursue expectant management, and she suggests that a policy of labor induction is to be preferred.

Each obstetrical department should establish the guidelines for labor induction based upon local resources. A recent Cochrane registry report suggests that induction of labor at 41 completed weeks of gestation is associated with fewer perinatal deaths, risk ratio (RR) of 0.31 (95% CI: 0.12–0.88) and significantly fewer cesarean deliveries (RR 0.89; 95% CI: 0.81–0.97) compared with expectant management.[13] Other benefits of induction include fewer cases of meconium aspiration syndrome.

- ACOG concludes that "Induction of labor between 41 0/7 and 42 0/7 weeks can be considered" and "Induction of labor after 42 0/7 weeks and by 42 6/7 weeks of gestation is recommended, given evidence of an increase in perinatal morbidity and mortality."
- SOGC says that induction of labor is offered between 41 and 42 weeks as the current evidence states decrease in perinatal mortality without increase in cesarean sections rates (Level I-A).

REFERENCES

1. International Statistical Classification of Diseases and Related Health Problems, 10th revision. Geneva (CH): World Health Organization, 2006
2. Martin JA, Hamilton be, Sutton Pd et al. Births: final data for 2005. Natl Vital Stat Rep. 2007; 56:1-103.
3. Hilder L, Costeloe K, Thilaganathan B. Prolonged pregnancy: evaluating gestation-specific risks of fetal and infant mortality. Br J Obstet Gynecol. 1998;105:169-73.
4. Boyd ME, Usher RH, Mclean FH, et al. Obstetric consequences of postmaturity. Am J Obstet Gynecol 1988;158:334.
5. Halloran DR, Cheng YW, Wall TC, et al. Effect of maternal obesity on postterm delivery. J Perinatol. 2012;32:85-90.
6. Kistka ZA, Palour L, Bosalaugh SE, et al. Risk of postterm delivery after previous postterm delivery. Am J Obstet Gynecol. 2007;196,241e1-241e6.
7. Laursen M, Bille C, Olesen AW, Hjelmborg J, Skythe A, Christensen K.Genetic influence on prolonged gestation: A population based Danish twin study. Am J Obstet Gynecol. 2004;190;489-94.
8. Suikkari Am, Jalkanen M, Heiskala H, Koskela O. Prolonged pregnancy: induction or observation. Acta Obstet Gynecol Scand Suppl 1983;116:58.
9. American College of Obstetricians and Gynecologists. Practice Bulletin. Management of postterm pregnancy. No. 55, 2004.
10. Royal College of Obstetricians and Gynecologists. Induction of labour. Evidence based clinical Guideline No. 9, June 2001. London: RCOG.
11. Mitchell MD, Flint APF, Bibby J, Brunt J, Anderson ABM, Turnbull AC. Rapid increase in plasma prostaglandin concentrations after vaginal examination and amniotomy. Br Med J. 1977;2:1183-5.
12. Feldman GB. Prospective risk of stillbirth. Obstet Gynecol. 1992;79:547-53.
13. Gülmezoglu AM, Crowther CA, Middleton P, Heatley E. Induction of labour for improving birth outcomes for women at or beyond term. Cochrane Database Syst Rev. 2012 Jun 13;6:CD004945. doi: 10.1002/14651858.CD004945.pub3.

Antepartum Hemorrhage

Gauri Gandhi, Snigdha Pathak, Divya Singh

Definition of antepartum hemorrhage (APH): It is the bleeding from or into the genital tract from 24 weeks of pregnancy till birth of the baby.[1]

Incidence: 3–5% of all pregnancies[2]

The bleeding may be from the placental site or extraplacental in origin.

The main causes of placental site bleeding are:
1. From abnormally situated low lying placenta (placenta previa).
2. Due to separation of a normally situated placenta (abruption placentae or accidental hemorrhage).

Together these two conditions are responsible for more than half of APH cases.

CASE SCENARIO

A 28 years old G3P2 at 34 weeks gestation with complaint of painless bleeding per vaginum for 2 hours.

On examination, patient is conscious, oriented, vitals— pulse rate-94/minute BP—124/80 mm Hg.

Per abdomen-uterus around 32–34 weeks, relaxed, lower segment cesarean section (LSCS) scar present, no scar tenderness uterine contour maintained, fetal heart present regular.

Q1. What are the causes of APH and their incidence?

Causes

- Placenta previa—31%
- Abruptio placentae—22%
- Unclassified—47%
  - Uterine rupture
  - Marginal—60%
  - Show—20%
  - Cervicitis—8%
  - Trauma—5%
  - Vulvovaginal varicosity—2%
  - Genital tumor—0.5%
  - Genital infection—0.5%
  - Hematuria—0.5%
  - Vasa previa—0.5%
  - Others—0.5%.

Q2. What do you understand by indeterminate APH?

It is not uncommon to fail to identify a cause for APH when it is described as 'indeterminate APH'.

Q3. What important points should be elicited in history?

History of Current Episode of Bleeding

Bleeding Per Vaginum

- Amount of bleeding—soaked how many garments/pads, passage of clots
- Painless or associated with pain abdomen
- Color of blood—bright red or dark altered
- Whether first incident or recurrent
- Whether the bleeding stopped on its own or still continuing
- Any inciting factor—history of intercourse, trauma, fall.

Pain Abdomen

- Is bleeding associated with pain?
- Character of pain—intermittent, colicky or constant, continuous
- Any reduction in pain
- Association of pain with membranes rupture—blood stained liqor is suggestive of revealed abruption.

In placenta previa: Bleeding is usually unprovoked, painless, causeless and recurrent. It is bright red in color and may have been initiated by coitus sometimes. Usually, the initial episode is small and stops completely on its own. It is a warning hemorrhage which should not be ignored.

In abruption: Bleeding is usually associated with pain abdomen. It may be concealed or revealed and color of blood is dark and altered by the time it trickles down.

In concealed abruption, the pain may be severe and continuous due to uterine stretching by uteroplacental blood accumulation.

In uterine rupture: Bleeding is fresh, red and associated with severe pain which dramatically subsides once rupture occurs.

In show: intermittent, colicky pain (labor) is associated with blood mixed mucus.

Sometimes, confusion in diagnosis can be due to onset of labor pains following bleeding in placenta previa. Also, 10% of women with placenta previa can have coexisting abuption thus presenting with abdominal pain.

Fetal Movements

Any history of loss of fetal movements associated with episode of hemorrhage.

In placenta previa: When bleeding is small in amount, the fetal condition usually is not compromised. In severe bleeding or shock due to excessive bleeding, fetal condition can be compromised.

In abruption: Fetal condition depends on extent of placental separation. If moderate to severe, there will be fetal distress or even fetal demise.

In uterine rupture: Fetus may be in distress or may already be dead.

Symptoms of Preeclampsia/Impending Eclampsia
- Any history of raised BP records in this pregnancy
- Any complaint of headache, blurring of vision, right upper abdomen pain, leg edema, facial puffiness or sudden weight gain, tightening of rings, etc.
- Any history of convulsions, symptoms of preeclampsia can be found in 15–30% women with abruption.

History of Overdistended Uterus
(Hydramnios, Multiple Pregnancy), followed by rupture of membranes

Abruption can be caused by sudden decompression of overdistended uterus.

History of Sudden Membrane Rupture
- PPROM (preterm premature rupture of membranes) can cause placental abruption. (usually if associated with an overdistended uterus)
- If APH is associated with spontaneous or iatrogenic rupture of fetal membranes, bleeding from ruptured vasa previa should be considered.

History of Uterine Manipulation (Rare Causes)
- External cephalic version can cause abruption or even uterine rupture in some cases of scarred uterus leading to APH.
- Or any history of sudden trauma or physical abuse.

Obstetric History

Multiparity: It is a risk factor for both placenta previa and placental abruption.

History of Previous Abortions (Spontaneous or Induced)
The greater the number of surgical abortions, greater is the risk of placenta previa and morbidly adherent placenta.

History of Previous Cesarean Section
- With increase in number of prior cesareans, there is increased risk of placenta previa:[1]
  No previous cesarean—0.26%
  Previous 1 cesarean—0.65%
  Previous 2 cesareans—1.5%
  Previous 3 cesareans—2.2%
  Previous 4 cesareans—10%
- Chances of morbidly adherent placenta (accreta) are higher in patients with placenta previa and a scarred uterus.
- Risk of uterine rupture is also greater in patient with previous cesareans.

History of APH in Earlier Pregnancy
- In case of placenta previa in previous pregnancy, there is 12 times increased risk of recurrence
- In case of placental abruption in previous pregnancy, recurrence risk is 6–16% after 1 such pregnancy and 25% after 2 such pregnancies.

Past History/Medical History
- History of hypertension, diabetes mellitus, heart disease
- History of bleeding diathesis or thrombophilias.

Family History
- History of hypertension, diabetes
- History of any bleeding diathesis or thrombophilias.

Personal History

Smoking and drug abuse (cocaine) are etiological factors for placental abruption.

Q4. What important points should be elicited in examination?

General Physical Examination
- General condition of patient—good or poor
- Whether patient is conscious, oriented or confused or in shock
- Check the pulse, blood pressure, respiratory rate and temperature.
  - Presence of pallor, tachycardia, hypotension are directly proportional to amount of blood loss
  - Concealed abruption may present with shock which is out of proportion to visible blood loss
  - Edema and hypertension can be associated with abruption wherein hypertension may mask the true hypovolemia
- Rough estimation of amount of blood loss (to assess need for blood transfusion)
- Assess for pallor, icterus, cyanosis, peripheral edema.

Systemic Examination
Respiratory and cardiovascular systems are duly examined to rule out underlying disease.

Abdominal Examination

Fundal Height

- If corresponds to period of gestation—placenta previa likely
- If more than period of gestation—abruption likely (retroplacental blood accumulation).

Uterine Contour, Consistency and Presence of Tenderness

- In placenta previa—uterine contour is maintained, uterus is relaxed and fetal parts are easily palpable
- In abruption—uterine contour is maintained, but uterus is tense, tender, rigid and fetal parts are felt with difficulty
- In uterine rupture—uterine contour may be distorted, fetal parts may be felt easily and abdomen will be tense, tender with presence of free fluid.

Presentation

Malpresentations and free floating head—common in placenta previa.

Multiple pregnancy

Number of fetuses with their lie and presentation to be noted as multiple pregnancy is a risk factor for both placenta previa and abruption.

Fetal heart sounds

- In placenta previa—usually present (unless severe shock)
- In abruption—depending on the severity, there may be fetal distress or fetal demise
- In uterine rupture—absent or there may be severe fetal distress or fetal demise.

Local Examination
Note for color of bleeding, amount of bleeding, presence of any signs of active bleeding or associated trauma, etc.

Speculum Examination
Useful to identify cervical dilatation or to identify a local cause for APH—cervical ectropion, cervicitis, cervical polyp, cervical malignancy, trauma, etc.

Vaginal Examination
Not to be done in Placenta Previa

If placenta previa is a possible diagnosis (Example—low lying placenta on previous scan, high presenting part on per-abdominal examination, or painless causeless bleeding), PV should be avoided till a scan has ruled out placenta previa.

Q5. How do you assess the severity of blood loss in a case of antepartum hemorrhage?

- It is difficult to assess the severity of blood loss as the blood pressure and pulse remain normal despite significant blood loss in a pregnant patient because of hypervolemia
- It is important to know the clinical condition before the onset of bleeding
- For purpose of uniformity, severity of bleeding can be classified into four groups.[3]

Loss of blood volume	Systolic BP	Signs and symptoms	Obsteric shock index	Degree of shock and urgency
500–1000 mL 10–15%	Normal SBP	Palpitation, mild tachy and dizziness	<1	Compensated Grade 4
1000–1500 mL 15–30%	Slight fall in SBP, increase diastolic	Weakness, marked tachy and sweating	>1	Mild Grade 3
1500–2000 mL 30–40%	Moderate fall (70–80 mm Hg)	Restlessness, marked tachy, pallor and oliguria	>1.5	Moderate grade 2
>2000 mL >40%	Marked fall (50–70 mm Hg)	Collapse, air hunger and anuria	>2	Severe grade 1

Q6. What are the important investigations in a case of APH?

Investigations to be done after initial resuscitation and stabilization of the patient.

Blood Tests

- ~20 mL blood sample taken for:
  - Blood grouping and cross-matching. Blood to be arranged as per estimated losses. (In cases of major/massive hemorrhage, 4 units of blood should be cross-matched. Also, the initial hemoglobin may not reflect the amount of blood lost, therefore clinical judgment should be used when calculating the amount to be transfused)
  - Hemogram with hematocrit and platelet counts
  - Bleeding time, clotting time
  - Coagulation profile (with abruption in mind)—Prothrombin time, activated partial thromboplastin time. (A coagulation screen is not indicated till the platelet count is abnormal).[1]
  - Investigations to rule out disseminated intravascular coagulation (DIC), if suspected—Serum fibrinogen, fibrinogen degradation products (FDPs), D-dimer.
  - Blood urea, serum creatinine, serum electrolytes; Liver function tests
- Urinalysis—for presence of proteins, sugar
- KB Test (Kleihauer Betke) in Rh negative women to quantify fetomaternal hemorrhage to gauge the dose of anti-D Immunoglobulin required.
- *Ultrasonography:* Most essential for placental localization.
  - Can be transabdominal (TAS) or transvaginal scan (TVS). TVS is safe and also superior to TAS
  - Can be used to diagnose placenta previa, but does not exclude abruption as USG has only limited sensitivity in identifying retroplacental clots (RPC).

Q7. What are the complications associated with antepartum hemorrhage?

Maternal Complications

- Hemorrhage (antepartum, intrapartum or postpartum) resulting in hypovolemic shock
- Disseminated intravascular coagulation as a result of massive hemorrhage
- Complications of blood transfusion
- Anemia
- Infection
- Renal tubular necrosis
- Anesthetic and surgical risks especially during emergency cesarean section
- Prolonged hospital stay
- Recurrence of placenta previa in future pregnancies.

Fetal Complications

- Fetal hypoxia
- Small for gestation age
- Fetal restriction
- Prematurity (iatrogenic or spontaneous)
- Fetal demise
- Common association of placenta previa with congenital malformations (usually of CNS, CVS, gastrointestinal and respiratory systems)
- Vasa previa rupture can result in fetal anemia.

Placenta Previa

Q8. What are the risk factors for placenta previa?

Risk factors are:[1]

- Previous placenta previa
- Prior cesarean section
- Prior dilatation and curettage
- Increased maternal age (>40 years)
- Multiparity
- Multiple gestation
- Deficient endometrium due to the presence/history of:
  - Uterine scar
  - Endometritis
  - Manual removal of placenta
  - Submucus fibroid.

Q9. What other things can one look for in ultrasound after localizing placenta?

- Retroplacental clots to be excluded
- Signs of placental separation (in case of associated abruption)
  Note: Negative findings on USG do not exclude placental abruption as diagnosis of abruption is primarily clinical
- Morbid adherence of placenta can be suspected on USG and further confirmed with the help of color Doppler and MRI
- Other findings to note are—cardiac activity, presentation, estimated fetal weight and gestational age, amount of liqor and to rule out congenital anomalies.

Q10. Is it possible to prevent APH in placenta previa?

It is considered good practice to avoid PV and PR examinations in known placenta previa cases. Also, these women should be advised to avoid sexual intercourse.

RCOG guidelines[4] indicate no role of cervical circlage or prophylactic tocolytics to prevent APH in women with placenta previa.

In acute episodes of APH, bed rest and bed pan facility should be made available to the patient.

After hemorrhage has settled, strict bed rest is also not mandatory and limited activity is permissible.

Q11. Do patients of placenta previa with APH always require hospitalization?

All women with placenta previa should remain in hospital till bleeding has stopped.

Where the bleeding has been spotting and has settled, and tests of maternal and fetal well-being are reassuring, the woman can go home after the counseling regarding symptoms and signs of emergency (labor pains, bleeding p/v, and decreased fetal movements) and to report stat.

Q12. Should steroid cover be given to women who present with APH before term?

A single course of corticosteroids should be given to women between 24^{+6} and 34^{+6} weeks of gestation[5] who are at risk of preterm birth (iatrogenic or spontaneous). Antenatal corticosteroids are associated with a significant reduction in the rate of neonatal death, respiratory distress syndrome and intraventricular hemorrhage.

Q13. How should patient of APH be managed when USG facility is unavailable?

If USG facility is unavailable or USG findings are inconclusive for placenta previa, the patient can be taken for examination in operation theater called as.

Double Setup Examination

- It is a PV examination in the OT to assess the relationship of lower placental edge with the cervical os
- Done only when delivery is planned
- Full preparation for immediate cesarean to be done along with second obstetrician who is scrubbed and ready to operate, should the need arise
- Anesthestist and pediatrician should be present
- Cross-matched blood should be available
- The patient is put in lithotomy position, cleaned, draped and bladder emptied
- A per-speculum examination is done to rule out local cause for bleeding
  Note: if cervix dilated with visible placenta → immediate LSCS.
- Gentle PV done with two fingers:
  – Each fornix is palpated to feel for presence of placenta ahead of the presenting part. There is a feeling of bogginess if placenta is present
  – If fornices are empty, the index finger is gently introduced into the os and surrounding felt for placental edge
  – If placental edge felt or os is closed or brisk vaginal bleeding occurs during the procedure → immediate LSCS
  – If no placental edge is felt and no bleeding is provoked, membranes should be ruptured in preparation for vaginal delivery. But, if there is bright red persistent bleeding after membrane rupture → go for immediate LSCS.

Q14. What are the contraindications for a double setup examination?

- Sonographic evidence of major degree placenta previa
- Fetal distress
- Profuse hemorrhage where immediate delivery is required
- Any contraindication to vaginal delivery.

Q15. What should be the management of placenta previa with reference to this case?

Women with placenta previa should be managed at centers with facilities for blood transfusion, intensive care and performing emergency operative delivery.

Management can be expectant or active depending upon:
- Severity of blood loss and whether it is ongoing
- Condition of mother
- Condition of fetus and gestational age
- Onset of labor.

Expectant Management

Aim of management in placenta previa is to allow the pregnancy to progress as close to term as is possible to allow for fetal lung maturity and then to terminate by elective cesarean section.

Only hemodynamically stable patients who are remote from term should be managed expectantly.

Note: In case of low lying placenta (more than 2 cm from os), vaginal delivery can be allowed after ruling out other obstetrical contraindications.

Q16. What protocol is to be followed during expectant management?

Initial treatment includes the following:
- Admit patient in labor room, give sedation, keep NPO and give IV fluid as necessary

- Take blood sample for blood grouping, cross-matching and relevant investigations
- Monitor vitals—pulse rate, blood pressure every 15 minutes till there is active bleeding and then half hourly after initial stabilization
- Record hourly output and maintain I/O chart
- Assess blood loss and transfuse accordingly especially if loss is severe or the patient was already anemic prior to episode
  Note: Aim is to maintain Hb above 10 g% and hematocrit above 30%.
- Maintain 4 hourly symphysio-fundal height (SFH) and abdominal girth (AG) chart to rule out abruption and concealed hemorrhage
- Monitor fetal heart sound by intermittent auscultation or preferably continuous electronic fetal heart monitoring
- Steroid cover is must for fetal lung maturity: injection Dexamethasone 12 mg IM 2 doses 24 hours apart. 1st dose to be given at admission Rh negative women ideally require a Kleihauer Betke (KB) test every time there is fresh bleeding and appropriate Anti-D prophylaxis depending on amount of exposure
- Patient may be shifted to maternity ward after bleeding has stopped for 24 hours. In the ward:
  - Allow restricted activity
  - Bed-pan facility
  - Correct anemia—transfusion or oral/injectable iron depending on degree of anemia
  - Intercourse, vaginal douching and suppositories are contraindicated
  - A gentle per-speculum examination can be done after bleeding has stopped for 48 hours to rule out local cervical pathology.

Q17. When should expectant management be terminated?

- When pregnancy reaches term
- There is severe bout of bleeding at any time
- Fetus is dead or malformed
- Onset of labor or rupture of membranes
- When abruption is suspected.

Q18. What is active management in a case of APH?

- It is the decision to terminate the pregnancy immediately after resuscitating and stabilizing the mother.
  Note: Coagulation profile must be corrected before any operative intervention.
- It is to be considered when:
  - Fetus is mature
  - Fetus is dead or has anomaly incompatible with life
  - There is maternal risk due to ongoing blood loss
  - Patient is in labor
  - Abruption is suspected.

Protocol for Active Management

- Resuscitate the patient—IV fluids, blood transfusions
- Correct coagulation profile—FFP (as per lab reports)
- Counsel relatives about high risk to mother and fetus
- Take informed consent about need for CS and possibility of hysterectomy in case of uncontrolled PPH
- Arrange operation theatre; shift patient to OT
- Keep adequate blood and blood products ready
- Double setup examination in OT in case of doubt of placenta previa OR cesarean straightaway in confirmed cases or when there is profuse bleeding.

Q19. Is technique of performing cesarean section different in case of placenta previa?

Yes, some important points to be kept in mind are:

- It is best to plan an elective cesarean section for major degree placenta previa as it results in less morbidity and mortality.
- Senior obstetrician should perform the cesarean section as there is a greater risk of complications in such a case
- The uterus is opened by a transverse incision in the lower segment. At times, the lower segment may not be well formed, or may be very vascular which can give rise in problems at the time of the incision
- After giving the transverse incision, the baby is delivered by either going by the side of the placenta and rupturing the membranes to extract the fetus or by going through the placenta and delivering the baby
- Early cord clamping to be done to prevent fetal exsanguination
- In case of preoperative or intraoperative suspicion of morbidly adherent placenta previa, upper segment cesarean section is better so as to avoid cutting the placenta.

Q20. What steps can be taken to control the bleeding from lower segment following cesarean?

In a case of placenta previa, intraoperative hemorrhage is very common as lower segment is less muscular and contraction and retraction do not completely occlude placental bed sinuses. Also, atonic uterus with large surface area of the placenta can result in excessive bleeding.

Few measures can be taken to control this bleeding. They are:
- Active management of third stage of labor and liberal use of oxytocics to counter atonicity.
- Intermittent mattress sutures on the placental bed to stem the bleeding
- **Stepwise devascularization:** Uterine artery ligation can be done. And if bleeding still not controlled then internal iliac artery ligation can be done
- Cho sutures—which are interrupted square-shaped sutures can be applied on the lower segment above and below the incision
- Balloon tamponade can be considered
- When conservative approaches fail, hysterectomy can be done as a last resort
- Uterine/Internal iliac artery embolization can be planned in the preoperative period in selected cases where morbid adherence of placenta is suspected. After discussion with the interventional radiologist preoperatively, the catheters are placed before starting the cesarean and embolization done soon after the baby is delivered
- Most importantly, adequately replace blood and blood products and correct coagulopathy.

Q21. What is the optimal mode of anesthesia for women with APH?

Regional anesthesia is recommended for operative delivery unless there is specific contraindication.

In a case of APH where maternal or fetal condition is compromised (for example, maternal cardiovascular instability and coagulopathy) and cesarean section required, general anesthesia to be considered to facilitate control of maternal resuscitation and expedite fetal delivery.

A consultant anesthesia should be involved in intrapartum care of women with APH with associated compromise.

Q22. Should Rh negative women presenting with APH, be given anti-D immunoglobulin (Ig)?

Anti-D immuglobulin should be given to all non-sensitized Rh negative women with APH, irrespective of routine prophylactic anti-D.

In non-sensitized Rh negative women with recurrent vaginal bleeding after 20 weeks, anti-D should be given at 6-weekly intervals.[6]

CASE SCENARIO

Mrs X 24 years lady primigravida at 34 weeks period of gestation presented in gyne casualty with complaints of pain abdomen and bleeding per vaginum with history of soakage of 4–5 pads over a period of 4–5 hours and history of passage of small clots

On Examination

Pallor ++, PR-104/min, BP-150/100 mm Hg, urine albumin is 2 +.

Abdominal Examination

Uterus is tense and tender, term size, uterine contour maintained, fetal parts cannot be appreciated and the fetal heart sound is not localized.

Q1. What is your diagnosis and how will you manage this case?

- In this scenario, the immediate need is resuscitation of the patient
- Alongside we should ascertain the amount of bleeding, take a quick history and examine the patient so as to reach a provisional diagnosis and further manage accordingly.

Q2. What is your provisional diagnosis and why?

The most likely diagnosis in this patient is *Abruptio placentae* because
- There is pain abdomen associated with bleeding
- Increased BP records with a urine albumin of 2 +
- Uterus is tense and tender
- Size of the uterus is greater with the period of gestation
- Pallor and vitals out of proportion to the blood loss.

Q3. What are your differential diagnosis?

With this clinical picture
- Ruptured uterus
- Associated placenta previa.

Q4. Why is this not a case of uterine rupture?

- Primigravida, no history of any scarring of uterus
- No evidence of a prolonged labor
- Uterine contour maintained, and is tense and tender
- Fetal parts not appreciated.

Q5. What are the required investigations in this patient?

- The history and examination is crucial to reach a final diagnosis

- Next all investigations need to be done
  - Blood grouping and cross-matching of blood and products
  - CBC—hemoglobin, hematocrit, platelet
  - Coagulation profile—bleeding time (BT), clotting time (CT), catheter-related thrombosis (CRT), prothrombin time (PT), activated partial thromboplastin time (APTT), fibrin degradation products (FDP), Fibrinogen, D-dimer
  - Liver function test (LFT), kidney function test (KFT), SE, blood sugar and urine analysis
  - Ultrasonography.

Q6. What is the importance of doing coagulation profile in this patient?

It is important to know that if there is evidence of DIC which need to be managed.

Normal Values
- Fibrinogen—150-600 mg/dL
- Prothrombin time—11-16 seconds
- Partial thromboplastin time (APTT)—22-37 seconds
- Platelet count—120,000-350,000/mm^3
- D-dimer—<0.5 mg/L.

Q7. How does a ultrasonography helps you in this patient?

- Placenta previa needs to be excluded as a cause of antepartum hemorrhage by an ultrasound
- If the patient is stable and immediate delivery is not intended it can be done in abruptio placenta as it has a poor sensitivity for Abruption (24%)
- Retroplacental clot can be identified in the ultrasound, a large retroplacental clot can be misinterpreted as a thick placenta
- A resolving clot will become sonolucent in 2 weeks
- Ultrasound will help in assessing the fetal presentation, weight, cardiac activity and help us make a plan for termination of pregnancy
- Also ultrasound can be helpful to asses and rule out if rupture uterus is present.

Q8. What is abruptio placenta?

- Separation of placenta partially or totally from its normal implantation site before delivery is called abruptio placentae.[7]
- Initiated by hemorrhage in decidua basalis.
- *Incidence*—0.5% or 1 in 200 deliveries
- Histological incidence is 4.5%
- Incidence increases with gestational age
- Abruption presents as vaginal bleeding in 78% cases—revealed or concealed type where no overt bleeding is seen
- Uterus is tense (characteristic woody consistency) and tender, with abdominal and backache
- Size of the uterus is more than the period of gestation
- Shock which is out of proportion to the apparent blood loss
- Fetal death is reported in 25-35% cases
- Presence of one or rarely all features help in the diagnosis of abruptio placenta
- The concealed type in which there is no vaginal bleeding is the more severe form of the disease, which is usually associated with disseminated intravascular coagulation (DIC).

Q9. What are the risk factors for abruption?

- Preexisting hypertensive disorders of pregnancy
- Cigarette smoking increases the risk up to 90%
- Abdominal trauma due to any cause
- Sudden decompression of an overdistended uterus for example in rupture of membranes in polyhydramnios, multiple pregnancy
- External cephalic version
- *Coagulation disorders:* Acquired and inherited thrombophilias—factor V leiden mutation, the prothrombin gene mutation, antiphospholipid syndrome, antithrombin III deficiency, protein C and protein S deficiency
- Preterm premature rupture of membranes especially if bleeding occurs before rupture of membranes
- Uterine malformations and uterine leiomyomas
- Substance abuse—cocaine.

Q10. What are the conditions associated with placental abruption?

- Gestational hypertension disorders
- Advanced maternal age
- Increasing parity
- Presence of multiple gestations
- Polyhydramnios with sudden rupture membrane
- Chorioamnionitis
- Trauma
- Possibly thrombophilias
- Maternal use of recreational drugs, such as cocaine
- Maternal smoking.

Q11. Does folic acid supplementation has any proved benefit to prevent placental abruption?

A systematic review of folic acid supplements in pregnancy (involving a re-analysis of a large randomized controlled trial and update of a Cochrane review) found no conclusive evidence of benefit (including risk of placental abruption) in women who took folic acid supplements.[7]

Q12. How do you grade abruptio placenta?

Grading[8]

- *Grade 0:* Patient asymptomatic diagnosed incidentally on seeing retroplacental clots after delivery of placenta.
- *Grade 1:* Hemorrhage with pain and irritable uterus no fetal or maternal compromise
- *Grade 2:* No maternal compromise but evident fetal distress
- *Grade 3:* Uterine tetany, maternal compromise and fetal demise.
  DIC and renal shut down are important complications. Average retroplacental blood loss >2500.

Q13. How will you manage this case?

The four pillars of management here are:
1. Call for help
2. Resuscitation
3. Monitoring and investigation
4. Arrest bleeding by arranging delivery of the fetus.

Management in abruptio placenta is guided by
- Grade at presentation
- Gestational age
- Presence of complications.
  The objective in this case as there is fetal demise with severe abruption is to decrease maternal morbidity and mortality which can be achieved by delivery of fetus.

In cases when there is fetal demise is dead it is seen that
- Placental separation is more than 50%
- Coagulopathy is associated with 50% cases
- Renal failure in about 10%.

Resuscitation Measures

- Assess airway, breathing and circulation
- Oxygen by mask at 10–15 liters/minute
- Intravenous access (2 wide bore)
- Investigations send
- Left lateral tilt position
- Monitors attached
- Catheterize the bladder
- Keep the woman warm using appropriate available measures.

Fluid Resuscitation

- Until blood is available, infuse up to 3.5 liters of IV fluids; Ringer's lactate (2 liters) and/or colloid (1–2 liters) as rapidly as required
- Fluid replacement should be done 3 times the estimated blood loss
- Fluid replacement—crystalloid or colloid
- 1 liter RL expand intravascular volume by approx 250 mL
- Crystalloid upto 2 liter. Colloid 1–2 liter
- Packed RBC and specific blood components according to HB
- Platelet transfusion if platelets are < 50,000/mL
- Fresh frozen plasma 4 units of FFP (12–15 mL/kg or total 1 liter)
  - For every 6 units of red cells or
  - If prothrombin time and/or activated partial thromboplastin time (PT and aPTT) >1.5 x mean control.

The aim is to maintain a hematocrit of 30% and an output of 30 mL/hour.

Q14. How is DIC associated with abruptio placenta?

DIC in abruption occurs due to massive release of thromboplastin into the circulation leading to:
- Intravascular fibrin formation
- Coagulation factors consumption
- Activation of the fibrinolytic system.

Q15. How do you make a diagnosis and manage coagulopathy?

- DIC profile is done
- There is a drop in fibrinogen level to 100 mg/dL or less
- PT and PTT is prolonged
- Reduction in platelet count
- Increased D-Dimer levels.

Correction of coagulopathy is by transfusing platelets, fresh frozen plasma and cryoprecipitate.

- No surgical intervention should be undertaken before correcting coagulopathy
- Usually coagulopathy subsided in the postpartum period but the high levels of FDP can interfere with myometrial contractility and cause postpartum hemorrhage.

Q16. How and when do you transfuse cryoprecipitate?

Patients with fibrinogen levels of less than 100 mg/dL should be transfused with 10–20 units of cryoprecipitate in a dose of 10–20 units immediately before and during caesarean section.

Q17. What will be the mode of delivery in your case?

As there is fetal demise in this case:
- If there is fetal demise, vaginal delivery is preferred
- If there is cephalic presentation factors are favorable for a vaginal delivery within 4–6 hours and fetal if heart is steady vaginal delivery can be planned with strict monitoring
- CS should be done if
  - Any other obstetric indicator
  - Massive abruption
- Vaginal delivery is preferred unless
- Malpresentation that requires caesarean section
- Massive hemorrhage that needs an immediate cesarean section
- Any other absolute indication for cesarean section.

Amniotomy should be performed at the earliest following which oxytocin drip should be started.

The outcome in the mother depends on adequate fluid and replacement of blood and blood products rather than interval to delivery.

Q18. How will your management change if this was a live fetus?

The management will be different as now both mother and fetus lives are at risk.

Alive Fetus and Rigid Uterus
- There can be two scenarios now
- Alive fetus and rigid uterus
- In these cases on most occasions, the abruption is large but less than 50%
- These patients are at very high risk of having fetal distress during labor
- Hence mostly emergency cesarean is planned except when the maternal condition is unstable and worsen with surgery or the fetal prognosis is poor.

Alive Fetus and Soft Uterus
- Here the abruption is less severe and mostly less than 25%.
- We can plan induction of labor for these patients and can normally undergo vaginal delivery
- Close monitoring should be done and emergency cesarean needs to be done if there is fetal distress at any occasion.

Q19. Do you consider conservative/expectant management in placental abruption?

- If there is mild abruption and pregnancy is <34 weeks and the condition of the mother and fetus is stable
- To prolong the duration of pregnancy for fetal lung maturity
- We need to monitor closely the maternal as well as fetal parameters
- Pregnancy may be terminated if there is derangement.

Q20. What are the risks in abruption placenta?

Maternal Riks
- Risk of disseminated intravascular hemorrhage in view of excessive blood loss. There can be fulminant DIC which can occur within 1–2 hours of abruption and is seen in 40% cases with fetal demise
- Hypovolemic shock in view of concealed hemorrhage
- Acute renal failure
- Postpartum hemorrhage mainly due to development of coagulopathy
- Amniotic fluid embolization
- Puerperal sepsis
- Risk of alloimmunization is increased
- Pulmonary edema, anemia, and caesarean section
- Recurrence in future conception.

Fetal Risks
- High perinatal morbidity and mortality in view of prematurity, fetal growth restriction (80%), congenital anomalies (4.4%) and associated maternal risks like hypertension
- Fetal anemia due to fetal blood loss and deranged hematology
- Respiratory distress syndrome and fetal hypoxia
- Hyperbilirubinemia
- Hypovolemic shock of the newborn
- Neurological deficits in the newborn post-delivery.

Q21. What is the risk of recurrence for abruption and the prognosis in future pregnancies?

- Recurrence rate is 6–17% after the 1st pregnancy and after 2 pregnancy it increase to 25%
- Cases with severe abruption has a similar outcome in next pregnancy in about 7% cases. 14% cases end up with abortions and almost 30% cases do not have a living child.

REFERENCES

1. RCOG Green Top Guideline No.63. Nov 2011.
2. Calleja-Agius J, Custo R, Brincat MP, et al. Placental abruption and placenta previa. Eur Clin Obstet Gynecol. 2006;2:121-7.
3. James DK, Weiner CP, Steer PJ, et al. Bleeding in late pregnancy. High Risk Pregnancy Management options. 2006;1259-75.
4. Royal College of Obstetricians and Gynaecologists. Placenta Praevia, Placenta Praevia Accreta and Vasa Praevia: Diagnosis and Management. Green-top Guideline No. 27. London: RCOG;2011.
5. Royal College of Obstetricians and Gynaecologists. Antenatal Corticosteroids to Reduce Neonatal Morbidity. Green-top Guideline No. 7. London: RCOG;2010.
6. Royal College of Obstetricians and Gynaecologists. The Use of Anti-D Immunoglobulin for Rhesus D Prophylaxis. Green-top guideline No. 22. London: RCOG;2011.
7. Williams obstetrics. 24th edn; 2014.
8. Charles DH, Ness AR, Campbell D, et al. Folic acid supplements in pregnancy and birth outcome: re-analysis of a large randomised controlled trial and update of Cochrane review. Paediatr Perinat Epidemiol. 2005;19:112-24.

CHAPTER 17

HIV with Pregnancy

Pushpa Mishra, Priyanka Chaudhary

CASE SCENARIO

A 25 years old female, Mrs A, wife of Mr X, resident of Shastri Park, homemaker, G2P1L1 with five months amenorrhea came to ANC OPD on 19/08/2017 for routine antenatal checkup and was diagnosed HIV positive during routine antenatal investigations. Her LMP was 02/04/2017 making her period of gestation (POG) 20 weeks on 19/08/2017. She has been married for 4 years, a non-consanguineous marriage, had full term normal vaginal delivery 3 years back. Her husband is a truck driver by occupation. Rest history and examination findings were unremarkable. How will you proceed in this case?

Q1. How to counsel a pregnant woman to get HIV test done? What is prenatal HIV screening? What is opt-out approach? How is HIV testing done?

- HIV testing is the first step towards prevention of parent to child transmission directed towards reduction of pediatric HIV infections.
- All pregnant women should be counseled to undergo HIV testing, whenever they come in contact with the healthcare system.

Pre-test Counseling Includes
- Confidentiality
- The test and the testing procedure
- Assessment of risk behavior
- Risk reduction strategies
- Abstinence and safe sex practices (including free condoms)
- Couple counseling
- Behavior change communication for high risk woman and her partner
- Repeat HIV testing considering window period if spouse is positive or she or he has high risk behavior. Regarding prenatal HIV screening, WHO recommends provider initiated HIV testing and counseling as a standard part of antenatal, intrapartum and postnatal care.

The CDC (2006, 2010a); AAP and ACOG 2011; USPSTF 2012 recommend prenatal HIV screening based on an **opt-out** approach. This means that the pregnant woman is told that HIV testing is included in a comprehensive set of antenatal tests but that testing may be declined. In areas of high HIV prevalence or in women at high risk of acquiring HIV infection during pregnancy, repeat testing in the third trimester is recommended (ACOG 2011).

Screening is performed using an enzyme-linked immunoassay (ELISA) with a sensitivity >99.5%. A positive test confirmation is done with either a western blot or immunofluorescence assay (IFA), both of which have a high specificity.

For acute primary HIV infection identification of viral p24 core antigen or viral RNA or DNA is possible.

Women with limited prenatal care or with undocumented HIV status at delivery should have a 'rapid' HIV test performed. These tests can detect HIV antibody in 60 minutes or less and have sensitivities and specificities comparable with those of conventional ELISA. A negative rapid test does not need to be confirmed, however, in a woman exposed to HIV within the last 3 months, repeat testing is recommended.

Testing Procedure
There are two categories of tests:
- Tests to identify the virus
- Tests to identify HIV antibodies

HIV diagnosis is commonly made through serological assays to detect HIV specific antibodies or by nucleic acid amplification test (NAAT) to detect HIV nucleic acids. Tests to identify the virus are very expensive and require specialized equipment and skills for testing, while tests to identify HIV antibodies are more cost effective.

Examples of antibody tests are the Western Blot, ELISA and Rapid Tests. Western Blot and ELISA are specialized tests done in laboratories, while Rapid Tests are simple, reliable tests that can be done at any clinic by doctors and paramedical staff. Additional tests available for antibody testing are: Chemiluminescence immunoassays (CIA), fluorescent immunoassays and line immunoassays. Nucleic acid amplification test (NAAT) uses DNA PCR (polymerase chain reaction) and p24 antigen detection for diagnosis of HIV.

The following tests are available for HIV testing:

1. *HIV EIA (Enzyme immunoassay):* Screening test for HIV infection. Sensitivity >99.9%. Reactive results must be confirmed with Western blot.
2. *Western blot:* Confirmatory test for HIV. Specificity when combined with ELISA >99.9%. Indeterminate results seen with early HIV infection, autoimmune disease, pregnancy and recent tetanus toxoid administration.
3. *Absolute CD4 lymphocyte count:* Most widely used predictor of HIV progression. Risk of progression is high with CD4 <200 cells/L. It is the best short-term predictor for development of opportunistic infections.
4. *CD4 lymphocyte percentage:* Useful in conjunction with CD4 count. Risk of progression is high with percentage <20%.
5. *Beta 2 microglobulin:* Cell surface protein indicative of macrophage-monocyte stimulation. Levels >3.5 mg/dL associated with rapid progression of disease.
6. *HIV RNA quantitative (viral load):* Most useful test for determining prognosis and monitoring therapy; can assist in drug selection prior to initial treatment for following therapeutic failure.
7. *HIV genotyping:* Useful for detection and assessment of resistance to antiretroviral therapy; can assist in drug selection.

Q2. If HIV test comes out to be positive, what other aspects should be covered in counseling such patients?

The following issues are covered if the HIV test results are positive:
- Emotional responses and concerns
- Psychosocial support (individual support and support group)
- Disclosure to family
- Safe sex practices, couple counseling, HIV testing of spouse and other living children
- Information on positive living, nutrition, contraception, disease progression, the immune system, CD4 viral load, opportunistic diseases and antiretroviral treatment
- Nutritional support and counseling
- Counseling on choices of continuation or medical termination of pregnancy (MTP) preferably within 3 months of pregnancy only.
- Screening for tuberculosis and other opportunistic infections
- Screening and treatment for STIs
- Linkage to ART services
- Complete physical examination and a staging assessment according to WHO criteria
- Follow-up CD4 testing
- Need for ART regardless of clinical stage and CD4 count
- Family planning services
- Infant feeding support through home visit
- The importance of annual PAP smears for HIV positive women

Q3. What are the modes of HIV transmission? What percentage of perinatal HIV transmission occur in absence of any intervention?

Modes of transmission of HIV (as per NACO annual report 2009-2010):

1. Heterosexual   87.4%
2. Parent to child transmission   5.4%
3. Homosexual/bisexual   1.3%
4. Injecting drug use   1.6%
5. Blood and blood products 1.0%
6. Unknown   3.3%

- Mother to child transmission is the most common cause of pediatric HIV infections. 15-40% of neonates born to nonbreastfeeding, untreated, HIV infected mothers get infected.
- It has been estimated that 20% of perinatal HIV transmission occurs before 36 weeks, 50% near term and 30% intrapartum.
- Intrapartum transmission can occur during labor through maternal-fetal exchange of blood or by contact of the infant's skin or mucous membranes with infected blood or other maternal secretions during delivery.
- **Estimated risk of perinatal HIV transmission in the absence of interventions:**

1.	During pregnancy	5–10%
2.	During labor and delivery	10–15%
3.	During breastfeeding	5–20%
4.	Overall without breastfeeding	15–25%

Q4. What are the various stages of disease in HIV infection?

Clinical Stages of HIV-AIDS[1]

1. *Stage 1:* Asymptomatic persistent generalized lymphadenopathy (PGL)—Painless enlarged lymph nodes >1 cm in two or more non-contiguous sites (excluding inguinal) in the absence of known cause and persisting for three months or more.
2. *Stage 2:* Mild symptoms
    - Moderate unexplained weight loss (<10% of presumed or measured body weight)
    - Recurrent respiratory tract infections
    - Herpes zoster
    - Angular cheilitis
    - Recurrent oral ulcerations (Aphthous ulcer)
    - Papular pruritic eruptions
    - Seborrheic dermatitis
    - Fungal nail infections of fingers
3. *Stage 3:* Advanced symptoms (opportunistic infections) appear.
    - Severe weight loss (>10% of presumed or measured body weight)
    - Unexplained chronic diarrhea for longer than a month
    - Unexplained persistent fever for more than a month
    - Oral candidiasis
    - Oral hairy leukoplakia
    - Pulmonary TB diagnosed in last two years
    - Severe bacterial infections (e.g. pneumonia, empyema, pyomyositis, bone or joint infection, meningitis, bacteremia)
4. *Stage 4:* AIDS—rapid decline in the number of CD4 cells. Opportunistic infections become severe and cancer may develop.
    - HIV wasting syndrome
    - Pneumocystis pneumonia
    - Recurrent severe or radiological bacterial pneumonia
    - Chronic herpes simplex infection
    - Esophageal candidiasis
    - Extrapulmonary TB
    - Kaposi sarcoma
    - CNS toxoplasmosis
    - HIV encephalopathy.

Q5. What are the factors that affect mother to child transmission of HIV?

The following factors affect mother-to-child transmission of HIV infection:[2-9]

Viral
- Viral genotype and phenotype
- Viral resistance
- Viral load

Transmission is increased in
- high levels of maternal viremia.
- advanced disease and at the time of seroconversion
- increase maternal viral load. More than half of the women with viral loads of >50,000.

RNA copies per mL at the time of delivery have been shown to transmit the virus.

Maternal
- Maternal immunological status
- Transmission from mother to child is more likely with decreased maternal immune status, reflected by low CD4+ counts, low CD4+ percentages or high CD4+/CD8 ratios.
- Maternal nutritional status
- Serum vitamin A levels and micronutrients (zinc)
- Maternal clinical status
- Behavioral factors

An increased rate of transmission from mother to child seen with:
- Cigarette smoking and maternal hard drug use.
- Unprotected sexual intercourse during pregnancy

A transmission rate of 30% was shown in women who had more than 80 episodes of unprotected sex during pregnancy compared with 9.1% in patient who used barrier.
- Antiretroviral treatment

Obstetrical
- Prolonged rupture of membranes (>4 hours)
- Mode of delivery
- Intrapartum hemorrhage
- Obstetrical procedures (CVS, amniocentesis)
- Invasive fetal monitoring

Fetal
- Prematurity
- Genetic
- Multiple pregnancy

Infant
- Breastfeeding
- Gastrointestinal tract factors
- Immature immune system

Q6. Does pregnancy affect the course of HIV infection? What is the effect of HIV infection in pregnancy?

Pregnancy does not have any adverse effect on the natural course of HIV infection but HIV can affect pregnancy in various ways.

Effect of HIV infection on pregnancy:
1. Spontaneous abortion
2. Ectopic pregnancy
3. Stillbirths
4. Preterm labor
5. Low birth weight
6. Infections
7. Behavioral problems

Q7. What important points have to be elicited in history and examination in such patient?

The following points are important in history and examination in such patient:

- Details and duration of presenting complaints if any:
  - Prolonged history (> 1 month) of the following symptoms—fever (intermittent or continuous), cough, diarrhea, weight loss(> 10% of body weight)
  - Associated symptoms—acquiring infections early.
- Obstetric history
  - Parity: if multiparous woman presents in first trimester, MTP can be offered.
  - Record of HIV testing in previous pregnancy
  - HIV status of children
- Past history: any prolonged illness, blood transfusion, surgical intervention or any tattooing
- Family/sexual/personal history
  - Husband HIV status (if known)
  - Sexual contact (self/partner)
  - Drug abuse/alcohol intake/smoking
- Vaccination history
  - BCG
  - Hepatitis A and B vaccines

Clinical Examination

Clinical examination should include general physical examination followed by systemic and local examination with emphasis on the following:

General Physical Examination

- General build and nutritional status (weight and height)
- Generalized lymphadenopathy
- Fundus examination (CMV retinitis) skin examination for lesions or abnormal patches (opportunistic infections)
- Mouth—for inspection of oral candidiasis

Systemic Examination

- CNS: Visual fields and signs of neuropathy, focal neurological deficit
- Respiratory system: Opportunistic infections
- Per abdomen: Hepatosplenomegaly

Local Examination

Per speculum and per vaginum examination: To rule out other STDs, look for bacterial vaginosis, candidiasis, and cervical cancer.

Q8. What investigations would you like to do for this patient?

Routine

Blood group, complete blood count, glucose tolerance test, VDRL (for both partners), urine routine and microscopy, ultrasound (to confirm gestational age, screen for anomalies, placental localization)

HIV Related

Hepatitis A, B, C serologies; liver and renal function tests; PAP smear; tests for STIs; CXR with abdominal shield.

HIV Specific

Absolute CD4 count; CD4 lymphocyte percentage; HIV viral load tests; p24 antigen.

Q9. What is PPTCT program?

- The prevention of parent to child transmission of HIV/AIDS (PPTCT) program was launched in the country in the year 2002 following a feasibility study in 11 major hospitals in the five high HIV prevalence states.[10]
- As on 31st August 2016 in India there are 20,756 Integrated Counseling and Testing Centers (ICTC), most of these in government hospitals, which offer PPTCT services to pregnant women.[10]
- The NACO Technical Estimate Report (2015) estimated that out of 29 million annual pregnancies in India, 35,255 occur in HIV positive pregnant women. In the absence of any intervention, an estimated (2015) cohort of 10,361 infected babies will be born annually.[10]
- The PPTCT program aims to prevent the perinatal transmission of HIV from an HIV infected pregnant mother to her newborn baby. The program entails counseling and testing of pregnant women in the ICTCs.[10]
- With effect from 1st January 2014, pregnant women who are found to be HIV positive are initiated on lifelong ART irrespective of CD4 count and WHO clinical staging.
- Newborn (HIV exposed) babies are initiated on 6 weeks of Syrup Nevirapine immediately after birth so as to prevent transmission of HIV from mother to child.
- Nevirapine treatment is extended to 12 weeks if the duration of the ART of mother is less than 24 weeks.[10]

In line with WHO standards for a comprehensive strategy, the National PPTCT program recognizes the four elements integral to preventing HIV transmission among women and children.

These are:
- *Prong 1:* Primary prevention of HIV, especially among women of child bearing age.
- *Prong 2:* Preventing unintended pregnancies among women living with HIV.
- *Prong 3:* Prevent HIV transmission from pregnant women infected with HIV to their child.
- *Prong 4:* Provide care, support and treatment to women living with HIV, her children and family in women in child bearing age.

The National PPTCT program adopts a public health approach to provide these services to pregnant women and their children. This approach seeks to ensure equitable access to high-quality PPTCT services at the grass-root level while taking into account what is feasible on a large-scale within available health infrastructure, human and financial resources.

Q10. What are the goals of PPTCT?

Goals of national PPTCT Program in India are.[11]

1. Primary prevention of HIV, especially among women in child-bearing age.
2. Integration of PPTCT services with general health services
   - Basic antenatal care (ANC), natal and postnatal services
   - Sexual reproductive health and family planning
   - Pediatric ART
   - Adolescent reproductive and sexual health (ARSH), TB and STI/RTI services
3. Strengthening postnatal care of the HIV-infected mother and her exposed infant
4. Provide the essential package of PPTCT services.

Q11. What are the technical guidelines summarized under national PPTCT program? Establish HIV status of pregnant women:[11]

1. Known HIV infected case and already receiving ART: continue ART (as per guidelines)
2. HIV test negative: Repeat HIV test (as per guidelines for window period and history of risk factor
3. Newly detected HIV infection:

From ICTC collect the blood sample for CD4 and send it to ART center and refer women to ART center

↓

ART center: Initiate ART to HIV positive pregnant mother regardless of WHO clinical stage and CD4 count results; preferred regimen: TDF+3TC+EFV; ART center will collect sample for baseline and other investigations

↓

Mother: Continue ART during labor, delivery and thereafter lifelong

↓

Mother: Continue ART lifelong

Infant

Daily NVP from birth until minimum 6 weeks of age, and then stop; EBF (exclusive breastfeeding) or ERF (exclusive replacement feeding).

Q12. What are the criteria for ART initiation in a pregnant woman?

- According to recent NACO guidelines lifelong ART should be initiated in all pregnant women with confirmed HIV infection regardless of WHO clinical stage or CD4 cell count. **TDF+3TC+EFV is the recommended first line ART regimen in pregnant and breastfeeding women (including pregnant women in the first trimester of pregnancy and women of childbearing age).**[11]
- ART shall be started only at ART center

CASE SCENARIO

A 21 years old female, Mrs F, wife of Mr Y, resident of Jharkhand, housewife, primigravida with nine months amenorrhea, unbooked and uninvestigated pregnancy came to gyne casualty on 15/08/2017 with false labor pains and was diagnosed HIV positive on rapid HIV kit. Her history and examination findings were unremarkable. False labor pains subsided with sedation.

Q1. What is the protocol for pregnant woman presenting in labor (unbooked cases) with HIV seropositivity?

Pregnant women coming directly in labor

↓

Found HIV positive using whole blood finger prick testing in labor room/ delivery ward

↓

Collect blood sample for CD4 and send the sample next day to ART center; Initiate maternal ART (TDF+3TC+EFV)

↓

Counseling and confirmation of HIV status and blood sample collection for CD4 testing

↓

Mother: continue ART after delivery; Link with ART center to continue ART as soon as possible

↓

Infant: Daily syrup nevirapine from birth until 6 weeks.[11]

Q2. What are the safer delivery techniques that are needed to be followed in a HIV positive pregnant woman?

Mother-to-child transmission risk is increased by:[11]
1. Prolonged rupture of membranes
2. Repeated per vaginum examinations
3. Assisted instrumental delivery
4. Invasive fetal monitoring procedures (scalp/ fetal blood monitoring)
5. Episiotomy
6. Prematurity

While delivering HIV infected women, following precautions should be observed:
1. Follow standard/universal work precautions
2. Avoid artificial rupture of membranes as long as possible
3. Minimize vaginal examination and use aseptic techniques
4. Avoid invasive procedures and instrumental deliveries; if indicated, low cavity outlet forceps is preferable to vacuum as it is generally linked with lower rates of fetal trauma than vacuum.
5. Suctioning the newborn with a nasogastric tube should be avoided unless there is meconium liquor staining.
6. Use of 'dry' hemostatic techniques to minimize bleeding.
7. During cesarean section, wherever possible, the membranes are left intact until the head is delivered through the surgical incision; the cord should be clamped as early as possible after delivery.
8. Use of round tip blunt needles for C-section; do not use fingers to hold the needle; use of forceps to receive and hold the needle; use of container while transferring sharps to surgical assistant.
9. Standard waste disposal management guidelines should be followed.

Q3. What are indications for cesarean section in a HIV positive pregnant woman?

- As per **ACOG 2010**, Scheduled cesarean delivery, defined as cesarean delivery performed before the onset of labor and before rupture of membranes, is advised for prevention of perinatal transmission of HIV in women with HIV RNA levels >1,000 copies/mL near delivery and for women with unknown HIV RNA levels.
- In cases of cesarean delivery performed to prevent transmission of HIV, ACOG suggests scheduling cesarean delivery at 38 weeks' gestation in order to reduce the likelihood of onset of labor or rupture of membranes before delivery.
- Cesarean section in HIV positive pregnant women should be performed only for obstetric indications as per latest NACO guidelines for PMTCT(2013).

Q4. How will you manage this patient in postpartum period?

- Within an hour of delivery: Infants born to HIV infected mothers should receive NVP prophylaxis immediately after birth
- Mother to be counseled to take ART regularly
- Follow-up of infants for immunization/EID(HIV exposed infant diagnosis)/CPT (cotrimoxazole therapy) initiation and continuation upto 18 months.

Q5. What ARV prophylaxis be given to infant born to HIV positive mother? What are the recommendations for breastfeeding for a HIV positive patient?

Infant ARV prophylaxis is required for all infants born to HIV infected women receiving ART to further reduce perinatal HIV transmission.

Based on WHO guidelines, daily nevirapine prophylaxis should be given from birth to 6 weeks minimum irrespective of whether exclusively breastfed or exclusively replacement fed (may be extended to 12 weeks, if mother has not received ART for adequate duration).[11]

Dose and duration of infant daily NVP prophylaxis is as follows:
1. Infants with birth weight <2000 grams : NVP 2 mg/kg once daily or 0.2 mL/kg once daily*.
2. Birth weight 2000–2500 grams: 10 mg once daily or 1 mL once daily*.
3. Birth weight >2500 grams: 15 mg once daily or 1.5 mL once daily*.

*Considering the content of 10 mg NVP in 1 mL suspension.

CASE SCENARIO

A 33 years old female; Mrs A, wife of Mr Z, resident of Seelampur, housewife, G4P2L1A1 with known case of HIV positive with CD4 count 200/mm³, presented to antenatal OPD at 34 weeks for routine antenatal checkup. Her obstetric history: married for 6 years, non- consanguinous marriage

Para 1: 5 years back, full term normal vaginal delivery at home, baby was female, birth weight not known, 6 months breast-fed, baby alive and healthy. Her HIV status was not known in this pregnancy.

Abortion 1: 4 years back, induced abortion at 2 months amenorrhea (UPT positive, USG not done), took MTP pill, not followed by evacuation.

Para 2: 2 years back, preterm vaginal delivery (at 35 weeks) at private nursing home, baby was male, birth weight 1.3 kg, expired 5 days after birth due to pneumonia. she was diagnosed HIV positive in this pregnancy and started on ART since then.

Q1. How would you assess the HIV status of her children?

Testing for HIV by rapid test is to be performed if positive a confirmation test has to be done.

Q2. Comment on the prevalence of HIV infection in India and worldwide?

- As per NACO technical report 2015, national adult (15-49 years) HIV prevalence is estimated at 0.26% (0.22%-0.32%) in 2015.
- In 2015, adult HIV prevalence is around 0.30% among males and at 0.22% among females. Among the States/Union territories in 2015, Manipur has shown the highest prevalence of 1.15% followed by Mizoram (0.80%), Nagaland (0.78%), Andhra Pradesh and Telengana (0.66%), Karnataka (0.45%), Gujarat (0.42%) and Goa (0.40%).
- The total number of people living with HIV (PLHIV) in India is estimated at 21.17 lakhs (17.11 lakhs-26.49 lakhs) in 2015.
- Children (<15 years) account for 6.54%, while two fifth (40.5%) of total HIV infection are among females.
- Based on the estimated HIV infections among adult females and assumptions on the effect of HIV on fertility and parent to child transmission rates, it is estimated that around 35 thousand HIV-positive pregnant women needed PPTCT services in 2015.
- According to UNAIDS data 2017; PLHIV (people living with HIV) in 2016 country-wise prevalence:
  1. East and southern Africa: 19.4 million
  2. Western and central Africa: 6.1 million
  3. Asia and pacific: 5.1 million
  4. Western and Central Europe and North America: 2.1 million
  5. Latin America and Caribbean: 2.1 million
  6. East Europe and Central Asia: 1.6 million
  7. Middle East and North Africa: 230,000

Q3. How will you monitor a pregnant women receiving ART?

Assess	Baseline	2 weeks	4 weeks	8 weeks	12 weeks	Every 6 months	Comment
Clinical Evaluation	Yes	Yes	Yes	Yes	Yes	Yes	Every month
Adherence	Yes	Yes	Yes	Yes	Yes	Yes	Every month
Hb	Yes	Yes	Yes	Yes	Yes	Yes	Re-check at
LFT	Yes	Yes	-	-	-	Yes	as and when

Contd...

Assess	Baseline	2 weeks	4 weeks	8 weeks	12 weeks	Every 6 months	Comment
Urinalysis	Yes	-	-	-	-	Yes	Specifically for TDF based
CD4	Thereafter every 6 months as per guidelines						
KFT	Yes	-	-	-	-	Yes	
BG/Rh	Yes	-	-	-	-	-	
HBV/HCV	Yes	-	-	-	-	-	
RPR/VDRL	Yes	-	-	-	-	-	
Blood	Yes	-	-	-	-	-	Repeat every 6 months if started on LPV/based
Lipid profile	Yes	-	-	-	-	-	
Weight	Yes	Yes	Yes	Yes	Yes	Yes	Every month

Q4. What is the indication for initiation of cotrimoxazole prophylactic therapy in HIV positive pregnant woman?

CPT (cotrimoxazole prophylactic therapy) should be started if CD4 count is <250 cells/mm^3 and continued through pregnancy, delivery and breastfeeding as per national guidelines.

Q5. What are the different ART regimen for HIV positive pregnant woman? What are the dosage schedule and side effects of commonly used ART drugs?

Preferred first line regimen: **TDF (tenofovir)+3TC (lamivudine)+EFV (efavirenz)**[11]

Alternative regimens:
- AZT (zidovudine) +3TC (lamivudine)+EFV (efavirenz)
- AZT (zidovudine)+3TC (lamivudine)+NVP (nevirapine)
- TDF (tenofovir)+3TC (lamivudine)+NVP (nevirapine)

Dosage schedule and side effects of commonly used ART drugs:

1. *Tenofovir Disoproxil Fumarate (TDF):* 300 mg once daily/side effects: nephrotoxicity, hypophosphatemia
2. *Lamivudine (3TC):* 300 mg once daily/side effects: hypersensitivity, rarely pancreatitis.
3. *Efavirenz (EFV):* 600 mg once daily/side effects: neuropsychiatric symptoms like hallucinations, nightmares, suicidal ideations, vivid dreams etc.
4. *Lopinavir/ritonavir (LPV/r):* LPV(200 mg)/r(50 mg)- 2 tablets BD/side effects: GI disturbances, lipodystrophy, glucose intolerance, hyperlipidemia.

Q6. What ART regimen is followed for a pregnant woman having prior exposure to NNRTIs for PPTCT?

The TDF+3TC+EFV regimen may not be fully effective due to persistence of archived mutation to NNRTIs in a pregnant women having prior exposure to NNRTIs for PMTCT. So such women require protease inhibitor based regimen: TDF+3TC (1 tablet daily)+LPV/r (lopinavir 200 mg/ritonavir 50 mg: 2 tablets BD)

Q7. What information has to be given regarding family planning in such patient? What are the various contraceptive methods available for HIV positive patients?[11]

- Information about effective contraceptive methods to prevent pregnancy
- The effects of progression of HIV disease on the woman's health
- Importance of family planning and birth spacing
- Risk of HIV transmission to uninfected partner while having unprotected intercourse
- Risk of transmission of HIV to infant and benefits of ARV prophylaxis
- Information on the interaction between HIV and pregnancy (including adverse pregnancy outcomes).

Contraceptive Methods

- Dual protection with condom use helps in prevention of cross infection of HIV virus to the partner as well as STIs
- DMPA is safe to use in women living with HIV as well as those on ART
- In women living with HIV (CD4 is >350 cells/mm^3), hormonal contraception is safe
- COCs are not recommended for women taking ritonavir-boosted PIs due to the potentially decreased efficacy of the contraception
- LAM (lactational amenorrhea method) does not protect against STIs, pregnancy and HIV
- Male sterilisation (using no scalpel vasectomy).

Q8. How are you going to manage a discordant couple and how to counsel them?

- A discordant couple is a couple, where only one partner is HIV positive. Women are more prone to infection in such a case.
- If a woman is HIV positive, then artificial insemination around ovulation is an option for the couple.
- If a woman is HIV negative but her husband is HIV positive, then by limiting the sexual intercourse around ovulation can reduce the risk of transmission.
- Sperm washing is a technique where spermatozoa is separated from the surrounding HIV infected seminal plasma by sperm swim up technique.
- This technique can also be tried in discordant couple where husband is HIV positive.

REFERENCES

1. WHO case definitions of HIV for surveillance and revised clinical staging and immunological classification of HIV-related disease in adults and children. Geneva: World Health Organization; 2007.
2. Goedert JJ, Mendez H, Drummond JE, et al. Mother-to-infant transmission of human immunodeficiency virus type 1: association with prematurity or low anti gp-120. Lancet. 1989; 2:1351-54.
3. Shearer WT, Kalish LA, Zimmerman PA. CCR5 HIV-1 vertical transmission. Women and Infants Transmission Study Group. J Acquir Immune Defic Syndr Hum Retrovirol. 1998; 17(2): 180-81.
4. Mtimavalye L, Biggar RJ, Taha TE, et al. Maternal-infant transmission of HIV-1. N Engl J Med. 1995, 332:890-91.
5. Ryder RW, Behets F. Reasons for the wide variation in reported rates of mother-to-child transmission of HIV-1. AIDS. 1994;8:1495-97.
6. Nieburg P, Hu DJ, Moses S, et al. Contribution of breastfeeding to the reported variation in rates of mother-to-child HIV transmission. AIDS. 1995;9(4):396-97.
7. Hengel RL, Kennedy MS, Steketee RW et al. Neutralizing antibody and perinatal transmission of human immunodeficiency virus type 1. New York City Perinatal HIV Transmission Collaborative Study Group. AIDS Res Hum Retroviruses. 1998;14(6):475-81.
8. Newell ML. Mechanisms and timing of mother-to-child transmission of HIV-1. AIDS. 1997;12:831-37.
9. Butlerys M, Lepage P. Mother-to-child transmission of HIV. Curr Opin Ped, 1998;10:143-50.
10. National AIDS control organization, MoHFW,GoI, national informatics centre(NIC);December 2016.
11. Updated guidelines for prevention of parent to child transmission (PPTCT) of HIV using multidrug antiretroviral regimen in India, December 2013 and NACO 2015 Guidelines.

18 CHAPTER

Pregnancy with Heart Disease

Chetna Arvind Sethi

CASE SCENARIO

G1 with 8½ months amenorrhea with heart disease.

Mrs X, 23 years old, wife of Mr Y resident of a village came to gyne casualty on 3/7/17 at 12:13 AM as a known case of heart disease with amenorrhea 8½ months. She complained of progressive breathlessness along with easy fatigability for 2–3 months. Her LMP was 1/11/16 making her period of gestation 34 weeks and 6 days on 3/7/17 and her EDD was 8/8/17.

History of Presenting Complaints

Patient is a booked antenatal case at private nursing home since 5 months of amenorrhea with poor compliance and only 3 visits to the center so far. She had her first antenatal visit at 5 months of amenorrhea when she went to the private nursing home with complaints of breathlessness on exertion (NYHA Class II). There she underwent a 2D Echo and was diagnosed to have rheumatic valvular heart disease (RHD) with mitral valve stenosis (MS) (as shown in records). All other antenatal investigations were normal. She was also put on some medication which she never took regularly (no records).

Her breathlessness had worsened over the last 2–3 weeks and was now comfortable only at rest. She is not able to do her day-to-day activities. She was referred to tertiary hospital.

- There was no history of significant fever with joint pain and limitation of activity or rash in the childhood or in recent past.
- There was no history of palpitations, orthopnea, chest pain, paroxysmal nocturnal dyspnea, syncope, hemoptysis and cough with expectoration.
- No specialist cardiac opinion had been taken and there was no advice regarding any surgical intervention.

Course in the Hospital

She was admitted to the high dependency unit for stabilization and was put to:
- Bed rest
- Propped-up position
- Oxygen by mask
- Diuretics were started to reduce preload (Injection Lasix 40 mg IV followed by 20 mg 8 hourly)
- Baseline blood investigations, ABG, urine routine and microscopy (R/M), C/S were sent
- Urgent cardiac consultation was taken and her ECG revealed sinus tachycardia and 2D Echo showed RHD with severe MS (MVA 0.6 cm^2) with severe MR/TR with severe PAH with normal systolic LV function EF 60%.
- She was stabilized and put on close fetomaternal monitoring for about a month then she went into spontaneous labor and delivered vaginally, uneventfully.

Diagnosis on History

G1 with 34 weeks + 6 days with Rheumatic heart disease, NYHA class III.

On Examination

General Physical Examination

- Patient is conscious-oriented and is in propped-up position.
- She is tachypneic and on oxygen by mask.
- She is average in built and nutrition, height—152 cm, weight—58 kg, pre-pregnancy weight was not known therefore BMI not calculated.
- No pallor, no cyanosis, no clubbing, no icterus, orodental hygiene is fair, no stomatitis or glossitis
- Thyroid not enlarged, no palpable lymph nodes pregnancy.

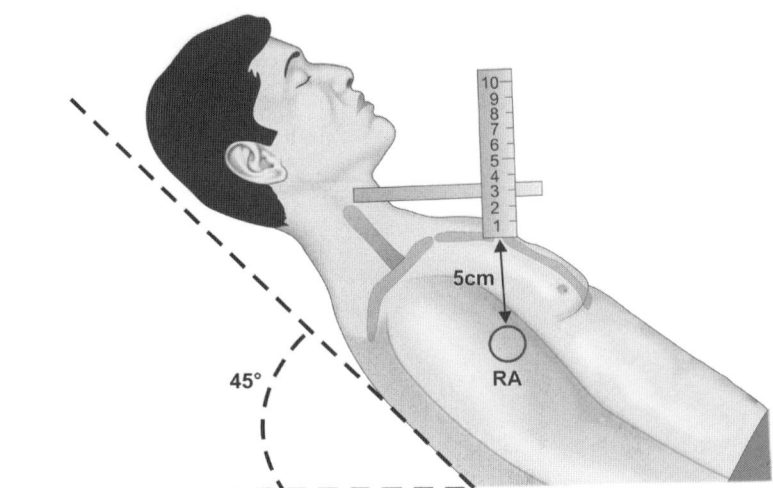

Fig. 1: Measurement of jugular venous pressure (JVP)

- JVP (Fig. 1) is raised to 8 cm. Trachea is central, mild pitting pedal edema.
- Afebrile.

RR: 25/min

PR: 100/min, regular, rhythmic, good volume, no radiofemoral delay, all peripheral pulses palpable.

BP: 100/60 mm Hg in right arm in sitting position.

No signs of rheumatic activity (arthritis, erythematous rash, subcutaneous nodules, abnormal movements).

Bilateral breasts show normal secondary changes of pregnancy.

Systematic Examination

Respiratory System

- **RR:** 25/min
- Bilateral air entry is normal with normal vesicular breath sounds.
- No basal crepitation or adventitious sounds.

Cardiovascular System

- *Inspection*: Normal precordium, no visible pulsations, no dilated veins/scars, no scoliosis, no signs of infective endocarditis.
- *Palpation*: Apex beat is in the 5th intercostal space in mid clavicular line, no heaving, P2 is palpable, no palpable S3 or S4, no palpable thrill, grade II left parasternal heave, no epigastric pulsations.
- *Percussion*: Right margin of cardiac dullness is retrosternal, left margin confirms to the apex.

Auscultation (Fig. 2)

- *Apex*: S1 is loud and tapping, opening snap followed by a long mid-diastolic rumble, best heard on left lateral position. No change with respiration or passive leg rising. Mid diastolic murmur heard at apex with radiation to axilla. No S3/S4 audible.
- *Tricuspid area*: S1 loud, no audible S3/S4. Grade III pansystolic murmur, no radiation of murmur, better heard in inspiration and during passive leg rising.
- *Aortic area*: S1 loud, S2 normally split, no S3/S4, no murmur.
- *Pulmonary area*: S1 loud, S2 normally split (A2—P2) with P2 loud, no S3/S4, no murmur.

Abdominal Examination

- *Inspection*: Uniformly distended with longitudinal ovoid, all quadrants moving well with respiration, linea nigra and stria gravidarum are present. Umbilicus central and flat, no scar marks, no dilated veins. All hernial are sites free.
- *Palpation*: No organomegaly noted
- Fundal height is 32 weeks, symphysiofundal height of 32 cm, and abdominal girth of 32 inches.
- *Fundal grip*: Soft broad irregular, ballotable part felt at fundus suggestive of breech.
- *Lateral grip*: Smooth curved structure felt on right lateral side of the abdomen suggestive of back, multiple knobby parts felt on the left side, suggestive of limbs
- Adequate liquor
- Estimated fetal weight approximately 2.2–2.4 kg
- *Pelvic grip*: First a hard, smooth, globular structure felt indicative of head, 2nd not engaged

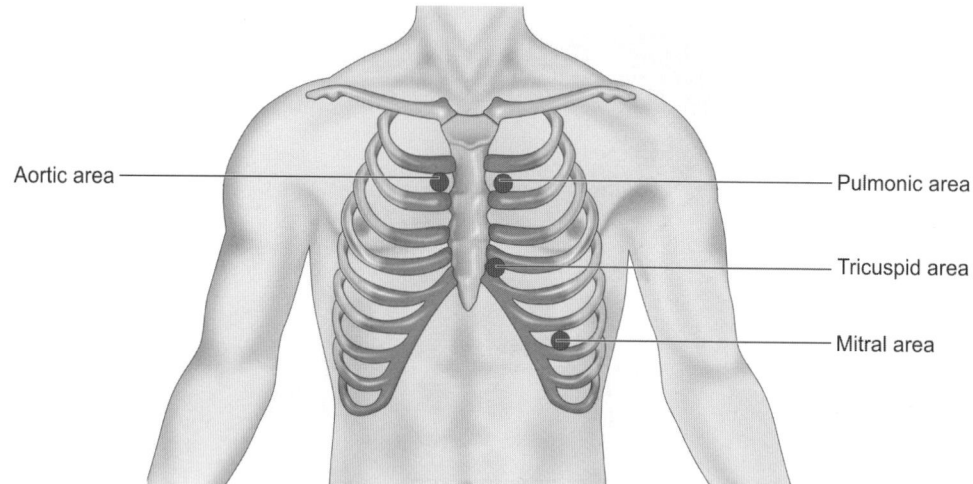

Fig. 2: Areas of cardiac auscultation.

- *Auscultation*: FHS right side, 130 bpm, and regular.
- *Perineal and per speculum examination*: Unremarkable.

Diagnosis after History and Examination

G1 with 34 weeks + 6 days with rheumatic valvular heart disease with mitral stenosis (MS)/mitral regurgitation (MR), NYHA class III, no atrial fibrillation (AF), with normal sinus rhythm, not in failure with single live fetus appropriate for gestational age (AGA), in cephalic presentation, not in labor.

Final Diagnosis after Investigations

G1 with 34 weeks + 6 days with rheumatic valvular heart disease with severe MS/moderate MR, severe TR, severe PAH, with normal biventricular function. NYHA class III, no AF, not in failure with single live fetus, AGA, in cephalic presentation, not in labor.

Q1. What are the hemodynamic changes in pregnancy?

Significant hemodynamic changes occur during pregnancy including:[1,2]
- Reduced peripheral vascular resistance (PVR)
- Reduced pulmonary vascular resistance
- Reduced oncotic pressure
- Increased heart rate
- Increased cardiac output (CO)

These changes begin by 10th week of gestation and peak at about 24–28 weeks.
- Increase in intravascular volume is the most important determinant of increase in CO. In a singleton pregnancy this raise may be up to 50% at 32–36 weeks.
- It is clinically indicated by a benign grade II/III ejection murmur heard parasternally.
- Despite so much increase in intravascular volume, central venous pressure (CVP) does not get affected due to associated reduction in PVR. This is clinically manifested as reduced systemic mean and diastolic pressures.
- Another physiologically important change is increase in aortic root compliance and its size. This may predispose to aortic dissection in patients with pre-existing Marfan's syndrome.

Q2. How does cardiac disease affect pregnancy?

- Pre-existing cardiac disease has profound effects on pregnancy and its outcomes.[3,4] Severity of the cardiac ailment and its resultant functional impairment along with chronic tissue hypoxia determines the risk of fetal morbidity and mortality.
- There is increased risk of IUGR, prematurity, abortion and inheritance of congenital heart disease.
- Maternal congenital heart disease increases the incidence of fetal congenital heart disease by about 8 fold (i.e. 4.5% versus 0.6% in overall population).[3]
- Poor fetal outcome can however be minimized by preconceptional counseling, adequate prenatal care, intensive management of acute heart failure and prolonged hospitalization.
- Risk of fetal mortality remains highest in mothers with cyanotic heart disease. Increased maternal and fetal mortality is associated with Marfan's syndrome due to risk of aortic dissection.

Q3. How does the pregnancy affect cardiac disease?

- The hemodynamic changes occurring during pregnancy increase cardiac work. When this exceeds the limited functional capacity, it may result in congestive heart

failure (CHF) and even death. Maternal mortality risk is up to 15% in severe cardiac ailments.[3]
- Acute decompensation is more likely to occur in association with physiological hemodynamic changes especially around 12–16 weeks of gestation.
- Other most risky period is about 28–32 weeks of gestation when cardiac activity is at its peak.
- Parturition also increases the risk of acute decompensation as each uterine contraction during labor injects 300 to 500 mL of blood into maternal circulation, this increases the cardiac output by about 15–20%. Along with this during 2nd stage of labor, maternal pushing reduces venous return to the heart, thus compromising the cardiac output.
- Another risky period is immediately after delivery and during placental separation when suddenly with release of pressure on the IVC, there is sudden increase in venous return and thus predisposing the heart to acute decompensation.
- Final dangerous period is around 4–5 days after delivery.
- Pulmonary hypertension patients, Eisenmenger's syndrome and cyanotic heart disease may be able to withstand pregnancy, labor and delivery, however they stand an additional risk of sudden death in early postpartum period.

Q4. How are the cardiac lesions stratified according to risk and predictors of cardiac events in pregnancy?

Modified WHO classification of maternal cardiovascular risk:[5]

Risk class	Risk of pregnancy by medical condition
I	No detectable increased risk of maternal mortality and no/mild increase in morbidity.
II	Small increased risk of maternal mortality or moderate increase in morbidity.
III	Significantly increased risk of maternal mortality or severe morbidity. Expert counseling required. If pregnancy is decided upon, intensive specialist cardiac and obstetric monitoring needed throughout pregnancy, childbirth, and the puerperium.
IV	Extremely high risk of maternal mortality or severe morbidity; pregnancy contraindicated. If pregnancy occurs termination should be discussed. If pregnancy continues, care as for class III.

Conditions[5]

WHO I
- Uncomplicated, small or mild
  - Pulmonary stenosis
  - Patent ductus arteriosus
  - Mitral valve prolapse
- Successfully repaired simple lesions (atrial or ventricular septal defect, patent ductus arteriosus, anomalous pulmonary venous drainage).
- Atrial or ventricular ectopic beats, isolated.

WHO II
(if otherwise well and uncomplicated)
- Unoperated atrial or ventricular septal defect
- Repaired tetralogy of Fallot
- Most arrhythmias

WHO II–III (depending on individual)
- Mild left ventricular impairment
- Hypertrophic cardiomyopathy
- Native or tissue valvular heart disease not considered WHO I or IV
- Marfan syndrome without aortic dilatation
- Aorta <45 mm in aortic disease associated with bicuspid aortic valve
- Repaired coarctation.

WHO III
- Mechanical valve
- Systemic right ventricle
- Fontan circulation
- Cyanotic heart disease (unrepaired)
- Other complex congenital heart disease
- Aortic dilatation 40–45 mm in Marfan syndrome
- Aortic dilatation 45–50 mm in aortic disease associated with bicuspid aortic valve.

WHO IV (pregnancy contraindicated)
- Pulmonary arterial hypertension of any cause
- Severe systemic ventricular dysfunction (LVEF <30%, NYHA III–IV)
- Previous peripartum cardiomyopathy with any residual impairment of left ventricular function
- Severe mitral stenosis, severe symptomatic aortic stenosis
- Marfan syndrome with aorta dilated >45 mm
- Aortic dilatation >50 mm in aortic disease associated with bicuspid aortic valve
- Native severe coarctation.

Q5. What are the features suggestive of heart disease in this patient?

Features suggestive of heart failure in this patient include gradually progressive dyspnea and palpitations, NYHA class III on presentation. On examination raised JVP, loud

S1 and P2, mid-diastolic rumble and grade III pan-systolic murmur.

Q6. What are the various differential diagnosis you will consider in this patient?

The differential diagnosis would include:
- Normal pregnancy changes
- Heart disease (most probably RHD with MS/MR)
- Respiratory disease
- Hyperthyroidism

Q7. How would you classify heart disease patients on the basis of NYHA?

NYHA Classification

- **Class I:** No limitation of physical activity. Ordinary physical activity does not cause undue fatigue, palpitation, dyspnea.
- **Class II:** Slight limitation of physical activity. Comfortable at rest. Ordinary physical activity results in fatigue, palpitation, dyspnea.
- **Class III:** Marked limitation of physical activity. Comfortable at rest. Less than ordinary activity causes fatigue, palpitation, or dyspnea.
- **Class IV:** Unable to carry on any physical activity without discomfort. Symptoms of heart failure at rest. If any physical activity is undertaken, discomfort increases.

Q8. When does a pregnant lady with pre-existing heart disease require hospital admission?

- Advanced heart disease, i.e. NYHA class III and IV patients require hospitalization.
- NYHA class I and II need only frequent OPD follow-up. Hospitalization may also be required in pregnant women with heart disease due to:
  - Associated anemia
  - Acute septic conditions
  - Worsening of functional class.

Q9. How do you manage heart failure in this patient?

- Typical symptoms of heart failure are breathlessness, palpitations, anxiety and chest-pain.
- Patient presented as heart failure requires immediate admission and management by a multispeciality team including a senior obstetrician, an anesthetist and a cardiologist.[6,7]
  - Bed rest is of prime importance to reduce the workload of the heart.
  - Propped-up
  - Oxygen by mask, continuous or intermittent
  - Heart rate reduction by beta blockers
  - Calcium channel blockers or digoxin along with diuretics for reduction of preload, i.e. intravenous Furosemide 20 to 40 mg in two to three daily doses.
- Basic cardiac condition may require additional pharmacological agents for management of heart failure, stenotic lesions generally respond to the above management and do not require additional support, whereas regurgitant lesions further require afterload reduction by nitroglycerine or sodium nitroprusside in order to reduce the cardiac workload. In situations where cardiac contractility is reduced, low dose dobutamine helps to improve circulation by its inotropic effect.

Intensive care management may be required in severe heart failure conditions.

Q10. How do you classify mitral stenosis (MS) on the basis of severity?

On the basis of severity MS is classified as:[8]

Stage	Class	Anatomy on ECHO
A	At risk of MS	Rheumatic involvement of the valve, however no significant stenosis
B	Progressive MS	Valve area > 1.5 cm^2
C	Asymptomatic severe MS (Very severe MS)	Valve area < 1.5 cm^2 (valve area < 1.0 cm^2)
D	Symptomatic severe MS (Very severe MS)	Valve area < 1.5 cm^2 (valve area < 1.0 cm^2)

Symptoms include easy fatiguability/decreased exercise tolerance and exertional dyspnea.

Q11. When does such a patient with stenotic lesion require operative cardiac intervention?

- Stenotic lesions, most commonly mitral stenosis may require nonpharmacological intervention which is recommended during the 2nd trimester (20–24 weeks of gestation). Usually mild to moderate mitral stenosis (valve area >1 cm^2) is managed conservatively as discussed above with close follow-up.[8]
- Severe valvular stenosis (i.e valve area <1 cm^2) may not always be manageable with drugs and supportive management and thus may require mechanical relief from stenosis by BMV (balloon mitral valvotomy).
- Surgical valve replacement is indicated in heavily calcified valves, or in those associated with significant valvular regurgitation and or presence of large atrial thrombi.
- Postoperative cases require additional care and need frequent monitoring for recurrence of symptoms and comorbidities like anemia or hyper/hypothyroidism.

- Valve replacement patients require prolonged anticoagulation through the pregnancy and beyond.

Q12. What is the role of induction of labor in such a patient?

- Induction of labor has a limited role in cardiac patients.[2] Concentrated oxytocin and artificial rupture of membrane (ARM) are indicated when Bishop's score is favorable, though ARM should be done in carefully selected cases under strict asepsis.
- Long induction time should be avoided, it increases risk of emergency cesarean section and risk of infection.
- Dinoprostone may be used for induction of labor in selected cases (NYHA I and II).
- In higher class (NYHA III and IV)—improve cardiac condition and review decision for induction.
- Mechanical methods like Foley's catheter for induction of labor may be used in selected cases.

Q13. How would you manage labor in this patient?

First Stage

- First stage is to be managed conservatively with patient kept in left lateral position with frequent vitals monitoring.
- Oxygen/propped up/optimum sedation and analgesia/hydration
- Periodic chest auscultation to pick up signs of heart failure is required. Restriction of IV fluids and to avoid tocolytics.
- Strict intake output monitoring, to avoid fluid overload, is to be done.
- Prophylactic antibiotics may be given as appropriate.
- Periodic assessment of fetal wellbeing is to be done.
- Continuous pulse oxymetry and CVP monitoring may also be required in advanced heart failure.
- Per vaginal examination, if required, is to be done under strict asepsis and artificial rupture of membranes is to be delayed or avoided.
- Adequate pain management with opioids (tramodol/morphine) is appropriate to allay anxiety and to reduce sympathetic drive. Care should be taken to check the availability of Naloxone in situations of overdose/effect of morphine so as to prevent fetal respiratory depression.

Second Stage

- In second stage of labor all these intensive monitoring and care should be continued.
- Its duration definitely needs to be cut short. Assisted vaginal delivery by either vacuum or forceps may be done as required.

Third Stage

- Third stage of labor is the most dangerous period for development of acute pulmonary edema especially in cases with mitral stenosis as well as those with compromised LV systolic function. Hence timely administration of diuretics (furosemide 20–40 mg IV 8 hourly) is essential and adequate pain management with sedation and opioids is required. It is recommended to avoid methergin during this stage in patients with heart disease to prevent sudden cardiac overload.
- Immediate postpartum period also requires strict monitoring to prevent and manage heart failure.

Q14. What are the indications of caesarean section in such a patient?

- Vaginal delivery is the preferred in majority patients.
- Cesarean section is required:[7]
    - All obstetric indications
    - Coarctation of aorta
    - Marfan's syndrome (aortic root > 45 mm)
    - Patients with acute decompensations
    - Preterm patients going into labor while on anticoagulation with warfarin can be considered for LSCS to prevent intracranial hemorrhage in preterm baby.
- In some centers a cesarean section is preferred in cases of:
    - Severe aortic stenosis
    - Severe PAH and
    - Acute heart failure.

Q15. How would you manage if there was AF in this case?

- AF presents as palpitation, chest pain, sweating, anxiety. In presence of mitral stenosis it can cause deranged hemodynamic changes as tachycardia, reduces diastolic filling time in an otherwise low output state and further compromises LV filling.
- Patient should be optimized with drugs to stabilize cardiac rhythm.[8]
- ECG, Echo, ABG, serum electrolytes should be done promptly to rule out clots in atrium and other reasons for the symptoms.
- Preferred strategy in such cases is rate control instead of rhythm control with target heart rate of 60–70 bpm.
- Anticoagulation is also recommended in severe cases with AF with complications.

Q16. Does this patient require Infective endocarditis prophylaxis (IE)?

- There is no recommendation to give routine endocarditis prophylaxis to this patient during labor or cesarean, as

per the latest guidelines. It is no longer recommended for gastrointestinal or genitourinary procedures.[7,8]
- Only specific groups considered high risk for IE require routine prophylaxis, these include:[7,8]
  - Patients with prosthetic valves.
  - Patients with history of previous IE.
  - Patients with congenital heart disease only for:
    - Unrepaired cyanotic CHD and those with palliative shunts/conduits
    - Completely repaired defects with prosthetic material or device during first 6 months postprocedure
    - Repaired CHD with residual defects, at the site or with prosthetic material.
  - Cardiac transplant recipients with valve disease
- Antibiotics routinely given for prophylaxis are given 30 to 60 minutes prior to the procedure.
- These include oral amoxicillin 2 g or clindamycin 600 mg in those sensitive to penicillin.
- In patients unable to take orally, intravenous 2 g ampicillin or 1 g cefazolin/ceftriaxone can be given and intravenous clindamycin 600 mg in those sensitive to penicillin and cephalosporin.

Q17. What are the recommendations for secondary prevention of rheumatic fever?

- Secondary prevention is required for established rheumatic valvular heart disease for 10 years or up to the age of 40 years (whichever is longer).[8]
- It is done by injection penidura 1.2 million units, deep IM every 3–4 weeks.
- In those intolerant to penicillin, macrolides, i.e. erythromycin 250 mg twice daily can be safely used as an alternative with similar efficacy.

Q18. What is the role of anticoagulation?

- Anticoagulation is indicated in this patient complicated by occurrence of AF or those having a mechanical prosthetic valve.[8]
- Oral anticoagulants (OACs), due to their efficacy are preferred over UFH (unfractionated heparin) and low molecular weight heparin (LMWH) for prevention of thrombotic events in pregnancy.
- UFH and LMWH are not used throughout pregnancy even though they are safer for fetus, because of the high-risk of thrombosis.
- However, if dose of Warfarin is ≥5 mg and that of Acitrom is ≥2 mg daily, patient should be shifted to heparin between 6–12 weeks of pregnancy because of risk of embryopathy (like nasal hypoplasia, hypertelorism, frontal bone prominence, short stature, CNS abnormalities and stippling of epiphysis).
- In the last 4 weeks OACs are again switched over to UHF/LMWH, so as to prevent bleeding complications in both mother and newborn.

Q19. Management of labor in patient already on anticoagulation?

- During labor the anticoagulation effect needs to be reversed with fresh frozen plasma in patients who have been taking OACs right through. Vitamin K may also be given if vaginal delivery is imminent.
- Although fetal risk of anticoagualtion persists for up to 1 to 2 weeks after discontinuation of the drug. Newborn may require replacement with FFP and vitamin K.
- Unfractionated heparin on the other hand requires to be discontinued 4 to 6 hours prior to the labor to reverse its effect and LMWH requires to be discontinued 12 hours prior to labor.
- For patients going into labor or requiring cesarean without discontinuation of heparin, protamine sulfate (1 mg for every 100 IU of heparin) is to be administered as an antidote.

Q20. What is the role of preconceptional counseling in a woman with cardiac ailment?

- Preconceptional counseling has a very important role in optimizing the maternal and fetal outcomes in women with cardiac ailment.[3,4,9]
- All women with cardiac disease in the reproductive age group should be enquired about their desire to conceive whenever they come in contact with health system.
- Counseling may be provided by an obstetrician, a medical specialist and a cardiologist.
- It is imperative to first evaluate her present cardiac condition, classify her functionally and stratify her into disease risk category as per modified WHO classification of maternal cardiovascular risk.
- She should be counseled regarding need of extensive investigations during pregnancy, increased number of hospital visits, prolonged hospital stay and need for strict compliance with management.
- Her cardiac condition needs to be optimized before conception which may require need for cardiac surgical procedures, modification of medication to safer drugs in pregnancy with nonteratogenic and lesser detrimental effects on the fetus.

- She should be explained about the need for anticoagulation and IE prophylaxis as and when required.
- Women with complex cardiac lesions need to be booked and delivered at tertiary centers with multidisciplinary care.
- She also needs to be counseled regarding the risks of worsening of cardiac condition and obstetric complications during antenatal, intrapartum and postpartum period.
- Risk of fetal transmission in case she suffers from congenital heart disease is to be assessed by involving geneticist and counseling done accordingly.
- Women with maternal cardiovascular risk category IV need to be informed of the very high risk of adverse outcome, counseled to avoid pregnancy and consider the option of adoption.

Q21. What contraceptive method is ideal for your patient?

CDC in 2010 has modified the MEC for contraception use by WHO in patients with cardiovascular diseases (CVDs).[2]

- Natural methods, like calendar method or withdrawal method are safe but ineffective due to higher failure rates.
- Condoms/barrier method are highly safe in cardiac patients and are recommended.
- Combined OCPs are not recommended (WHO-MEC-3) in cardiac patients due to high-risk of thromboembolic events.
- DMPA are not recommended in patients with heart failure due to risk of retention of fluid.
- Progesterone only implants/LNG IUCDs are considered safe and most efficient option for women having PAH and cyanotic heart disease, but to be applied in hospital settings due to risk of vasovagal reactions in complex CVD.
- Copper IUCD is an accepted option in mildly cyanotic and acyanotic disease. Routine IE prophylaxis is not advised for insertion or removal of implant/IUCDs.
- Sterilization is a safe method used at family completion, preferably by mini-laparotomy.
- Vasectomy of husband is an effective option but one should also keep in mind the longterm prognosis of the female with heart disease.

CASE SCENARIO

G2P1L1A0 with 8 months amenorrhea

Mrs A, 25 years old, wife of Mr B, resident of Loni, a housewife, came to gynecology casualty on 10/07/2017 with complaints of:
- Amenorrhea 8 months
- Breathlessness since 10 days
- Palpitations since 10 days
- Leg swelling since 10 days

Her LMP was 15/11/2016 so making her period of gestation 33 weeks and 5 days on 10/7/2017.

History of Present Pregnancy

Spontaneous conception, planned pregnancy. Pregnancy confirmed by UPT on day 7 of missed period. Patient was booked antenatal case at private hospital since 4 months amenorrhea. She got all her routine antenatal investigations done at 5 month amenorrhea including level II USG which were normal. She was compliant with oral iron tablets and calcium supplementation and immunized with two doses tetanus toxoid. The patient had an uneventful antenatal period until last 10 days when she started having sudden onset respiratory discomfort which had progressed to breathlessness at rest with orthopnea and paroxysmal nocturnal dyspnea since last 3 days. She also complained of palpitations and progressive bilateral leg swelling since 10 days. No associated complaint of chest pain, hemoptysis. She did not give history of any underlying medical ailments or allergies, fever, cough with or without expectoration, any blood loss, joint swelling, urinary or bowel complaints.

Course in the Hospital

- She was admitted to high dependency unit (HDU) after her general physical and abdominal examination.
- Her blood samples complete blood count, arterial blood gas analysis, liver function test, kidney function test, serum electrolytes was taken.
- ECG, chest X-ray with abdominal shield, and 2D echo-were done. Nonstress test for fetus was done.

She was put on:
- Bed rest
- Prop-up position
- Oxygen by mask
- Injection Lasix 40 mg IV given
- Urgent physician and cardiologist consultation was taken.

Obstetric History

Married since 5 years.

G2P1L1A0

- G1: Booked at private hospital in Loni at two month amenorrhea, immunized, had an uneventful antenatal period, went into spontaneous labor 2 days prior to expected date of delivery had a normal vaginal delivery with episiotomy. Delivered a baby girl weighing 2.7 kg, postnatal period was uneventful. Discharged in satisfactory condition on the second postpartum day.
- G 2: Present pregnancy

On Examination

Patient is conscious, oriented, dyspneic.
- GC: Poor
- Weight: 62 kg.
- Height: 154 cm.
- BMI: Not calculated as prepregnancy weight is not known.
- Pallor: Absent
- Icterus: Absent
- Cyanosis: Absent
- Clubbing: Absent
- Pedal edema: Pitting 3+.
- Pulse rate: 120 per minute, regular, rhythmic, all peripheral pulses palpable, no radiofemoral delay.
- Respiratory rate: 34/min.
- Thyroid: Normal
- JVP: Raised up to 8 cm
- Lymph nodes: Not palpable.
- Respiratory system: Patient was dyspneic with respiratory rate of 34/minute, trachea central, bilateral crepts with decreased air entry at the lung bases.

Cardiovascular System

- *Inspection*: Hyperkinetic precordium, no visible pulsations, no dilated veins/scars, no scoliosis, no signs of rheumatic activity (arthralgia/arthritis, erythematous rash, subcutaneous nodules, abnormal movements), no signs of infective endocarditis.
- *Palpation*: Apex beat is in the 6th intercostal space lateral to mid clavicular line, palpable S3, no S4, no palpable thrill, no left parasternal heave, no epigastric pulsations.
- *Percussion*: Right margin of cardiac dullness is retrosternal, left margin confirms to the apex.

Auscultation

- *Apex*: S1 is soft, audible S3, no murmur, no adventitious sounds.
- *Tricuspid area*: S1 soft, no audible S3/S4. No murmur.
- *Aortic area*: S2 normal intensity, normally split, S3 gallop present. No S4, no murmur.
- *Pulmonary area*: S2 normally split (A2-P2) normally split, no S3/S4, no murmur.

Abdominal Examination

Within normal limits.

Diagnosis after Examination

G2P1L1A0 with POG 33 week 5 days with single live fetus, cephalic presentation with peripartum cardiomyopathy NYHA class IV.

Investigation Reports

- Electrocardiography revealed sinus tachycardia, nonspecific ST segment and T wave abnormalities.
- Echocardiography showed global hypokinesia with dilated left ventricle with severe systolic left ventricular dysfunction, ejection fraction 30%.
- Chest radiograph (with abdominal shield) showed cardiomegaly, pulmonary edema, with bilateral pleural effusion.

Q1. What are the differential diagnosis in this case?

The differential diagnosis include:
- Peripartum cardiomyopathy (PPCM)
- Acute pulmonary embolism
- Acute pulmonary edema
- Acute viral fevers
- Acute lung conditions—pneumothorax.

Q2. What are the diagnostic criteria for PPCM?

Peripartum cardiomyopathy is a diagnosis of exclusion, with no other identifiable cause for heart failure. The diagnostic criteria are:
- Systolic dysfunction leading to heart failure in the later part of pregnancy or in the first 5 months postpartum
- No known cardiac ailment before the presentation in last trimester
- 2D echo shows features of global hypokinesia with left ventricular ejection fraction of <45%, may or may not show dilatation of left ventricle.

This condition should also be thought of when the cardiac parameters do not revert back to normal prepregnancy state after delivery.

Q3. What are the probable causes and risk factors for PPCM?

- The causes of peripartum cardiomyopathy largely remain unclear though infections, inflammation, and autoimmune causes are thought to play some role.
- PPCM is thought to be the resultant effect of unbalanced oxidative stress ending in proteolytic breakdown of prolactin hormone to angiostatic and pro-apoptotic products.
- Predisposing factors[10] are:
  - Multiparity
  - Family history
  - Ethnicity
  - Diabetes
  - Hypertensive disease
  - Preeclampsia
  - Extremes of reproductive age groups (teenage/advanced age)
  - Malnutrition.

Q4. How will you manage this case of PPCM?

- Mainstay of management in such a case is treating heart failure:
  - The prime therapy starts with bed rest, avoiding supine position, adequate oxygenation, restricting fluid intake.
  - Diuretics are administered to reduce preload, i.e. injection furosemide (Category C) 40 mg IV followed by 20 mg IV 8 hourly.
  - Low dose beta-blockers are of benefit to control heart rate and reduce cardiac workload.
  - After load reduction is done by reducing systemic vascular resistance and achieving vasodilatation with agents like hydralazine (Category B), as ACE inhibitors and ARBs are contraindicated in pregnancy.
  - Inotrops may be required to improve cardiac contractility in cases with hemodynamic instability. Digoxin (Category C) can also be used in partly compensated patients, after ruling out arrhythmias.
- Anticoagulation is considered in patients with LVEF of <25% or in cases with thrombotic event.
- Steroid cover is given for fetal lung maturity.
- Close maternal and fetal monitoring is required and patient is to be kept in HDU/ICU.
- Patients who worsen despite medical therapy require invasive monitoring (right heart catheterization) and should be delivered irrespective of fetal maturity.
- Vaginal delivery is recommended for pregnant patients who develop serious heart failure in the third trimester.
- Cesarean section is reserved for obstetric indications only.

Q5. How will you prognosticate this patient?

- The prognosis of patients with PPCM is directly related to the improvement in LVEF.
- The risk of mortality ranges between 25% to 50 % and half of these occur within a period of three months after delivery.
- Cardiomegaly and cardiac congestion resolve in half of the patients with PPCM by 6 months postpartum with almost 100% survival chances.
- On the other hand, in cases with persisting cardiomyopathy even after 6 months, there is a very high 5 year mortality rate of up to 85%.

Q6. How will you counsel this patient for future pregnancy?

- Future pregnancy has a high-risk of recurrence for PPCM, up to 30% to 50 %. In cases where there has not been a complete resolution of cardiac congestion and recovery of LV function, patients should be discouraged for subsequent conception.[11]
- Where the EF is fully normalized, patient should be counseled as there is a risk of recurrence with next conception.

CASE SCENARIO

A 25 years old female, married for 2 years, primigravida, a diagnosed case of VSD with Eisenmenger's syndrome since 10 years, NYHA III, presented to the OPD at 28 weeks of pregnancy with a single live intrauterine fetus appropriate for gestational age.

On Examination

- Patient has cyanosis, clubbing and pedal edema.
- Her pulse rate is 108 per minute, low volume, regular and synchronous
- Blood pressure is 100/70 mm Hg, respiratory rate of 27/min.
- Precordial examination is unremarkable on inspection.
- On palpation apex beat is in 6th intercostals space lateral to mid-clavicular line (evidence of cardiomegaly), there is grade II parasternal heave with palpable

P2. Percussion confirmed the cardiac borders. On auscultation the S1 is normal. P2 is loud with a short early diastolic murmur in pulmonary area.

2D echocardiography done 2 days back showed dilated LA/LV. Large VSD with bidirectional flow, severe PAH, mild PR with normal biventricular function. O_2 saturation is 86% on room air.

Q1. How will you prognosticate and manage a woman with Eisenmenger's syndrome in pregnancy?

- Women with Eisenmenger's syndrome have a very poor fetomaternal outcome with a high maternal mortality rate of up to 20–50% and fetal live birth occurs only in <12% of pregnancies if the maternal oxygen saturation <85%. The woman in such a case should be advised termination of pregnancy if she is in the first trimester of pregnancy. However, if she decides to continue pregnancy or comes in her second or third trimester, she needs special care and fetomaternal monitoring in consultation with the cardiologist.
- The management includes:
  - Bed rest to reduce workload
  - Avoiding supine position
  - Avoidance of hemoconcentration by adequate hydration
  - Supplemental oxygen
  - Diuretics to be used judiciously, avoiding hemoconcentration
  - Anticoagulants, with caution as there is a tendency for hemoptysis and thrombocytopenia
  - Digitalis in case of ventricular dysfunction to improve contractility.
- There is a tendency of iron deficiency anemia, hence special care needs to be taken for oral iron supplementation and if required parenteral therapy be given.
- The cardiac condition is monitored by frequently measuring oxygen saturation and complete blood counts.
- Fetal growth restriction and poor fetal outcomes are common to this condition due to reduced uteroplacental perfusion and low maternal oxygen saturation. Hence fetal growth monitoring is mandatory, as is administration of antenatal corticosteroids for fetal lung maturity anticipating need of early delivery.
- Delivery should be electively planned with avoidance of prolonged induction and labor with epidural analgesia. Vaginal delivery is a safer option but cesarean may be required in cases with extreme growth restriction or sudden deterioration.
- Despite all precautions and monitoring there is a high-risk of sudden death during labor and early postpartum phase due to thromboembolic event, hypovolemia, right heart failure and arrhythmias.
- Role of antenatal sildenafil, prostanoids and phophodiesterase inhibitors and intra-partum nitric oxide inhalation, PGE1 nebulization have shown better outcomes in few case reports.[12,13]

Q2. What is the risk of inheritance of congenital heart disease in the offspring?

- The risk of inheritance of congenital heart disease is much higher than in general population. It varies between 3% and 50% depending upon the underlying maternal cardiac lesion.[14]
- The autosomal dominantly inherited defects like Marfan's syndrome and hypertrophic cardiomyopathy have a inheritance risk of 50%.
- Every woman with a congenital heart disease should undergo a fetal echocardiography between 18 weeks and 22 weeks of pregnancy to rule out cardiac defects in the baby.
- Genetic counseling is done to assess risk of inheritance, testing with dual marker, nuchal translucency scan and if required invasive testing may be offered as per the merit of the case.

Q3. What are the factors affecting pregnancy outcome in patients with congenital heart disease?

- The outcome of pregnancy in women with congenital heart disease is determined by various factors like:
  - Complexity of underlying heart disease
  - Ventricular function
  - Valvular condition
  - Functional class of the woman
  - Presence of cyanosis
  - Severity of associated PAH
  - Previous cardiac corrective surgery
  - Development of pregnancy related complications like preeclampsia.
- Maternal cardiac adverse events are seen to occur in around 12% completed pregnancies.[15]
- The fetal and neonatal complications occur frequently and mortality is reported to be around 4%.
- Women with uncorrected lesions, cyanosis with saturation of <85%, severe PAH, severe left outflow obstruction have poor fetomaternal outcomes and should be advised against conception.

REFERENCES

1. Cunningham GF, Leveno JK, Bloom LS, et al. Williams obstetrics, 24th edition. Cardiovascular disorders. 973-99.
2. Regitz-Zagrosek V, Blomstrom CL, Borghi C, et al. ESC guidelines on the management of cardiovascular diseases during pregnancy. Eur H J. 2011;32:3147-97.
3. Phadke SM, Jaiswal RV. Cardiac disease and pregnancy, Arias' practical guide to high risk pregnancy and delivery. 2014; 268-85.
4. De Swiet's Medical Disorders in Obstetric Practice. Heart disease in pregnancy. Wiley-Blackwell. 2015;5:118-52.
5. Thorne S, MacGregor A, Nelson-Piercy C. Risks of contraception and pregnancy in heart disease. Heart. 2006;92:1520-5.
6. William Ledger, Clark J. Recent advances in Obstetrics & Gynaecology. 25, 2015.
7. Nanna M, Kathleen Stergiopoulos K. Pregnancy Complicated by Valvular Heart Disease: An Update. J Am Heart Assoc. 2014; 3: e000712.
8. Nishimura RA, Otto CM, Bonow RO, et al. 2014 AHA/ACC Guideline for the Management of Patients With Valvular Heart Disease. J Am Coll Card. (2014). doi: 10.1016/j.jacc.2014.02.536.
9. Cardiac disease in pregnancy: Good practice guidelines. Green-top guidelines No.13, RCOG. June 2011.
10. Sliwa K, Fett J, Elkayam U. Peripartum cardiomyopathy. Lancet. 2006;368:687-93.
11. Habli M, O'Brien T, Nowack E, et al. Peripartum cardiomyopathy: prognostic factors for long-term maternal outcome. Am J Obstet Gynecol 2008;199:415 e411–e5.
12. Cartago R, Alan PA, Benedicto J. Pregnancy outcomes in patients with severe pulmonary hypertension and Eisenmenger syndrome treated with sildenafil monotherapy. Chest. 2014;142(4)(suppl):999A.
13. Siddiqui S, Latif N. PGE1 nebulisation during caesarean section for Eisenmenger's syndrome a case report. J Med Case Rep. 2008;2:149.
14. Pierpont ME, Basson CT, Benson DW Jr, et al. Genetic basis for congenital heart defects: current knowledge: a scientific statement from the American Heart Association Congenital Cardiac Defects Committee, Council on Cardiovascular Disease in the Young: endorsed by the American Academy of Pediatrics. Circulation. 2007;115:3015-38.
15. Balint OH, Siu SC, Mason J, et al. Cardiac outcomes after pregnancy in women with congenital heart disease. Heart. 2010;96:1656-61.

19
CHAPTER

Thyroid Diseases in Pregnancy

Deepti Goswami, Chinmoyee Sonowal

HYPOTHYROIDISM IN PREGNANCY

CASE SCENARIO

Mrs RB aged 34 years, a homemaker, educated till 12th class, resident of a colony near Lok Nayak Hospital, New Delhi has presented to the antenatal clinic with 4 months of amenorrhea (period of gestation by USG done at 6 weeks—15 weeks 3 days).

Brief Details of this and Previous Pregnancies

- This is her fourth pregnancy. She had uneventful first trimester with occasional complain of nausea. She was taking one tablet of folic acid daily as per the advice of her local doctor.
- Her first pregnancy resulted in a normal term vaginal delivery in January 2014. She had a spontaneous abortion at three months of gestation in her second pregnancy in March 2016. Her third pregnancy also ended in a spontaneous abortion at two months of gestation in December 2016.
- She reports history of prolonged menstrual cycle of 45-60 days after first childbirth. She had breastfed her first born for six months after birth.
- She had never used any contraceptive.
- She has no known medical or surgical disorder.

Examination

- Her vital signs (normal blood pressure), general physical and systemic examinations were unremarkable.
- Abdominal examination showed gravid uterus with fundal height corresponding to 16 weeks of gestation.

Investigations

Apart from the ultrasound report other investigations done so far were:
- Blood group: B+
- Hb: 12 g%
- Hematocrit: 37
- Blood glucose random: 85 mg%
- Infection screen (HIV, HBsAg, VDRL): negative
- Serum TSH: 10.5 mIU/L (normal range, 0.4–5.0 mIU/L)
- Urine (routine, microscopy, culture): No abnormality detected.

Q1. What is your diagnosis?

This woman is 15 weeks pregnant with hypothyroidism.

Q2. How common is thyroid disease in reproductive age group women?

Thyroid disease is the second most common endocrinological disorder in women of reproductive age group; first being diabetes mellitus.

Q3. How is hypothyroidism diagnosed in pregnancy?

Hypothyroidism is diagnosed during pregnancy by measuring serum thyroid stimulating hormone (TSH) level. If the TSH level is abnormally high, free T4 concentration should be measured. A high TSH and a low free T4 levels are diagnostic of overt hypothyroidism. Ideally, when available, pregnancy and population specific reference levels should be referred to.

Previous recommendations based on initial studies in the US and Europe:
- 1st trimester —0.1–2.5 mU/L
- 2nd trimester—0.2–3.0 mU/L
- 3rd trimester—0.3–3.0 mU/L

Latest recommendations of American Thyroid Association (ATA), 2017;[1]

These recommendation take into consideration:
a. The published studies from India, China, Korea and the Netherlands.
b. Observation that reduction in FT4 occurs only when the serum TSH is more than 4.8 mU/L

Recommendation for first trimester:
- Lower reference range for TSH can be reduced by 0.4 mU/L
- Upper reference range for TSH can be reduced by 0.5 mU/L

In absolute terms:
- First trimester (from 7–12 weeks onwards)—upper-reference limit for TSH to be 4.0 mU/L
- Second and third trimester—gradual return towards the non-pregnant range

Elevated TSH and decreased serum T4 and T3 levels indicate overt hypothyroidism while isolated raised TSH and normal serum thyroxine (total or free T4) indicate sub-clinical hypothyroidism.

Indian studies have reported different trimester specific values of TSH.[2]

Q4. What is the incidence of various thyroid disorders in pregnancy?

Overt hypothyroidism affects 1% of pregnant women while subclinical hypothyroidism affects 3–15% of pregnancies. Overt hyperthyroidism affects 0.2% of pregnant women and 95% of them have a diagnosis of Grave's disease. Subclinical hyperthyroidism is found in 1.7% of pregnant women.

Q5. How does a pregnant woman with hypothyroidism present?

The woman may be asymptomatic or may report nonspecific symptoms which are often confused with that of normal pregnancy.

The signs and symptoms are as follows:

Symptoms	Signs
Fatigue	Goiter
Weakness	Hypothermia
Weight gain	Bradycardia
Constipation	Hyporeflexia
Cold intolerance	Prolonged relaxation phase of deep tendon
Dry skin	Reflexes
Hair loss	Periorbital edema
Hoarseness of voice	Edema
Edema	Enlargement of tongue
Muscle cramps	Diastolic hypertension
Intellectual slowness	Enlargement of tongue
Insomnia	Hair loss
Depression	Pleural and pericardial effusion
Paresthesias	Carpal tunnel syndrome
Dry gritty feeling eyes	

Q6. What are the causes of hypothyroidism?

The various causes of hypothyroidism are as follows:

Primary Hypothyroidism
- Autoimmune hypothyroidism (Hashimoto's thyroiditis, atrophic thyroiditis)
- Iodine deficiency
- Drugs (lithium, amiodarone, antithyroid medications, p-aminosalicylic acid, etc.)
- Subacute de Quervains thyroiditis
- Postpartum thyroiditis
- Following thyroidectomy, radio-iodine therapy, external irradiation of neck for thyroid tumors
- Congenital hypothyroidism.

Secondary Hypothyroidism
- Hypothalamic or pituitary tumor, surgery, radiation
- Sheehan's syndrome
- Lymphocytic hypophysitis.

Hashimoto's thyroiditis is an autoimmune disorder characterized by glandular destruction by autoantibodies, particularly antithyroid peroxidase (anti-TPO) and anti-thyroglobulin (anti-Tg) antibodies. There is diffuse atrophy of the gland, which is replaced by dense fibrotic bands of collagen.

Q7. What are the risks associated with hypothyroidism in pregnancy?

The risks are maternal as well as fetal

Maternal	Fetal
Spontaneous abortion	Fetal growth restriction/low birthweight babies
Gestational hypertension preeclampsia, eclampsia	Congenital malformation
Abruption	Fetal death
Preterm delivery	
Anemia	
Myxedema coma	

Q8. What is the risk of fetal loss in hypothyroidism in pregnancy?

Women with inadequately treated overt hypothyroidism carry 60% risk of fetal loss.[3]

Q9. What is the incidence of gestational hypertension in hypothyroidism?

One of the studies has reported this incidence to be 22% in overt hypothyroidism and 15% in subclinical hypothyroidism as compared to 7.6% in general population.[4]

Q10. What is the most serious complication of hypothyroidism in pregnancy?

Myxedema coma is the most serious complication of hypothyroidism but is a rare medical emergency in pregnancy. It has a mortality rate of 20%. Clinical picture may comprise of feature of hypothyroidism along with altered consciousness, hyponatremia, hypoglycemia, hypoxia, hypercapnia. Once diagnosis is made, treatment should begin immediately with supportive care and thyroid hormone replacement. Symptoms usually improve after 12 to 24 hours of therapy.

Q11. What are the long-term effects on the children of women with hypothyroidism in pregnancy?

Thyroid hormone plays important role in neuronal migration and myelination during fetal brain development and postnatally. Delayed mental and motor development at 1 and 2 years of age was reported in children of women with hypothyroxinemia at 12 weeks of gestation.[5] Impaired neuropsychiatric development and low IQ at 8 ± 1 years of age has been reported in the offspring of hypothyroid mothers and treating maternal hypothyroidism in the first 12 weeks of pregnancy improves the outcome.[6] Cretinism characterized by deaf mutism, spastic motor disorder and hypothyroidism is a severe form of brain damage caused by severe maternal iodine deficiency.

Q12. How will you manage a case of hypothyroidism in pregnancy?

Overt hypothyroidism is treated with the oral levothyroxine in dose of 1–2 μg/kg daily or an initial dose of 12.5–25 μg/day (FDA category A).[7] Patients with pre-existing hypothyroidism in whom thyroid assessment cannot be done immediately should increase the dose of levothyroxine by 30% when pregnancy is diagnosed (2 additional tablet/week, i.e. 9 tab/week instead of 7).

Therapy is monitored by measuring TSH levels (instead of free T4) every 4 to 6 week. The levothyroxine dose is increased by 25 to 50 μg increments until normal TSH values are achieved. The aim is to maintain maternal TSH concentration below 2.5 mIU/L. If TSH levels are stable on treatment, checking thyroid function in each trimester will suffice. If dosage changes are implemented then TSH levels should be measured after 4 to 6 weeks. More frequent testing every 2 weekly may be required for poor control.

Q13. What all should be explained to the woman regarding treatment with levothyroxine?

It should be administered preferably on an empty stomach 30–45 minutes before breakfast since food, caffeine, milk, sucralfate, proton pump inhibitors, iron and calcium supplements decrease its absorption. Oral levothyroxine and iron supplements intake should be separated by at least 4 hours.

Iodine rich foods should be consumed which include seafood, milk and milk products, eggs, banana, green leafy vegetables, sweet potato along with iodized salt. The Institute of Medicine recommends daily dietary intake of 150 μg of iodine for reproductive age group women, 220 μg for pregnant women and 290 μg for lactating women.[8]

Q14. Is there a role of termination of pregnancy?

There are no recommendations for termination of pregnancy at any gestation even if patient is severely hypothyroid.

Q15. How will you manage her after delivery?

Following delivery, levothyroxine should be reduced to the patient's preconception dose in case of pre-existing hypothyroidism. In case of hypothyroidism diagnosed during pregnancy, dose of levothyroxine is to be reduced by 30% or 2/3rd of the final dose that she was taking during pregnancy. Thyroid function should be tested at 6 weeks postpartum.

Q16. What is subclinical hypothyroidism? What is its significance in pregnancy?

Subclinical hypothyroidism (SCH) describes those patients who have high TSH and normal thyroxine concentration with no obvious symptoms or signs of thyroid dysfunction.

It is increasingly appearing in literature because of a suggested association with adverse obstetric outcome. Stagnaro Green reported that subclinical hypothyroidism with elevated TSH (>3 mIU/L) was associated with increased risk of very preterm delivery (<32 weeks).[9] Negro et al. reported that SCH with antibody positive not on treatment had a higher pregnancy complication rate (pregnancy loss—13.8%, preterm delivery—22.4%) than those on treatment (3.5%). Hypertension, pre-eclampsia, placental abruption did not vary between the groups. They concluded that T4 supplementation should occur early.[10] Reports from other studies did not find any association between SCH in 1st or 2nd trimester with adverse obstetric outcome.[11] An RCT of 21,800 pregnant women with untreated subclinical hypothyroidism found no effect on cognitive function of children at 3 years of age.[12] Data from RCTs are lacking regarding whether or not intervention improved outcome in SCH.

Q17. Should women be tested universally for thyroid function before or during pregnancy?

There has been a difference of opinion regarding whether universal screening should be recommended for thyroid dysfunction in pregnancy. The American Thyroid Association (ATA) and American Association of Clinical Endocrinologists (AACE) recommend selective screening and not universal screening.[1] The ACOG and the Society for Maternal-Fetal Medicine are against universal screening for thyroid disease in pregnancy. Cochrane review states that universal screening does not clearly impact maternal and infant outcomes (Table 1).

The ATA recommends that all patients seeking pregnancy or newly pregnant should undergo clinical evaluation. If any of the following risk factors are present, testing for serum TSH is recommended:

- A history of hypothyroidism or hyperthyroidism or current symptoms or signs of thyroid dysfunction.
- Known thyroid antibody positivity or prior thyroid surgery
- History of head or neck radiation or prior thyroid surgery
- All women >30 years old
- Type I diabetes or other autoimmune disorders
- History of pregnancy loss, preterm delivery, or infertility
- Multiple prior pregnancies (>2)
- Family history of thyroid disease or autoimmune disorders
- Morbid obesity (body mass index >40 kg/m^2)
- Use of amiodarone or lithium or recent administration of iodinated radiologic contrast
- Residing in an area of known moderate to severe iodine insufficiency.

Table 1: Recommendations of various professional bodies regarding universal screening for thyroid dysfunction in pregnancy

Professional source	Recommendation
American Thyroid Association[1], 2017	Selective screening
The Endocrine Society,[13] 2012	• Two versions since concensus could not be reached: • Some members recommended universal screening of all pregnant women (serum TSH) by the ninth week or at first antenatal visit. (USPSTF recommendation level: C) • Other members were neither or nor against universal screening, however they strongly supported aggressive case finding to identify and test high-risk women
Society for Maternal-Fetal Medicine,[14] 2014	• Routine thyroid screening in pregnancy is not recommended • Thyroid testing in pregnancy should be conducted for women "at risk," including known thyroid disease • Symptoms of overt thyroid disease, suspected goiter, autoimmune medical disorders such as Type 1 diabetes mellitus
ACOG,[15] 2015	Universal screening for thyroid disease in pregnancy is not recommended because identification and treatment of maternal subclinical hypothyroidism has not been shown to result in improved neurocognitive function in offspring. Thyroid function testing is indicated for women with a personal history of or symptoms of thyroid disease
COCHRANE Review,[16] 2015	Universal screening for thyroid dysfunction does not clearly impact (benefit or harm) maternal and infant outcomes

HYPERTHYROIDISM IN PREGNANCY

CASE SCENARIO

A primigravida presents at 20 weeks of pregnancy for antenatal checkup. She complains of heat intolerance and palpitations.

Examination

- Pulse: 105/min
- Blood pressure: 130/80 mm Hg
- General and systemic examination: unremarkable
- Uterus enlarged corresponding to period of gestation.

Investigations

She had been investigated from elsewhere and carried a thyroid function report of:
- S-TSH: 0.033 mIU/L (normal range, 0.4 to 5.0 mIU/L)
- Free T4: 33 pmol/L (normal range, 7.7 to 15.4 pmol/L)
- Her other laboratory investigations were normal
- Ultrasound done two days back showed single live fetus of 19 weeks and no other abnormal finding.

Q1. What is your diagnosis? Why?

This patient is a primigravida with 20 weeks pregnancy and hyperthyroidism. She has elevated free T4 and suppressed serum TSH levels.

Q2. What are the causes of hyperthyroidism?

The causes of hyperthyroidism are as follows:

Primary Hyperthyroidism

- Grave's disease
- Toxic multinodular goiter
- Toxic nodule, adenoma
- Subacute thyroiditis
- Acute thyroiditis (de Quervain's viral or postpartum thyroiditis)
- Iodine treatment (Jod-Basedow phenomenon)
- Amiodarone therapy
- Ectopic thyroid tissue (functioning thyroid cancer metastases, struma ovarii)
- Excess thyroid hormone ingestion

Secondary Hyperthyroidism

- Pituitary tumor secreting TSH
- Very high hCG levels (hydatidiform mole).

Q3. What is the most common cause of hyperthyroidism in pregnancy?

Grave's disease comprises of 95% of cases of hyperthyroidism in pregnancy. It is an autoimmune disorder characterized by circulating IgG antibodies to the TSH receptor (TRAb), which stimulates thyroid hormone production and thyroid gland enlargement.

Q4. What are the symptoms and signs of hyperthyroidism?

Symptoms of hyperthyroidism may mimic that of normal pregnancy. Differentiating symptoms may be weight loss, tremor, lid lag, lid retraction, and persistent tachycardia > 100 beats/ min

Symptoms	Signs
Nervousness	Goiter
Irritability	Hair thinning
Insomnia	Eye signs—lid lag, lid retraction
Psychosis	Palmar erythema
Sweating	Tachycardia
Fatigue	Hypertension
Weight loss	Atrial fibrillation
Increased appetite	Dermopathy
Heat intolerance	Fine tremor
Palpitation	Proximal muscle weakness and wasting
Diarrhea	

Q5. What are the risks associated with hyperthyroidism in pregnancy?

Though rare, two most serious maternal complications of untreated hyperthyroidism are heart failure and thyroid storm that is a life-threatening condition with a maternal mortality rate of 25% even with appropriate management. Heart failure is more common out of the two (8%). It is caused by the long-term myocardial effects of T4 resulting in cardiomyopathy and pulmonary hypertension, which is intensified by other pregnancy conditions, such as preeclampsia, infection or anemia.

Other associations are as follows:
- Miscarriages
- Growth restriction
- Fetal deaths
- Preterm labor
- Placental abruption
- Gestational hypertension, pre-eclampsia
- Infection
- Increased perinatal mortality
- Chromosomal abnormalities.

Treatment improves outcome in these patients. Treatment decreases risk of stillbirth from 24% to 5–7% and incidence of prematurity from 53% to around 10%.

Q6. What are the fetal and neonatal risks associated with hyperthyroidism in pregnancy?

There is a risk of fetal and/or neonatal thyrotoxicosis due to the transplacental transfer of immunoglobulins in women with Grave's disease. Fetal thyrotoxicosis may be suspected in a fetus with a persistent tachycardia >160 beats/min, a goiter or growth restriction.

Fetal thyrotoxicosis may result in:
- Preterm delivery
- Hydrops fetalis
- Fetal craniosynostosis
- Hepatosplenomegaly
- Thrombocytopenia
- Exophthalmos
- Goiter with neck obstruction
- Polyhydramnios
- Growth restriction
- Neonatal features: Jaundice, poor feeding, poor weight gain and irritability.

Q7. How will you manage a case of hyperthyroidism in pregnancy?

Subclinical hyperthyroidism is not associated with adverse pregnancy outcome and treatment is not recommended, however, overt hyperthyroidism requires treatment. Therapeutic modalities for hyperthyroidism can be divided into the following:[7]

Thionamides

Mainstay of treatment during pregnancy. They act by competitively inhibiting the peroxidase catalyzed reactions necessary for iodine organification. They also block the coupling of iodotyrosine, especially di-iodothyronine formation. However, the clinical response is delayed until the preformed hormones are depleted which can take 3 to 4 weeks.

The ATA and US FDA recommend use of propylthiouracil be limited to first trimester only and that patients be switched to methimazole in second trimester. Both drugs cross the placenta. Methimazole is related to esophageal or choanal atresia, aplasia cutis in fetus and propylthiouracil is related to liver failure in adults. Methimazole is 20–30 times as potent as propylthiouracil. Therefore, the switch over balances the risk of the two rare adverse effects: methimazole embryopathy and propylthiouracil hepatotoxicity. Another disadvantage with propylthiouracil is that more frequent dosing is required than with carbimazole.

The dose of propylthiouracil is 50–150 mg orally three times daily to be initiated depending on the clinical severity. Methimazole is initiated at a dose of 10 – 40 mg orally in two or three divided doses initially which can be reduced to a single dose. Serum free T4 (not TSH) should be measured every 2–4 weeks and dose of drugs adjusted accordingly. The goal is to maintain free T4 slightly above or in the high normal range regardless of the TSH levels with the lowest possible dose of thionamides to avoid fetal hypothyroidism.

Propylthiouracil is still recommended in preference to methimazole in the setting of life-threatening thyrotoxicosis to take advantage of its ability to inhibit peripheral conversion of T4 to T3. Medication should be continued during lactation, as there is minimal excretion of drug in breast milk.

β-blockers

In those with troublesome autonomic (sympathetic) symptoms of palpitation, tachycardia and tremor, propranolol may be used for up to a month until longer term treatment with thionamides become effective. β-blockers have an additional beneficial action of reducing peripheral conversion of T4 into T3. Propranolol is used at a dose of 10–40 mg every 6 to 8 hours and gradually discontinued over 2–6 weeks. Longer treatment with β-blockers should be avoided because of the risk of fetal growth restriction, bradycardia and neonatal hypoglycemia.

Surgery

It is reserved for patients who do not respond to medication are intolerant or allergic to medication, or have compressive symptoms from a large goiter. When required, it is performed in the second trimester of pregnancy. Preoperatively maternal thyroid receptor antibody (TRAb) determination is recommended as there is a risk of fetal hyperthyroidism caused by high titers after withdrawal of antithyroid drugs following surgery. Preparation for surgery includes β-blocking agents and a short course of potassium iodide solution (50–100 mg/day) for two weeks. Thyroid surgery may be associated with hypothyroidism hypoparathyroidism, hypocalcemia and recurrent laryngeal nerve palsy postoperatively.

Fetal Surveillance

It is required in women with uncontrolled hyperthyroidism and in women with high TRAb levels. This involves ultrasound in the second and third trimesters to assess for fetal goiter, growth, amniotic fluid volume and heart rate.

Q8. How will you manage such a case in the postpartum period?

Antithyroid drugs are continued in postpartum period irrespective of breastfeeding status and thyroid function testing is done at 6 weeks postpartum.

Q9. What is thyroid storm? How will you manage a case of thyroid storm in pregnancy?

Thyroid storm is a hypermetabolic state that occurs due to excessive thyroid hormone. Labor, delivery, sepsis, pre-eclampsia, and anemia may precipitate thyroid storm in pregnant women with poorly controlled or untreated thyrotoxicosis. It may result in maternal heart failure. It is a medical emergency with a maternal mortality rate of 25% even with appropriate management. Fever, tachycardia, cardiac dysrhythmia, central nervous system dysfunction, gastrointestinal and hepatic disturbances may lead to multiorgan failure.

Awareness about this condition is essential for its diagnosis. Diagnosis is confirmed by measurement of serum free T4 and TSH levels. Management should be carried out in intensive care setting under supervision of an endocrinologist or a physician.

Management

- Inhibition of release of T3 and T4 by the thyroid gland:
  - Oral propylthiouracil 1000 mg loading dose, then 200 mg PO every 6 hours
  - Iodine administration 1–2 hours after propylthiouracil by:
    - Sodium iodide 500–1000 mg IV every 8 hours
      Or
    - Potassium iodide 5 drops PO every 8 hours
      Or
    - Lugol solution 10 drops PO every 8 hours
      Or
    - Lithium carbonate 300 mg PO every 6 hours (in case of iodine anaphylaxis)
- Blockage of peripheral conversion of T4 to T3:
  - Dexamethasone 2 mg IV every 6 hours for four doses
    Or
  - Hydrocortisone 100 mg IV every 8 hours for three doses
- β-blockers to control tachycardia—Propranolol, labetalol or esmolol may be used.
- Supportive measures like IV fluids, anxiolytics, antibiotics to control infection, treating fever, external cooling
- Treatment of precipitating cause.

- Avoid delivery in the presence of thyroid storm.
- Stabilization of maternal condition improves fetal status.

Q10. Should one assess for antithyroid peroxidase antibodies (TPOAb) in a pregnant woman?

The ACOG does not support routine testing for TPOAb since the results rarely lead to a change in management. However, women with subclinical hypothyroidism and positive antibodies are more likely to progress to overt hypothyroidism later on. The endocrinologists get it assessed to triage the management of women with borderline raised TSH values.

Q11. Are additional maternal or fetal testing or surveillance required in treated women with thyroid disease during pregnancy apart from thyroid function tests?

Additional surveillance is not recommended unless pregnancy is complicated by other conditions that require surveillance. However, TSH receptor antibody monitoring is required in cases of Grave's disease treated with ^{131}I ablation or surgical resection.

OTHER THYROID DISORDERS IN PREGNANCY

CASE SCENARIO

A 27 years old woman, gravida 5, para 4, presented to the emergency with a history of amenorrhea for two months and vaginal bleeding for one week.

Examination

She had tachycardia (108/min), and blood pressure of 126/76 mm Hg. She had moderate pallor. Her general physical and systemic examination was unremarkable. Uterus was enlarged corresponding to 24-week gestation.

Investigations

- Ultrasonography of her enlarged uterus revealed uterine cavity filled with small cystic material suggestive of complete molar pregnancy.
- Serum human chorionic gonadotropin (hCG) was reported as >10^5 mIU/L.
- Her thyroid-function tests were markedly deranged:
  - Serum TSH—0.005 mIU/L (normal range, 0.39 to 6.0 mIU/L)
  - Free thyroxine (FT4) 4.11 ng/dL (normal range, 1–2 ng/dL)
  - Free tri-iodothyronine (T3) 8.63 pg/mL (normal range, 3–7 pg/mL).
- Blood counts—hemoglobin of 8.1 g/dL, TLC—7800/mm^3 and platelet count—2.52 lakh/mm^3.
- Other biochemical investigations were normal.

Suction evacuation of the mole was done. The hCG values decreased to 54000 mIU/mL after 1 week and 3800 mIU/mL after 2 weeks of evacuation. Her Serum TSH improved to 0.02 mIU/mL three days after evacuation and was normal at 4 weeks of follow-up.

Q1. What is your diagnosis?

This patient had complete hydatidiform mole with markedly elevated serum hCG levels and thyroid function tests suggestive of hyperthyroidism. Post evacuation her thyroid functions normalized as her serum hCG levels got settled. These findings are suggestive of gestational transient thyrotoxicosis.

Q2. What is gestational transient thyrotoxicosis?

It is the result of TSH receptor stimulation by high concentration of human chorionic gonadotropin (hCG). hCG is only about 1/104 as potent as TSH therefore the thyroid function tests are mostly unaltered during pregnancy, however high levels of hCG as seen in molar pregnancy or multiple gestation can stimulate TSH receptors giving rise to this condition.

Q3. How common is this condition?

On review of the 196 patients with gestational trophoblastic neoplasia treated with chemotherapy in the United Kingdom between 2005 and 2010, biochemical hyperthyroidism was present in 7% and clinical hyperthyroidism in only 2%.[17]

Q4. What are the clinical features of gestational transient thyrotoxicosis and how is it managed?

This is a self-limited mild disorder of early pregnancy characterized by hyperemesis with no prior history of thyroid disease or stigmata of Grave's disease. A suppressed serum TSH and elevated free T4 or total T4 in the absence of TRAb usually excludes Grave's disease. Management is usually supportive-rehydration, and antiemetics if patient has hyperemesis. Antithyroid drugs are not recommended, β-blockers may be considered for symptomatic management.

Q5. What is postpartum thyroiditis? How will you manage it?

It is an inflammatory autoimmune condition characterized by thyroid dysfunction, excluding Grave's disease, in the first postpartum year in women who had normal thyroid functions prior to pregnancy. This condition is characterized by transient thyrotoxicosis followed by transient hypothyroidism with normalization of thyroid functions by the end of the year.

Treatment is usually symptomatic with β-blockers being used for symptomatic women in thyrotoxic phase. Antithyroid drugs are not recommended for thyrotoxic phase. Oral levothyroxine should be considered for symptomatic women in hypothyroid phase. TSH level should be monitored every 4–8 weeks until thyroid function normalizes followed by annually to evaluate for development of permanent hypothyroidism.

Q6. How will you assess a case of thyroid nodule or thyroid cancer during pregnancy?

A pregnant woman with a thyroid nodule should be assessed in the following manner:
- Complete history and physical examination
- Serum TSH testing
- Ultrasound of the neck—If features suspicious of malignancy (hypoechoic pattern, irregular margins and microcalcifications) are present, then fine needle aspiration may be recommended. Timing may be influenced by cancer risk assessment or by patient preference, although it is safe in any trimester.

Radionuclide scintigraphy or radio-iodine uptake determination is not recommended during pregnancy. Cytologically benign static nodules do not require surgery. If malignancy is diagnosed during the first or second trimester, thyroidectomy may be performed before the third trimester. If malignancy is diagnosed in the third trimester or it is a non-aggressive thyroid cancer, surgery can be deferred to the immediate postpartum period.

GENERAL QUESTIONS ON PHYSIOLOGY OF THYROID GLAND

Q1. Describe the physiology of the thyroid gland?

The thyroid gland is responsible for the secretion of three hormones—thyroxine (T4), triiodothyronine (T3) and calcitonin. It is made up of follicles and a single layer of follicular cells lines each follicle with a lumen containing colloid.

The iodine content of the thyroid gland regulates the uptake mechanism in the thyroid follicular cells. Dietary iodine occurs in the form of iodide in blood and its concentration is low (0.2–0.4μg/dL). Its uptake is the rate-limiting step in the thyroid hormone production and it occurs by an active transport process (Na^+: I^- symporter or NIS). This is called as iodide trapping and is stimulated by thyroid stimulating hormone that is secreted by the anterior pituitary gland. Iodide is carried across the apical membrane and oxidized by thyroid peroxidase into iodinium (I^+) ions. This combines with the tyrosil residues of thyroglobulin to form inactive monoiodotyrosine (MIT) and di iodotyrosine (DIT). This process is called the organification of iodide or iodination. Pairs of iodinated tyrosil residues couple together to form T3 and T4. This process is known as coupling and is catalyzed by thyroid peroxidase. The hormones remain stored in the thyroid colloid.

Production and secretion of thyroid hormones is regulated by the hypothalamopituitary axis. Thyrotrophin releasing hormone (TRH) is released from the paraventricular nucleus of hypothalamus. This reaches the anterior pituitary via the pituitary stalk and stimulates the production and secretion of TSH which stimulates the thyroid gland to produce and secrete thyroid hormones. TSH regulates all iodine uptake, oxidation and coupling. The stored hormones re-enter the follicular cells by endocytosis. Proteolysis by various lysosomal proteases liberates the hormones into the circulation.

Q2. What are the changes in the physiology of the thyroid gland during pregnancy?

More than 99% of all the thyroid hormones are bound to plasma proteins—thyroxine binding globulin (TBG), transthyretin and albumin (in the order of affinity). About 75% of all the thyroid hormones are bound to TBG. Only 0.03–0.08% of T4 and 0.2–0.5% of T3 are in the free form which is the active form that enters the target cells.

Pregnancy results in a rise in the levels of TBG and transthyretin due to the effects of estrogen favoring their increased synthesis and decreased hepatic clearance. This rise is present in the second week of gestation and peaks at 20 weeks and remains so till delivery.

There is a state of relative iodine deficiency during pregnancy secondary to the following:
- An increase in renal loss due to increased glomerular filtration rate in the early first trimester.
- Transfer of iodine to the developing fetus.
- Increase in type III 5-deiodinase due to increased placental mass leading to increased thyroid hormone destruction.
- The thyroid gland has to produce nearly 50% more thyroid hormones.

Thus, there is 50% increase in daily iodine requirement. In order to compensate, the thyroid gland increases its uptake of iodine from the blood, and if there is iodine deficiency, cellular hyperplasia and goiter will result. A physiologic goiter may be seen on ultrasound examination by a change in gland size of up to 10–20%, which is not clinically detectable. If clinically apparent, it suggests iodine deficiency or pathology.

TSH is a glycoprotein with α and β subunits. TSH and human chorionic gonadotropin (hCG) share a common α subunit. Serum hCG levels start rising in early pregnancy, progressively increase up to 9–12 weeks and stabilize thereafter. Raised hCG stimulates TSH receptor causing a rise in T4 with resulting suppression of TSH release. Initial rise in TSH peaks at 6 weeks and decreased thereafter, reaching nadir at 12 weeks and thereafter rises with advancing gestation (Fig. 1). This rise in T4 in early pregnancy has the advantage of providing the fetus with T4 before it becomes autonomous. Rise in T4 and T3 plateaus when hCG levels are maximum. However, free T4 concentration appears to be highest in the first trimester (but still lower than nonpregnant values) and falls with rising gestational age due to increased TBG. There is also an enhanced peripheral conversion of free T4 to free T3, which may be in preparation for exertions of labor and delivery.[18]

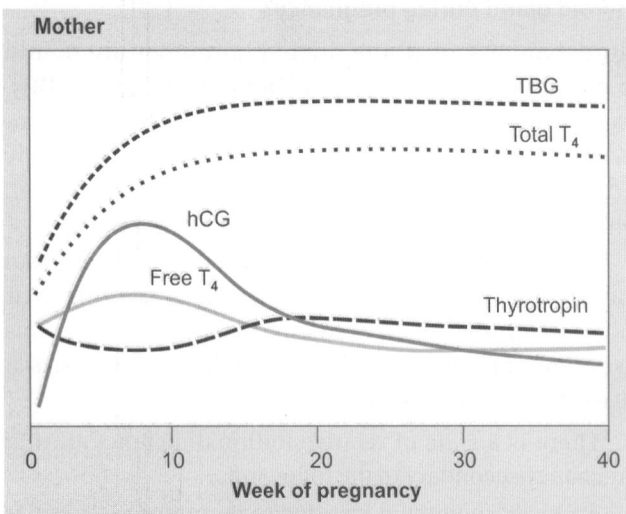

Fig. 1: Thyroid hormone profile in mother and fetus during pregnancy

Q3. What is the physiology of the fetal thyroid gland?

Fetal thyroid gland develops from the first pharyngeal arch by 5 weeks of pregnancy, migrates caudally and reaches its final position by 7 weeks of gestation. It matures and begins iodide trapping by 12 weeks. Fetal thyroid hormones (free and total T3, T4, TSH, TBG) can be detected in fetal blood from 12 weeks onwards, increasing with advancing gestation and reaching adult levels by 36 weeks. Fetal thyroid function comes under pituitary control by midgestation, hypothalamic TRH is detectable by 9 weeks and pituitary portal circulation is functioning by the end of the first trimester.

Thus the fetus is completely dependent on maternal thyroid hormones in the first trimester. Only maternal T4 and TRH are available for fetal use during first trimester and these are the only thyroid hormones that can cross the placenta. The fetal brain relies on its own conversion of T4 to T3, which occurs only in the fetal brain unlike adults due to the presence of type II deiodinase. Even after 12 weeks maternal T4 is important, as it comprises 30% in the fetal serum.

The initiation of neuronal development occurs early in the first trimester, the multiplication of neuroblasts in the fetal brain reaches its peak in the second trimester and then declines, during which neuroblasts develop into neurons, synapse formation occurs and extends into the postnatal life. Thyroid hormones are essential for timing this neuronal division, differentiation and maturation and their deficiency may result in inadequate development of the neuronal circuit.[19]

Thus, adequate supply of maternal thyroid hormones is necessary throughout pregnancy to ensure normal neurological development of the fetus.

REFERENCES

1. Alexander EK, Pearce EN, Brent GA, et al. 2017 Guidelines of the American Thyroid Association for the Diagnosis and Management of Thyroid Disease during pregnancy and the postpartum. Thyroid. 2017;27(3):315-99.
2. Marwaha RK, Chopra S, Gopalakrishnan S, et al. Establishment of reference range for thyroid hormones in normal pregnant Indian women. BJOG. 2008; 115(5):602-6.
3. Abalovich M, Gutierrez S, Alcaraz G, et al. Overt and subclinical hypothyroidism complicating pregnancy. Thyroid. 2002;12:63-8.
4. Leung AS, Millar LK, Koonings PP, et al. Perinatal outcome in hypothyroid pregnancies. Obstet Gynecol. 1993;81:349-53.
5. Pop VJ, Brouwers EP, Vader HL, et al. Maternal hypothyroxinaemia during early pregnancy and subsequent child development: a 3-year follow-up study. Clin Endocrinol. 2003;59(3):282-8.
6. Haddow JE, Palomaki GE, Allan WC, et al. Maternal thyroid deficiency during pregnancy and subsequent neuropsychological development of the child. N Engl J Med. 1999;341:549-55.

7. Tripathi KD. Thyroid Hormone and Thyroid Inhibitors. In: Essentials of Medical Pharmacology, 6th edn. New Delhi: Jaypee Brothers Medical Publishers; 2008.pp.242-53.
8. Institute of Medicine. Dietary reference intakes: the essential guide to nutrient requirements. Washington, DC: National Academies Press; 2006.
9. Stagnaro – Green A. Maternal thyroid disease and preterm delivery. J Clin Endocrinol Metab. 2009;94(1):21-5.
10. Negro R, Schwartz A, Gismondi R, et al. Universal screening versus case finding for detection and treatment of thyroid hormonal dysfunction during pregnancy. J Clin Endocrinol Metab. 2010;95(4):1699-707.
11. Cleary-Goldman J, Malone FD, Lambert MG, et al. Maternal thyroid hypofunction and pregnancy outcome. Obstet Gynecol. 2008;112(1):85-92.
12. Lazarus JH, Bestwick JP, Channon S, et al. Antenatal thyroid screening and childhood cognitive function. N Engl J Med. 2012;366(6):493-501.
13. De Groot L, Abalovich M, Alexander EK, et al. Management of thyroid dysfunction during pregnancy and postpartum: an Endocrine Society clinical practice guideline. J Clin Endocrinol Metab. 2012;97(8):2543-65.
14. Screening for thyroid disease in pregnancy. SMFM Consult. Contemp Obst Gynae. 2012;8:45-7.
15. The American College of Obstetricians and Gynaecologists Practice Bulletin: Thyroid Disease in Pregnancy; No. 148.2015; 125(4):996-1005.
16. Spencer L, Bubner T, Bain E, et al. Screening and subsequent management for thyroid dysfunction pre-pregnancy and during pregnancy for improving maternal and infant health. Cochrane Database Syst Rev. 2015; 9:CD011263.
17. Walkington L, Webster J, Hancock BW, et al. Hyperthyroidism and human chorionic gonadotrophin production in gestational trophoblastic disease. B J Can. 2011;104(11):1665-9.
18. Kenyon AP, Nelson-Piercy C. Thyroid disease. In: James DK, Steer PJ, Weiner CP, Gonik B (Eds). High Risk Pregnancy Management Options. 4th edn. Philadelphia,PA: Elsevier-Saunders; 2011.pp.813-25.
19. Patel J, Landers K, Li H, et al. Thyroid hormones and fetal neurological development. J Endocrinol. 2011:209;1-8.

Neurological Disorder in Pregnancy

Latika Sahu, Tarang Preet Kaur

CASE SCENARIO

Mrs X, 25 years old G4P1L1A2 at 35 weeks of pregnancy with BMI 20.8 with known case of seizure disorder came to OPD for regular ANC check-up.

Presenting Complaint
Patient was a booked antenatal case of the same hospital.

History of Present Pregnancy
She had spontaneous conception and it was an unplanned pregnancy.

1st Trimester
Pregnancy was confirmed at home by urine pregnancy test when she was overdue by 15 days. Patient had been taking her antiepileptic medication (valproate) regularly along with folic acid (5 mg) as prescribed by the neurologist before pregnancy. After confirmation of pregnancy, she went to her neurologist for reviewing her medicines and was advised to continue the same. She had one episode of spotting blood per vaginum at 3 months amenorrhea for which she had conservative management. She had no history of pain abdomen, discharge per vaginum, fever with rashes, bladder and bowel symptoms or radiation exposure. She had symptoms of hyperemesis which were relieved on taking medicine (doxylamine). She received her two doses of tetanus toxoid. She had no seizure episodes. She was followed up in high-risk antenatal clinic (ANC).

2nd Trimester
Quickening felt at around 5 months amenorrhea. Iron and calcium started. folic acid continued. She was regularly taking antiepileptic drug and was reviewed from the neurologist and was advised to continue the same drug and dosage. Blood and urine tests were done and patient was told all normal. Level II ultrasound was done in 5 month of pregnancy and placenta was found to be low lying partially covering os with no other abnormality. Her blood pressure was normal on all antenatal visits—she visited antenatal clinic 3 times in 2nd trimester. She had no history of polyphagia, polydipsia, polyuria. She had no bleeding per vaginum episodes in this trimester. She had no seizure episodes.

3rd Trimester
Repeat ultrasound for placental localization was done—placenta was not low lying. She was regularly taking her hematinics and antiepileptic drug. She had *one episode of seizure* at 7 and half months amenorrhea. Levetiracetam was added to valproate by the neurologist. No history of headache, epigastric pain, blurring of vision. No history of polydipsia, polyuria, poyphagia. No history of breathlessness, chest pain, pedal edema.

Obstetric History
She is married since 4 years. Nonconsanguineous marriage. G4P1L1A2

- G1 was 3 years back, supervised pregnancy, spontaneous, full term, normal vaginal delivery, at tertiary care centre, baby was female, 2.5 kg birth weight, 1 year breastfed. She had no episodes of seizure antenatally or posnatally. Discharged in safe condition postpartum day 2. Baby is alive and healthy with normal milestones, immunized till date
- G2 was 2.5 years back, patient had 2 episodes of seizure at 2 months amenorrrhea after she spontaneously aborted. Patient was admitted to the hospital in view of bleeding per vaginum and was diagnosed to be an incomplete

abortion. Evacuation and curettage was done. Patient was discharged the next day. No further episode of seizures
- G3: A2 was 2 years back. Patient again presented to the hospital with bleeding per vaginum and was diagnosed to be an incomplete abortion. Evacuation and curettage was done. No episodes of seizure during this pregnancy.
- G4: Present pregnancy.

Menstrual History

- Menarche—attained at 13-14 years. Last menstrual period (LMP)—30/10/16. Estimated date of delivery (EDD)—06/08/17
- Previous cycles were regular, 4–5 days of bleeding with 28–30 days cycles with normal flow
- No history of dysmenorrhea, menorrhagia
- Contraceptive history—barrier method. No history of pills intake for contraception or missed periods prior to conception.

Past History

- *Medical:* Patient is a known case of seizure disorder since 4 years when she was diagnosed to have tubercular granuloma in the left parietal area for which she was started on antituberculous treatment (ATT). Patient had completed her 6-month course. Patient was started on antiepileptic drug-valproate
  She had generalised tonic clonic seizures. She had her last seizure 2.5 years back
  Patient had been taking antiepileptic drug since then. No history suggestive of chronic hypertension, diabetes, asthma in the past. No history of blood transfusions
- *Surgical history:* No history of any surgical intervention.
- *Family history:* No history of tuberculosis (TB), hypertension, diabetes or epilepsy in the family
- *Personal history:* She is a housewife. She had normal bowel and bladder pattern with normal sleep pattern. Nonvegetarian. Nonsmoker, nonalcoholic and no other addictions
- *Socioeconomic history:* She lives in a nuclear family of 3 in a pucca house with MCD water supply with modern sanitation and electricity facilities. She belongs to lower middle class
- *Dietary history:* She is nonvegetarian by choice. Patient takes approximately 2,400 kcal as per 24 hours recall method. Her protein intake is approximately 60 g. Her diet is almost balanced
- *History summary:* G4P1L1A2 with 35 weeks of gestation with seizure disorder.

Examination

- Patient is conscious, oriented and sitting comfortably in bed
- Average built, normal hairline, average orodental hygiene.

General Physical Examination

- Pulse = 80/min, regular, no radio-radial or radiofemoral delay
- Blood pressure—120/80 (urine albumin—nil) in right arm in sitting position
- Respiratory rate—18/min
- Tempeature—98.6°F.
- Pallor—absent, pedal edema—present; icterus-absent, cyanosis—absent clubbing—absent, thyroid—normal.

Systemic Examination

- Respiratory—trachea centrally placed, bilateral air entry equal, no added sounds
- Cardiovascular system (CVS): S1S2 +, no murmur heard.

Neurological Examination

- *Higher mental functions:* It is considered sufficient if the patient is alert and oriented.
  In case of any suspicion of impaired cognitive functioning at present or in the past, assessment of consciousness level with Glasgow Coma Scale (Table 1) or more detailed mini mental state examination (MMSE) should be done
- *Glasgow coma scale:* E4V5M6[6]

Table 1: Glasgow coma scale

	1	2	3	4	5	6
Eyes	Does not open eyes	Open eyes in response to painful stimuli	Opens eyes in response to voice	Opens eyes spontaneously	N/A	N/A
Verbal	Makes no sounds	Incomprehensible sounds	Utters inappropriate words	confused, disoriented	Oriented, converses normally	N/A
Motor	Makes no movements	Extension to painful stimuli	Abnormal flexion to painful stimuli	Flexion/withdrawal to painful stimuli	Localizes painful stimuli	Obeys commands

Note: Score ranges from 3 (deep coma) to 15 (fully awake)

- *Mini mental state examination (MMSE):* The MMSE is a tool that can be used to objectively assess mental status. It is an 11-question measure that tests five areas of cognitive function: orientation, registration, attention and calculation, recall, and language. The maximum score is 30. A score of 23 or lower is indicative of cognitive impairment. The MMSE takes only 5 minutes to administer and is therefore practical for routine repeated use.

Cranial Nerve Examination (Table 2)

Table 2: Cranial nerve examination

Cranial nerve	Examination	Comments
1. Olfactory nerve	Sense of smell	Taste and smell is normal
2. Optic nerve	Visual acuity Visual fields Pupil shape and size Pupil light reflex Fundoscopy	No complain in vision Pupils—normal size, normal reacting
3. Oculomotor 4. Trochlear 5. Abducens	Eye position and movements	No ptosis, double vision movements in all directions normal
6. Trigeminal	Facial sensation	Bilateral sensation in upper, middle and lower face normal
	Corneal reflex	Both direct and consensual blinking present
	Muscles of mastication	Bulk—normal bilaterally no deviation of jaw on opening it against resistance
	Jaw jerk	Just present
7. Facial	Motor	No asymmetry in face patient is able to raise her eyebrows, tightly close eyes against resistance, able to show her teeth, able to blow out cheeks
	Taste over anterior 2/3rd of tongue	Able to differentiate sweet, sour, salt and bitter
8. Vestibulocochlear	Whisper and tuning fork tests	Hearing—normal
	Vestibular tests	No complain of vertigo, nystagmus
9. Glossopharyngeal 10-Vagus	Quality of voice Movement of palate	No dysarthria/dysphonia on saying aaah-palate and uvula looked normal

Contd...

Cranial nerve	Examination	Comments
11. Accessory	Trapezius and sternocleidomastoid	Patient is able to raise her shoulders and rotate the head left and right against resistance
12. Hypoglossal	Tongue appearance and movement	No wasting, fasciculations, involuntary movements of tongue On sticking out tongue—no deviation, involuntary movements, side- to-side movements present

Motor Examination (Table 3)

Table 3: Motor examination

Motor examination	Bulk		Tone		Power	
	Left	Right	Left	Right	Left	Right
Shoulder	N	N	N	N	5/5	5/5
Elbow	N	N	N	N	5/5	5/5
Wrist	N	N	N	N	5/5	5/5
Small muscles of hand	N	N	N	N	5/5	5/5
Hip	N	N	N	N	5/5	5/5
Knee	N	N	N	N	5/5	5/5
Ankle	N	N	N	N	5/5	5/5
Small muscles of foot	N	N	N	N	5/5	5/5

(N-Normal)

Medical Research Council Scale (MRCS) for Muscle Power (Tables 4 to 7)

Table 4: MRCS for Muscle power

0	No muscle contraction visible
1	Flicker of contraction but no movement
2	Joint movement when effect of gravity eliminated
3	Movement against gravity but not against examiner's resistance
4	Movement against resistance but weaker than normal
5	Normal power

Table 5: Deep tendon reflexes

Deep tendon reflexes	Brisk/normal/sluggish/absent
Biceps (C5,C6)	Normal
Supinator (C5,C6,C7)	Normal
Triceps (C6,C7,C8)	Normal
Knee (L2,L3,L4)	Normal
Ankle (S1,S2)	Normal

Superficial reflexes	Left	Right
Plantar reflex	Flexor response	Flexor response

Contd...

Table 6: Sensory examination

Sensory examination	Left	Right
Fine touch	Normal	Normal
Pressure	Normal	Normal
Pain	Normal	Normal
Temperature	Normal	Normal
Joint position	Normal	Normal
Romberg's test	Normal	Normal
Vibration	Normal	Normal

Table 7: Coordination examination

Coordination	Left	Right
Rebound phenomenon	Normal	Normal
Finger-nose test	Normal	Normal
Heel-shin test	Normal	Normal
Rapid alternating movements	Normal	Normal

- Stance and Gait: Normal
- Meningeal signs: Absent

Abdominal Examination

- *Inspection:* Abdomen is uniformly distended with all quadrants moving with respiration. Linea nigra, stria gravidarum present, no other scar marks are seen. Umbilicus is central and everted. All hernial sites are free
- *Palpation:* Fundal height—34 weeks. Symphsiofundal height—33 cm. Abdominal girth—33 inches
- *Fundal grip:* A soft broad non-ballotable structure felt at fundus suggestive of breech
- *Lateral grip:* Smooth and curved structure felt on the right lateral side of the abdomen suggestive of back. Multiple knobby structures felt on the left side suggestive of limbs
- *Pelvic grips:* A hard globular and smooth ballotable structure felt on palpation suggestive of head
- *On deep palpation:* Head was freely mobile and not engaged
- *Auscultation:* Fetal heart sound was heard at the right spinoumbilical line—134 beats per minute, regular
- *Perineal examination:* External genitalia normal.no bleeding and no leaking observed
- *Perspeculum examination:* os closed. Cervix-normal no discharge, bleeding or leaking observed.
- *Per vaginal examination:* Not done
- *Diagnosis:* Mrs X, G4P1L1A2 with 35 weeks with seizure disorder on tablet valproate 100 mg B.D. since 4 years. She has singleton live fetus in cephalic presentation.

CASE SCENARIO

Mrs X, 26 years old G3P2L1 at 33 weeks pregnancy with BMI 19 is a known case of seizure disorder (GTCS) came to Gynae casualty with following presenting complaints of-3 episodes of abnormal movements in last 30 minutes and was unconscious. She was throwing another episode of abnormal movements involving whole of the body when she arrived at the hospital. She had passed urine in her clothes and froth was coming out from her mouth. She had missed her antiepileptic drug dose the previous day.

History of Presenting Complaint

Patient was a booked antenatal case of the same hospital. Her each episode of abnormal movement lasted for a period of 1–2 minutes and she was unconscious in between the episodes. She was having episodes of abnormal movements every 10 minutes.

History of Present Pregnancy

Her pregnancy was spontaneous conception and unplanned pregnancy.

1st Trimester

Her urine pregnancy test was positive at home when she was overdue by 15 days.

Patient had been taking her antiepileptic medication (valproate and phenytoin) irregularly along with folic acid (5 mg) as prescribed by the neurologist before pregnancy. After confirmation of pregnancy, she stopped her medication on her own. She threw an episode of seizure at 2 months amenorrhea. Then she visited her neurologist and her antiepileptics were reviewed and clobazam was added. She started taking her antiepileptics regularly. She had no further episode in first 3 months.

She had no episode of spotting blood per vaginum. She had no history of pain abdomen, discharge per vaginum, fever with rashes, bladder and bowel symptoms or radiation exposure. She had no history of excessive vomiting. She received her two doses of tetanus toxoid. She had her first ANC visit.

2nd Trimester

Quickening felt at around 5 months amenorrhea. Iron and calcium started. folic acid continued. she was regularly taking all these drugs. She was regularly taking her antiepileptic drugs. She had 2 episodes of seizure for which she revisited her neurologist. Blood investigations were done and dosages of antiepileptic drugs were accordingly increased. Urine tests was done and patient was told all normal. Level II ultrasound was done in 6 month of pregnancy and it was told to be normal. Her blood pressure was normal on all antenatal visits—she visited antenatal clinic 3 times in 2nd trimester. She had no history of polyphasic, polydipsia, polyuria. She had no bleeding p/v episodes in this trimester.

3rd Trimester

She was regularly taking her hematinics and antiepileptic drugs. No history of headache, epigastric pain, blurring of vision. No history of polydipsia, polyuria, poyphagia. No history of breathlessness, chest pain, pedal edema. She was admitted from gyne casualty in view of multiple episodes of seizure at 33 weeks.

Obstetric History

She is married since 5 years. Nonconsanguineous marriage. G3P2L1.
- **G1** was a supervised pregnancy, spontaneous, full term, vaginal delivery, at tertiary care center, 3 years back, patient had an episode of seizure during labor. Baby was macerated with no sign of life, female, 2.5 kg birth weight. She had 4-5 episodes of seizure antenatally and 1 episode of seizures posnatally for which neurology referrals were taken. She was discharged in safe condition on 5th postpartum day.
- **G2** was also a supervised pregnancy, spontaneous, full term normal vaginal delivery, at tertiary care center, 2 years back. Baby was female, 2.2 kg birth weight, she had 2 episodes of seizure antenatally in third trimester and no episode of seizure postpartum. Discharged in safe condition on 2nd postpartum day.

Menstrual History

Normal

No history of pills intake for contraception or missed periods prior to conception.

Contraceptive History

She was using barrier method of contraception.

Past History

- *Medical history:* Patient was a known case of seizure disorder since 6 years of age. Patient had got her MRI done which was a normal study. She was started on tablet phenytoin 300 mg HS and tablet valproate 500 mg BD as prescribed by her neurologist. She had generalized tonic clonic seizures. Her last episode prior to pregnancy was 1 month back when she was involved in an argument with her husband over some personal matter. She had history of headache preceding an episode of abnormal movements when she faced some kind of stress

  No history suggestive of chronic hypertension, diabetes, asthma in the past. No history of blood transfusions
- *Surgical history:* No history of any surgical intervention
- *Family history:* No history of TB, hypertension, diabetes in the family
- *Personal history:* She is a housewife with normal bowel and bladder pattern with normal sleep pattern. Nonvegetarian. Nonsmoker, nonalcoholic and no other addictions
- *Socioeconomic history:* She lives in a nuclear family of 3 in a pucca house with MCD water supply with modern sanitation and electricity facilities

  She belongs to lower middle class as per modified Kuppuswamy scale
- *Dietary history:* She is vegetarian by choice. Patient takes approximately 2,400 kcal as per 24 hours recall method. Her protein intake is approximately 60 g. Her diet is almost balanced
- *History Summary:* G4P1L1A2 with 33 weeks with known case of seizure disorder with status epileptics.

Examination

- Patient is unconscious lying in bed and having abnormal movements of all the limbs.
- Froth was seen coming out her mouth. Average built, normal hairline, average orodental hygiene.

General Physical Examination

Pedal edema–present. Others normal

Systemic Examination

- Respiratory: Trachea centrally placed, bilateral air entry equal, no added sounds.
- CVS-S1S2 +, No murmur heard.

Neurological Examination

- Post-seizure episode
- Higher mental functions conscious, oriented to
- Glasgow coma scale E4V4M5.(Refer to Table 1)
- Mini mental state examination: Score 28, (Refer scoring system on page 164)
- Cranial nerve examination and motor function and muscle power—normal.

Her deep tendon reflexes and sensory examination was normal.

- Stance and gait: Normal
- Meningeal signs: Absent

Abdominal Examination

Single live fetus cephalic presentation

Diagnosis: G4P1L1A2 with 33 weeks with seizure disorder on tablet phenytoin 300 mg HS, valproate 500 mg BD and clobazam since 20 years. She has singleton live fetus in cephalic presentation.

Q1. How do you define seizure and epilepsy?

Seizure disorder is a condition characterized by the episode of abnormal, uncontrolled neuronal activity in the brain resulting in various manifestations ranging from dramatic convulsive activity, altered consciousness, abnormal sensations to experiential phenomena not readily discernible by an observer.[1]

Epilepsy is described by ILAE 2014 includes atleast 2 unprovoked (or reflex) seizures occurring more than 24 hours apart.

Q2. What is the latest classification of seizures?

See Flowchart 1.

Q3. What are the various antiepileptic drugs, their principal uses, typical doses, side effects and their FDA pregnancy categories?

Antiepileptic drugs commonly (Table 8) used are:

- *Classical (older):* Phenytoin, phenobarbital, primidone, carbamazepine, ethosuximide, valproate.
- *Newer:* Lamotrigine, felbamate, topiramate, gabapentin, tiagabine, vigabatrin, oxcarbazepine, levetiracetam, fosphenytoin.[1]

Q4. What are the drugs recommended for various types of seizures?[1]

Generalized-Onset Tonic-Clonic	Focal	Typical absence	Atypical absence, Myoclonic, Atonic
First line	First line	First line	First line
Valproic acid Lamotrigine Topiramate	Lamotrigine Carbamazepine Oxcarbazepine Phenytoin Levetiracetam	Valproic acid ethosuximide	Valproic acid Lamotrigine Topiramate
Alternatives	Alternatives	Alternatives	Alternatives

Contd...

Flowchart 1: Classification of seizure types extended version. [International League Against Epilepsy (ILAE) 2017]

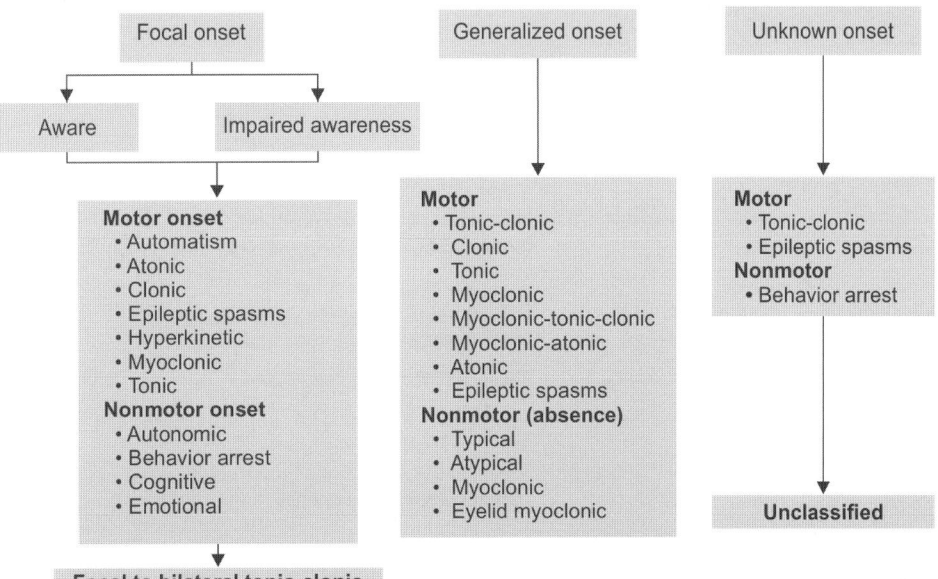

Contd...

Zonisamidea	Topiramate	Lamotrigine	Clona-zepam
Phenytoin	Zonisamide	Clonazepam	Felbamate
Carbamazepine	Valproic acid		
Oxcarbazepine	Tiagabine[a]		
Phenobarbital	Gabapentin		
Felbamate	Lacosamide		
	Phenobarbital		

Q5. Which antiepileptic drug is recommended for use in pregnancy?[2]

All the currently available antiepileptic drugs have teratogenic potential or the data available is limited about their safety in pregnancy. The commonly used drugs should follow the principle of:

- Older antipileplic drug (AED) preferred over newer
- Monotherapy over polytherapy
- Levetiracetam and lamotrigine have least teratogenic potential and are being promoted
- Avoid sodium valproate due to it teratogenic potential and long term effect on IQ.

Q6. What are the points of consideration in preconception counseling and management?

The main aim is to minimise the risk of congenital anomalies and adverse impact on long-term neurodevelopment of the newborn following in utero exposure to antiepileptic drugs.

- Women in preconceptional period should take high dose of folic acid 5 mg daily. They should start folic acid from 3 months prior to pregnancy and to continue its intake atleast till the end of first trimester to minimise the incidence of major congenital anomalies.[3]

Table 8: Various drugs commonly used for epilepsy in pregnancy, their uses, doses, side effect, pregnancy category and its effect with enzyme inducing drugs

Generic name	Principal uses	Typical dose; Dose interval	Side effects	US FDA pregnancy safety classification	Effects on drug levels with enzyme inducing drugs[a]
Phenytoin	Tonic clonic, Focal onset	300–400 mg/d (3–6 mg/kg, adult)qd-bid	Ataxia, dizziness, confusion, gum hyperplasia, hirsutism, osteomalacia, facial worsening, lymphadenopathy	D	Decreased
Carbamzepine	Tonic clonic, Focal onset	600–1800 mg/d;bd-qid	Ataxia, dizziness, diplopia, vertigo, aplastic anemia, leukopenia, gastrointestinal irritation, hepatotoxicity, hyponatremia	D	Decreased
Valproate	Tonic clonic, absence, Atypical-absence, Myoclonic, Focal-onset, Atonic	750–2000 mg/d (20–60 mg/kg); bd-bid	Ataxia, tremor, sedation, hepatotoxicity, thrombocytopenia, gastrointestinal irritation, weight gain, transient alopecia, hyperammonemia	D	Decreased
lamotrigine	Focal onset, Tonic clonic, Atypical absence, Myoclonic, Lennox-Gastaut syndrome	150–500 mg/d; bd	Dizziness, diplopia, sedation, ataxia, headache, skin rash, Stevens-Johnson syndrome	C	Decreased
Gabapentin	Focal onset	900–2400 mg/d; tds-qid	Sedation, dizziness, ataxia, fatigue, gastrointestinal irritation, weight gain, edema	C	No known significant interaction
Phenobarbital	Tonic clonic, Focal onset	60–180 mg/d; qid	Sedation, ataxia, confusion, dizziness, decreased libido, depression, skin rash		Level increased by phenytoin
Clonazepam	Absence, Atypical-absence, Myoclonic	1–12 mg/d; qd-tid	Ataxia, sedation, lethargy, anorexia	D	Decreased
Levetiracetam	Focal-onset	1000–3000 mg/d; qd-bid	Sedation, fatigue, incoordination, mood changes, anemia, leukopenia	C	No known significant interaction

- Neurologist should review the type of antiepileptic drug to be continued during pregnancy and try switching to monotherapy wherever possible. Dose of the antiepleptics should be minimized to the lowest effective dose for controlling seizures in a women planning pregnancy. Aim should be to avoid sodium valproate and polytherapy weighing the risks and benefits.[3]
- Prepregnancy withdrawal of antiepileptic drugs should be considered for women who have been seizure for many years on medication or those who have infrequent or mild seizures arising from small and contained focus with low-risk of seizure generalization. This is gradually done over 6 months prior to pregnancy although little information is available about the optimal approach of tapering and discontinuing AED. The risk of a recurrent seizure in the first 2 years off medications is 40% as compared to 20% for patients who remain on medications.[4,5]
- Women with epilepsy (WWE) demanding drug withdrawal before pregnancy should be explained about the possible risk of break through seizures and consequent effects.
- Detailed counseling should be done regarding the teratogenic potential of the antiepileptic drugs. They should be informed that the overall risk of congenital anomalies babies born to antiepileptic women is 5–6% compared to 2–3% in healthy women.[1]
- Genetic counseling should be offered in patients with genetically determined causes of epilepsies such as subependymal heterotopia.

Q7. What are the major congenital malformations associated with AED?[6]

The congenital malformation associated with commonly used drugs are:
- Phenytoin: Fetal hydantoin syndrome, congenital heart disease, facial clefts
- Valproate: Neural tube defects, craniofacial, skeletal, cardiovascular, cerebral defects. Language problems
- Carbamazepine: Neural tube defects, congenital heart defects, reduced growth, and hypospadias.
- Barbiturates: Congenital heart, craniofacial defects, limb abnormalities, growth deficiency
- Benzodiazepines: Orofacial clefts
- Lamotrigine: Weak evidence of non-syndromic facial cleft.

Q8. What are the most common presenting complaints of pregnant women with epilepsy?

Mostly they are asymptomatic. They may present with bleeding per vaginum, headache, depression.

Q9. What are important components of antenatal care in WWE?

The important measures to be considered in Ante natal care are:
- Baseline levels of AED especially in patients with recurrent seizure episodes
- Level 1 scan to look for nuchal thickness and nuchal body
- Serum alpha-protein and serum ACh
- Consider amniocentesis in patients with abnormal levels of ACh
- Level 2 scan to rule out congenital anomalies around 18–20 weeks
- Fetal echo in suspected level 2 scans—no studies available for role of fatal echo over level 2 scan for ruling out cardiac anomalies in baby
- Level 3 scan for fetal well-being.

Q10. How do you manage women with epilepsy in labor and during delivery[3]

Risk of seizures in labor: 3.5%[7]

So, the important measures to be considered while managing a women with epilepsy in labor are:
- Antiepileptic drug should be continued even in labor.
- Parenteral AED should be considered in case of excessive vomiting
- Adequate hydration should be maintained
- Pain relief: Transcutaneous electrical nerve stimulation, nitrous oxide and oxygen, regional anesthesia (spinal, epidural, combined) should be considered
- Cases with very high-risk for seizures—clobazam can be considered
- Injection vitamin K should be given to the newborn.

Q11. What are the precipitating risk factors for seizures in labor?

The precipitating factors for seizure in labor are:
- Sleep deprivation
- Stress
- Non-intake of AED doses
- Dehydration
- Pain.

Q12. How will you manage an acute episode of seizure?[1,3]

The basic principles for management of acute episode of seizure are:
- Establish the ABCs, and check vital signs, including oxygenation
- Assess the fetal heart rate or fetal status
- Rule out eclampsia
- Administer a bolus of lorazepam (0.1 mg/kg, i.e. 5–10 mg) at a rate of no more than 2 mg/min
- Diazepam 5–10 mg administered slowly intravenously is an alternative
- If seizures are not controlled then load phenytoin (20 mg/kg, i.e. 1–2 g) at a rate of no more than 50 mg/min, with cardiac monitoring, if above. If seizures are not controlled then load phenobarbital (20 mg/kg, i.e. 1–2 g) at a rate of no more than 100 mg/min
- Check laboratory findings, including electrolytes, AED levels, glucose, and toxicology screen
- If fetal well-being test results are nonreassuring, move to emergency delivery.[8]

Q13. What are the common indication for admission in WWE?

The common indications for admission to hospital in women with epilepsy are:
- Convulsions
- Gestational hypertension/severe preeclampsia
- Gestational diabetes mellitus
- Gross congenital anomaly in the baby
- Threatened abortion
- Antepartum hemorrhage.

Q14. What is important in postpartum care of WWE?[3]

The important things to be considered in postpartum care are:
- As immediate postpartum is a high-risk period for seizures due to stresss, sleep deprivation, dehydration, missed medication and anxiety, AED should be continued post-delivery. Women with history of seizures in the month prior are particularly at high risk
- Patient should be reviewed by the neurologist regarding AED dose and dose should be tapered in the first 10 days after delivery to avoid toxicity
- Neonatal general examination should be done to look for any gross congenital anomalies
- Breastfeeding should be encouraged as the prospective study has shown that the psychomotor development of the breastfed children was better at 6 and 18 months when compared with those of non-breastfed children.
- Screen for postpartum depression.

Q15. What is the safest choice of contraception for WWE on AED?[3]

The safer contraceptives are:
- Copper intrauterine devices
- Levonorgestrel-releasing intrauterine system
- Medroxyprogesterone acetate injection

These methods are not affected by the enzyme inducing AED (carbamazepine, phenytoin, phenobarbital, primidone, oxcarbazepine, topiramate, eslicarbazaepine).

Oral contraceptive pills (OCPs), Transdermal patches, vaginal ring, progestogen-only implants may be affected by the enzyme inducing AEDs and may lead to contraceptive failure.

WWE not on any AED/non-enzyme inducing AED (sodium valproate, levetiracetam, gapapentin, vigabatrin, tiagabine, pregabalin) may be offered all the methods of contraception.

Q16. What are the common complications associated with pregnancy?

The most common complications associated with pregnancy in women with epilepsy are:
- Threatened abortion
- Pregnancy induced hypertension
- Severe preeclampsia
- Gestational diabetes mellitus
- Antepartum hemorrhage
- Postpartum hemorrhage
- Congenital anomaly in baby.

Q17. What is the role of induction of labor and cesarean section?[3]

Seizure disorder per se is not an indication for induction of labor or cesarean section.

Pregnancy can be continued till term in uncomplicated cases of seizure disorder. They can be induced or cesarean section can be done as indicated in any obstetric complication.

Q18. What are the signs and symptoms of AED toxicity?

The common toxicity features of antiepileptic drugs are:
- *Central nervous system:* Ataxia, drowsiness, coma, convulsions
- *Gastrointestinal tract:* Nausea and vomiting
- *Cardiovascular:* Hypotension, arrhythmias.

Q19. What are the differential diagnosis of seizures in pregnancy?

Pregnancy related convulsions—eclampsia
- Convulsions not directly related to pregnancy
- Infections—meningitis, encephalitis, cerebral malaria, cerebral abscesss:

Febrile Convulsions

- Cerebrovascular accidents—venous thrombosis, infarction, hemorrhage
- Metabolic hypoglycemia, hyperglycemia, hyponatremia, hypocalcemia
- Trauma
- Drug withdrawal—cocaine, alcohol
- Paroxysmal nonepileptic seizures
- Organic—syncope, migraine, transient ischemic attacks
- Psychogenic.

Q20. What is psychogenic nonepileptic seizure?

Psychogenic nonepileptic seizures (PNES) or pseudo seizures or psychogenic seizures are often misdiagnosed as epileptic seizures; however PNES are psychological.[9]

- Seen in 20-30% of patients with refractory seizures[10]
- Considered as a part of conversion disorder
- Do not result from abnormal electrical discharge from the brain; they are a physical manifestation of a psychological disturbance
- Typically begin in young adulthood, more common in women
- Treatment: Behavior therapy.

Most of the patients are treated for epilepsy resulting in delay in the correct diagnosis. Duration of illness increases resulting in poorer prognosis. Thus obtaining a definite diagnosis early in the course of disease is critical.

Q21. What are the causes of headache in pregnancy?

Headache is the most common neurological complaint in pregnancy.[11]

- Primary headaches are more common than the secondary headaches in pregnant women.[12]
- International Classification of Headache Disorder, 3rd edition (beta version)-2013 classifies it as follows:

Primary Headaches

- Tension —type headache—most common[13]
- Migraine—2nd most common
- Trigeminal autonomic cephalgias
- Other.

Secondary Headaches

- Trauma—head and neck injury
- Vascular—Cranial and cervical vascular disorder
- Nonvascular intracranial disorder
- Substance use or its withdrawal
- Infection
- Disorder of homeostasis
- Psychiatric disorder
- Disorder of cranium, neck, eyes, ears, nose, sinuses, teeth, mother other facial or cervical structure
- Painful cranial neuropathies, other facial pains and other headaches

CASE SCENARIO

> A 25 years old primigravida at 35 weeks of gestation with history of Migraine headache since childhood has come to OPD with acute history of sudden episode of migraine since the day before.

Q1. Describe the characteristics of migraine in pregnancy.

Migraine is characterized as unilateral and pulsating, maybe associated with photophobia, nausea and exacerbation of physical activity.[14]

- Prevalence of migraine headache—2% in first trimester.[17]

Antepartum

- Usually improve during pregnancy (estrogen levels are higher and constant).[15,16]
- Women with severe migraine in first 8 weeks have slightly increased risk of limb reduction defects[18]
- Increased risk of preeclampsia and cardiovascular comorbidities.[19-21]

Postpartum

Recurrence has been observed due to fall in estrogen levels particularly in menstrual associated migraines[15,16]

Q2. Write the management of migraine in pregnancy.

The management of migraine in pregnancy includes-

Nonpharmacological[22] limited data about its use and effectiveness

- Biofeedback
- Acupuncture
- Transcranial magnetic stimulation

Pharmacological[24]

- Acute therapies
  - Nonsteroidal anti-inflammatory drugs (NSAIDs)
  - Acetaminophen (Category B drug)—first line[23]
  - Ibuprofen (Category B)
  - Caffeine (Category B)
  - Opioids (Category B/C)
  - Butalbital (Category C)
  - Sumatriptan (Category C)—in migraines refractory to first line drugs
  - Metoclopramide (Category B)—adjunctive therapy, effective in treating nausea and vomiting

- Prochlorperazine (category C)
- Promethazine (Category C)
- Ergotamines (Categories X)—causes uterine hypertony, abortions, hypoxic events in fetus
- Recurrent (3 or more migraines per month)/chronic migraines
- Antidepressants
  - Amitriptyline (Category C)
  - Nortryptyline (Category D)
- Beta blocker
  - Propranolol (Category C)
  - Metoprolol (Category C)
- Calcium channel blockers
  - Nifedipine (Category C)
  - Verapamil (Category C)
- Trimagneium Dictate (Category A)—some role
- In refractory migraines, corticosteroids (prednisone, methylprednisone) can be used.

CASE SCENARIO

A 22 years old primigravida at 30 weeks of gestation with history of Bells palsy since childhood has come to OPD for ANC.

Q1. Write regarding Bell palsy in pregnancy and its management.[11]

Bell palsy in pregnancy is:
- Incidence: 4 times more compared with non-pregnant women
- Characterized by facal nerve inflammation and often associated with reactivate of herpes virus or herpes zoster virus
- Usually it has an abrupt and painful onset
- Maximum facial nerve weakness reaches by 48 hours
- Effect of pregnancy on recovery of spontaneous facial nerve recovery: unclear
- Effect of Bell palsy on pregnancy—5 times increased risk of gestational hypertension or preeclampsia.

Management
- *Supportive care:* Facial muscle massage
- Eye protection from drying and corneal laceration
- *Pharmacological:* Prednisone (1 mg/kg orally for 5 days)
- Antiviral drug—Controversial.

CASE SCENARIO

A 28 years old primigravida at 32 weeks of gestation with prior history of multiple sclerosis for last 5 years has come to OPD for ANC.

Q1. Mutiple sclerosis in pregnancy and its management.

Incidence: 3.6 per 1,00,000 person-years (95% confidence interval (CI) 3.0-4.2) in women[25]
- Usually affects women in reproductive age group[11]
- Familial recurrence rate: 15%
- Incidence in offspring—increases 15-fold
- Clinical features: Sensory loss, visual symptoms from optic neuritis, weakness, paresthesias and other neurological symptoms depending upon organ involvement
- Effect of pregnancy on MS:[26] Reduction in relapse rate during pregnancy
- Increase in relapse rate during postpartum
- Effect of MS on pregnancy:[11] No adverse effects on pregnancy outcome in uncomplicated disease.
- Increased rate of induction of labor and hence increased cesariean delivery rate.

Management
- *Acute attack:*
  - High dose intravenous methylprednisone (500-100 mg daily) for 3-5 days followed by oral prednisone for 2 weeks
  - Plasma exchange
- *Preventing relapse*
  - Disease modifying drugs—interferons B1a (Category C) and interferons B1b (Category C), glatiramer acetate (Category B)
  - Natalizumab (Category C)
  - Fingolimad (data unavailable)
- *Symptomatic:* Analgesics, carbamazepine, phenytoin, amitriptyline(neurogenic pain), baclofen (spasticity), @2 adrenergic blockers for bladder neck relaxation, cholinergic and anticholinergic drugs to stimulate or inhibit bladder contractions
- *Prevention of prolapse postpartum:* Intravenous immunoglobalin (IVIG) (0.4 g/day) for 5 days during 1,6 and 12 weeks.

REFERENCES

1. Daniel H L, Denis LK, et al in Harrison's Principle of Internal Medicine. 19th edition, 2015, Part 17 Neurologic disorder, section 2 chapter 445 diseases of the CNS.2542-59.
2. Weston J, Bromley R, Jackson CF, et al. Monotherapy treatment of epilepsy in pregnancy:congenital malformation outcomes in the child. The Cochrane Library 2016.
3. RCOG Greentop Guidelines, No 68. Epilepsy in pregnancy. June 2016.
4. Medical research council Antiepileptic Drug Withdrawal Study Group. Randomised study of antiepileptic drug withdrawal in patients in remission. Lancet. 1991;337(8751):1175-80.

5. Specchio LM, Tramacere L, La Neve A, et al. Discontinuing antiepileptic drugs in patients who are seizurefree on mono therapy. J Neurol Neurosurg Psychiatry. 2002;72(1):22-5.
6. Bangar S, Shastri A, El Sayeh H, et al. Women with epilepsy: clinically relevant issues. Functional neurology. 2016; 31(3):127.
7. Pennell PB. EURAP outcomes for seizure control during pregnancy; useful and encouraging data. Epilepsy Curr. 2006;6:186-8.
8. National Institute for Health and Care Excellence. The Epilepsies: the diagnosis and management of the epilepsies in adults and children in primary and secondary care. NICE Clinical Guideline. 137. 2012.
9. LaFrance WC, Benbadis SR. Avoiding the costs of unrecognised psychological nonepileptic seizures. Neurology. 2006;66(11):1620-1.
10. Mellers JD. The approach to patients with non-epileptic seizures. Postgrad Med J. 2005;958:498-504.
11. Cunningham FG, Leveno KJ, Bloom SL, Spong CY, et al .William obstetrics 24th edition 2014, chapter 60 Neurological disorders, pp 1189-91.
12. Digre KB. Headaches during pregnancy. Clinical obstetrics and gynecology. 2013;56(2):317-29.
13. Goadsby PJ, Lipton RB, Ferrari MD. Migraine—current understanding and treatment. New Eng Medi. 2002;346(4): 257-70.
14. International Headache Society. The international classification of headache disorders: 2nd edition. Cephalalgia. 2004;24 (suppl 1):9-160.
15. Marcus DA. Interrelationships of neurochemicals, estrogen, and recurring headache. Pain 1995;62(2):129-39.
16. Melhado EM, Maciel JA Jr, Guerreiro CA. Headache during gestation: evaluation of 1101 women. Can J Neurol Sci 2007;34(2):187-92.
17. Chen TC, Leviton A. Headache recurrence in pregnant women with migraine. Headache: The Journal of Head and Face Pain. 1994;34(2):107-10.
18. Bánhidy F, Ács N, Horváth-Puhó E, et. al. Pregnancy complications and delivery outcomes in pregnant women with severe migraine. Eur J Obstet Gynecol Reprod Biol. 2007;134(2):157-63.
19. Facchinetti F, Allais G, Nappi RE, et al. Migraine is a risk factor for hypertensive disorders in pregnancy: a prospective cohort study. Cephalalgia. 2009;29(3):286-92.
20. Sanchez SE, Qiu C, Williams MA, et. al. Headaches and migraines are associated with an increased risk of preeclampsia in Peruvian women. Am J Hyperten. 2008;21(3):360-4.
21. Schürks M, Rist PM, Bigal ME, et al. Migraine and cardiovascular disease: systematic review and meta-analysis. BMJ. 2009;339:b3914.
22. Airola G, Allais G, Gabellari IC,et al. Non-pharmacological management of migraine during pregnancy. Neurol Sci. 2010;31(1):63-5.
23. Lipton RB, Stewart WF, Ryan RE, Jr., et al. Efficacy and safety of acetaminophen, aspirin, and caffeine in alleviating migraine headache pain: three double-blind, randomized, placebo-controlled trials.[see comment]. Arch Neurol. 1998;55(2): 210-7.
24. Powrie RO, Greene MF, Camann W. de Swiet's Medical Disorders in Obstetric Practice. 15th edition, Singapore: Wiley-Balckwell, 2010, chapter 35. Approach to headaches in pregnancy, 674-6.
25. Alonso A, Hernan MA. Temporal trends in the incidence of multiple sclerosis: a systematic review. Neurology 2008;71(2):129-35.
26. Vukusic S, Confavreux C. Pregnancy and multiple sclerosis: the children of PRIMS. Clinical neurology and neurosurgery. 2006;108(3):266-70.

21 CHAPTER

Renal Diseases in Pregnancy

Sangeeta Bhasin, Neelam Yadav

Though quite uncommon in pregnancy, obstetricians often come across renal disorders in the form of preexisting renal disease or a preexisting subclinical condition which gets uncovered during pregnancy. With continuous progress in obstetrics and neonatology and the appearance of high-risk pregnancy clinics there has been great improvement in both maternal and fetal outcome in pregnancies with renal disorders.

CASE SCENARIO

A 30 years old G2P1L1 at 30 weeks period of gestation presents with increased frequency of micturition and suprapubic pain.

Q1. What is your probable diagnosis? What points in history and examination will help you to come to your diagnosis?

The Lady Most Probably has Cystitis.
- Urinary tract infection (UTI) generally manifests itself in three clinical presentations; asymptomatic bacteriuria, cystitis or pyelonephritis
- Cystitis usually presents as abrupt onset frequency of micturition, urgency, dysuria, nocturia, suprapubic pain during and after voiding, microscopic or visible hematuria and offensive urine. Systemic symptoms like fever, costovertebral angle tenderness and leukocytosis are absent or slight
- A history of hematuria, flank pain colicky in nature radiating to lower back and groin and dysuria points to urinary calculus
- History of diabetes mellitus/recent antibiotic use/previous UTI/presence of renal calculi/use of diaphragm, spermicides like nonoxynol-9 increase *E. coli* vaginal colonization and are risk factors for developing UTI.

Q2. Why are pregnant women prone to UTI and pyelonephritis?

The anatomic and physiological alterations caused by pregnancy promote urinary stasis and increase susceptibility for UTI. The factors responsible are:
- Progesterone-induced ureteric dilatation causes static column of urine in ureter
- Gravid uterus displaces urinary bladder superiorly and anteriorly thereby causing urinary stasis
- Decreased bladder tone, increased bladder capacity, incomplete emptying all predispose to increased vesicoureteric reflux resulting in ascending bacterial infection
- Altered physical and chemical composition of urine in the form of increased excretion of bicarbonate and glucose favors bacterial multiplication
- In puerperium, bladder distension due to decreased sensitivity caused by nerve trauma during labor, discomfort due to painful episiotomy, catheterization may lead to frank infection.

Q3. What are the important physiological changes that occur in the kidney during pregnancy?

There are three important physiological changes that occur in the kidney during pregnancy.[1]
1. Renal plasma flow increases by 50–70% due to a combined effect of increased cardiac output and decrease in renal vascular resistance, reaching maximum of 80% above nonpregnant level in second trimester and falling to 50% in late third trimester.
2. Increase in glomerular filtration rate (GFR) as a consequence of increased renal plasma flow. GFR increases by approximately 25% as early as 3–4 weeks of conception and by 16 weeks GFR is 55% above nonpregnant level. Consequently, creatinine clearance increases from 100–180 mL/min to 150–200 mL/min.

Blood urea nitrogen and serum creatinine decline. A blood urea nitrogen (BUN) and serum creatinine value greater than 14 mg/dL and 0.9 mg/dL indicates preexisting renal disease or pregnancy, induced complications.
3. Changes in tubular reabsorption of glucose, sodium, amino acids and uric acid.

Q4. What are the anatomical changes that occur in the renal system during pregnancy?

The anatomical changes that occur in the renal system during pregnancy are:
- Each kidney increases in length by 1–1.5 cm
- Ureters dilate, elongate, widen and become more curved
- Urinary bladder is displaced upwards and flattened in anteroposterior diameter
- Elevated progesterone of pregnancy causes smooth muscles relaxing effect which contributes to these anatomical changes of pregnancy.

Q5. What is asymptomatic bacteriuria (ASB) of pregnancy and what is its significance?

Presence of significant bacteriuria (>10^5 cfu/mL) in the absence of clinical symptoms is known as asymptomatic bacteriuria. Though asymptomatic bacteriuria does not need to be treated outside pregnancy, it has been seen that if left untreated in pregnancy it will lead to ascending infection and pyelonephritis in 20–30% of cases.[2] Treatment of asymptomatic bacteriuria early in pregnancy decreases the incidence of pyelonephritis to 2–3%.

Therefore, American College of Obstetricians and Gynecologists (ACOG) recommends that all pregnant women be screened at least once at the end of first trimester or early second trimester for asymptomatic bacteriuria through urine culture and treated for the same. Women at high risk for developing pyelonephritis should be screened every 6 weeks throughout pregnancy.

In late pregnancy the condition is associated with prematurity, fetal growth restriction and neonatal death.

Q6. How will you confirm your diagnosis?

Confirmation is through urine examination.
- *Gross urine examination:* Cloudiness caused by presence of crystals and white blood cells, foul odor
- *Microscopic examination of urine*
  - Casts, crystals, red blood cells—chronic kidney disease (CKD)
  - White blood cells indicates cystitis (≥8–10 pus cells/hpf ≈ ≥10^5 cfu/mL)
  - Epithelial cells indicate contamination
  - Microscopic hematuria can be seen in acute cystitis, bladder calculus, bladder tumor
  - Microscopic pyuria can be seen in non-infectious condition like dehydration, stress, fever, neoplasm
  - Microscopic bateriuria >5 org/oil immersion field ≈ ≥ 10^5 cfu/mL
- *Urine culture sensitivity:* Midstream urine analysis detects the causative organism and also the antibiotics to which it is susceptible.

Q7. How will you treat asymptomatic bacteriuria?

Treatment aims to attain urine sterility with the shortest possible course of a safe antimicrobial. Seven day course of safe, susceptible antimicrobial which is excreted by kidney is the preferred regimen in pregnancy.

The common drugs used for a three-seven day course are: **amoxicillin** 500 mg TDS, **ampicillin** 500 mg QID, **cefixime** 200 mg BD, **cephalexin** 250 mg QID, **nitrofurantoin** 100 mg QID.

In an international double blinded, placebo-controlled randomized trial conducted by WHO, a 7-day oral regimen of nitrofurantoin 100 mg twice daily was found to be most effective in cases of ASB.[3] In case of repeated infection, low dose antibiotic suppression with nitrofurantoin 100 mg orally or cephalexin 250 mg orally daily should be continued till 4 weeks postpartum.[4]

Q8. The same patient presents with high grade fever with chills and rigor and generalized muscle pain, tachycardia and tachypnea after few days. What will be your clinical diagnosis and how will you manage the patient?

A diagnosis of acute pyelonephritis is made based on the following signs and symptoms: Acute onset pain in one or both loins radiating to iliac fossa, anorexia, nausea, vomiting, suprapubic pain, generalized muscular pain, fever with chills and rigor, tachycardia, hypotension, tenderness and guarding in costovertebral angles.

Management
- Intensive care and hospitalization
- Maintenance of adequate hydration—intravenous fluid to ensure urine output of >30 mL/hr
- Lowering of temperature by analgesic, hydrotherapy, broad-spectrum antibiotics
- Monitoring of vitals and close observation for early indication of shock
- Diagnostic investigations include:
  - Microscopy and culture of urine
  - Complete blood count (leukocytosis, thrombocytopenia), renal function test, creatinine

clearance, serum electrolytes, peripheral smear for hemolysis, lactate dehydrogenase (LDH), blood culture to detect septicemia
- Chest radiograph if dyspnea or tachypnea
- Renal tract ultrasound for excluding perinephric collection
- Antimicrobial therapy based on culture sensitivity—safety considerations make cephalosporin the drug of choice—ceftriaxone 1–2 g/day[5]
- Tocolysis with beta agonist to prevent premature contractions caused by bacterial endotoxins but care should be exercised to avoid pulmonary overload caused by sodium and water retaining property of beta agonist
- Once patient is asymptomatic for 24 hours she is shifted to oral antibiotics for 7–10 days
- Midstream urine analysis should be repeated 7–10 days after completion of antibiotic treatment.

CASE SCENARIO

A 25 years old primigravida at 32 weeks period of gestation presents to gyne casuality with history of pain abdomen and bleeding per vaginum. She is pale (clinically 6 g%), has pedal edema, BP = 160/110 mm Hg. Her abdomen is distended to 36 weeks, is tense, has a single fetus in cephalic presentation and fetal heart is not localized. On bladder catherization, only 5 mL urine is drained which shows 2+ urine albumin on dipstick testing.

Q1. What are the important relevant points in history and examination that will help you to come to a diagnosis?

- History of painful bleeding followed by intrauterine demise (IUD) and decreased urine output
- Symptoms of preeclmpsia or impending eclampsia—headache, pain in right hypochondrium, blurring of vision, edema of legs, puffiness of face, sudden weight gain, tightness of finger rings
- History of pre-existing renal disorder/any urinary complaint
- History of nephrotoxic drug intake
- General physical examination—general condition, level of consciousness, degree of pallor, edema, icterus, cyanosis, hydration status, temperature, pulse, blood pressure (BP), respiratory rate
- Systemic examination—cardiovascular system-associated heart disaese, volume overload
- Respiratory system—crepts (evidence of volume overload)
- Abdominal examination (inspection)—abdominal wall edema, fundal height more than period of gestation symptom of concealed abruption
- Palpation—uterine contour, consistency (tense tender and rigid uterus is feature of abruptio placentae), hepatosplenomegaly, palpable urinary bladder
- Auscultation—fetal heart
- Vaginal examination—after ruling out placenta previa—to do bishop scoring, pelvic assesment and deciding upon mode of delivery.

Q2. What is your diagnosis?

Primigravida with 32 weeks pregnancy with severe preeclampsia with abruptio placentae with intrauterine death with acute renal failure.

Q3. What is acute renal failure and how do you diagnose it?

Acute renal failure (ARF), acute kidney injury is defined as a sudden reduction in renal function, as evidenced by a rise in serum creatinine above normal, which results in accumulation of waste products of metabolism, retention of sodium and water and acid-base disturbances. It is characterized by:
- Abrupt decrease in GFR
- Urine output less than 400 mL in 24 hours
- Rising plasma urea and creatinine level.

Apart from the above factors, features of the associated clinical condition that has caused the kidney injury will help us to make a diagnosis of ARF, for example:
- Anorexia, fatigue, excessive nausea and vomiting, dehydration, mental status changes in hyperemesis
- Fever, foul smelling discharge, abdominal pain, peritonitis in sepsis
- Increased blood pressure, headache, epigastric pain blurring of vision, pulmonary edema, elevated right atrial pressure, shortness of breath in preeclampsia
- Painful bleeding, tense and tender uterus in abruption.

Q4. What are the renal biochemical parameters in normal pregnancy?

- Plasma urea—9–12 mg%
- Plasma creatinine—<1.0 mg%
- Urinary protein excretion—<300 mg/day
- Plasma sodium—130–140 mEq/L
- Plasma HCO_3—18–20 mEq/L
- Plasma albumin—2.5–3.5 g/dL.

Q5. What are the causes of acute renal failure in pregnancy?

The causes can be divided into pre-renal, renal and post-renal.

Pre-renal

- Severe hypovolemia resulting in reduced renal perfusion as in severe antepartum hemorrhage (APH)/postpartum hemorrhage (PPH), hyperemesis, diarrhea
- Sepsis leading to reduced renal perfusion from hypotension/fluid shift as in septic abortion/pyelonephritis/gram-negative sepsis/chorioamnionitis/puerperal sepsis.

Renal

- Microangiopathy from platelet fibrin thrombi occluding microvasculature as in preeclampsia/HELLP/TTP-HUS syndrome
- Acute tubular necrosis from toxic or ischemic insult to renal tubulointerstitium as in preeclampsia, acute fatty liver of pregnancy (AFLP), sepsis, drugs like aminoglycosides
- Glomerulonephritis as in systemic lupus erythematosus (SLE)/crescentic glomerulonephritis.

Post-renal

Extrinsic compression of ureters/kidney stones causing obstruction.

Q6. What is the pathogenic mechanism behind ARF?

- *Prerenal failure:* Moderate degree of ischemia
- *Acute tubular necrosis:* More prolonged ischemia (evidenced by persistent oliguria and rising serum creatinine despite intravascular volume and BP correction)
- *Acute cortical necrosis:* Follows severe renal ischemia.

Q7. What are the clinical phases of renal failure?

- *Oliguric phase:* Urine output ≤400 mL/hr
- *Polyuric phase:* Markedly increased urine output
- *Recovery phase:* Urine output reverts back with variable return of renal function.

Q8. What are the investigations one should proceed with?

- *Blood investigations:* Complete blood count, kidney/liver function tests, serum electrolytes, arterial blood gas (ABG), coagulation profile/smear for hemolysis/LDH
- *Urine investigations:* Microscopy for white blood corpuscles (WBCs)/red blood corpuscles (RBCs)/renal tubular cells, renal tubular cell cast, muddy brown pigment cast, osmolality, specific gravity, electrolyte concentration, protein excretion
- *Fractional excretion of sodium:* Fractional excretion of sodium (FENa).

Q9. How will you differentiate between pre-renal and renal ARF?

Urine analysis will help differentiate between the two[6] (Table 1).

Table 1: Differentiating features of pre-renal and renal failure

Parameter	Pre-renal failure	Renal failure /ATN
Urinary sodium	≤20 mEq/L	≥40 mEq/L
Urine osmolality	≥500	≤350
FENa	≤1%	≥2%
Urinary creatinine/plasma-creatinine ratio	≥40	≤20
Urinary sediment	Occasional hyaline/granular casts	Muddy brown granular casts/ tubular cell debris

Abbreviation: FENa, fractional excretion of sodium

Q10. How will you manage the patient with reference to renal failure?

Main aim of management is:

- Identification of the precipitating factor and its correction: In this patient, abruption has exacerbated the already constricted intravascular compartment caused by severe preeclampsia. The combined hypovolemic effect of these conditions has led to the development of ARF. Early termination of pregnancy along with strict control of BP through antihypertensives/prophylactic anticonvulsants/monitoring of LFT and coagulation profile and replacement with blood and blood products should be done.
- The mainstay of treatment is optimal fluid resuscitation:
  - Early phase hypovolemia with transient oliguria of <100 mL/4 hours is usually corrected by a fluid challenge with 500 mL isotonic saline given over 20 minutes after excluding signs of pulmonary edema
  - Inadequately treated hypovolemia leads to transient acute tubular necrosis (ATN) which may subsequently progress to bilateral cortical renal necrosis (CRN) and permanent renal damage. 50% of the ATN cases may be nonoliguric. About 20% of patients with ATN progress to CRN and CRN should be suspected when anuria persists for more than a week
  - In severe preeclampsia with serum creatinine above 1.3 mg%, fluid therapy should be guided by placement of a pulmonary artery catheter in the intensive care unit as central venous pressure monitoring alone is inaccurate in these patients due to the increased systemic vascular resistance (SVR) which results in disparate left and right ventricular function.[7] Appropriate treatment is then based on the invasive hemodynamic parameters (Table 2).

Table 2: Treatment based on the invasive hemodynamic parameters

Low PCWP and high SVR	Fluid at 250 mL/hr till PCWP is 10–12 mm Hg
Normal/high PCWP and normal SVR	IV hydralazine or low dose dopamine (2.5 µg/kg/min)
Markedly high PCWP and high SVR	Aggressive reduction of afterload with furosemide infusion 5 mg/h and fluid restriction

Abbreviatons: PCWP, pulmonary capillary wedge pressure; SVR, systemic vascular resistance; IV, intravenous

- Once the patient becomes euvolemic, volume of intravenous fluid replacement should equal previous hours output plus insensible loss—usually 30 mL/hour
- Invasive central hemodynamic monitoring should continue until the diuretic phase in postpartum period.
- Fluid replacement should include blood and isotonic sodium chloride or ringer lactate solution. Dextrose is hypotonic and may cause hyponatremia. Colloid solution may increase pulmonary capillary wedge pressure (PCWP) markedly
- Monitor pulse rate and volume/BP/respiratory rate/chest auscultation for evidence of fluid overload/strict input with hourly urine output record/twice daily kidney function test (KFT)/serum electrolytes/ABG.

Q11. What are the indications of dialysis in these patients?

The goal is to maintain maternal blood pH above 7.2 and dialysis should be started before symptoms of acidosis/electrolyte imbalance set in:

- Cardiovascular overload during oliguric phase of ATN
- Nonresponding hyperkalemia
- Uremic encephalopathy or metabolic acidosis
- Uremia—BUN ≥39 mg/dL, serum creatinine ≥5.65 mg/dL.

Q12. When will you suspect that renal cortical necrosis has set in?

- Anuria persisting for >a week
- Doubling of serum creatinine within 48 hours
- Diagnosis is confirmed by CT scan with contrast or selective renal angiography.

CASE SCENARIO

P2L2 with SLE in remission phase with blood pressure well controlled without drugs with moderate renal impairment is planning to conceive.

Q1. What prepregnancy counseling will you give her?

- Women with chronic kidney disease (CKD) with serum creatinine >2 mg/dL or when kidney function is impaired by >50% should ideally refrain from pregnancy. Risk of pregnancy complications, deterioration of renal function and low chances of successful pregnancy outcome have to be explained to patient before making a decision to conceive
- The diagnosis of pregnancy is delayed in these women as women with CKD have irregular menstrual cycles and impaired fertility. Also, hCG levels are raised in renal failure making the diagnosis of pregnancy uncertain. Therefore, an early dating USG should be done
- Periconceptional 400 µg folic acid per day
- Stop angiotensin-converting enzyme (ACE) inhibitors/angiotensin-receptor blocker (ARB) prior to conception.

Q2. What are the effect of chronic renal disease on pregnancy and vice versa?

- The major determinants of maternal and fetal outcome are the nature of renal disease, the level of renal impairment at the beginning of pregnancy, degree of hypertension, the presence of coexisting infection and proteinuria
- Chronic hypertension and preconception proteinuria worsen as pregnancy progresses. Perinatal mortality increases by 6-10 times. There is a 50% increased risk of preeclampsia
- The likelihood of accelerated renal damage and progression to end-stage renal disease increases with increasing baseline serum creatinine and varies with type of renal disease.
    - Mild renal impairment (serum creatinine ≤1.4 mg%)—there is normal intravascular volume expansion and increase in GFR. Risk of deterioration of renal function during pregnancy is 2%
    - Moderate renal impairment (serum creatinine 1.4–2.4 mg%)—40% women will show deterioration in renal function and in half of them deterioration will persist postpartum. 2% will rapidly decline to end-stage renal disease (ESRD).
    - Severe renal impairment (serum creatinine ≥2.5 mg%)—there is markedly attenuated increase in blood volume and no increase in GFR, 66% show deterioration in renal function that nearly always persists postpartum and progresses to ESRD within 6 months of delivery in 23% of cases.
- Chronic kidney disease is associated with increased incidence of spontaneous abortion, therapeutic pregnancy termination on medical grounds, preterm labor—both spontaneous and iatrogenic, fetal growth restriction secondary to hypertension and uremia, osteomalacia due to maternal disturbance of calcium metabolism, a higher perinatal mortality and a higher cesarean section rate of around 60%.

Q3. What are the effects of prepregnancy renal function on pregnancy outcome and maternal renal function?

Table 3: Effects of prepregnancy renal function on pregnancy outcome and maternal renal function

Aggressive reduction of afterload with furosemide infusion 5 mg/hr and fluid restriction	Fetal growth restriction (%)	Preterm delivery (%)	Pre-eclampsia (%)	Perinatal deaths (%)	Loss of >25% renal function during pregnancy	Loss of >25% renal function postpartum	End-stage renal disease after 1 year
<1.4	25	30	15–22	1	2	0	0
1.4-2	40	30–60	40	5–15	40	20	2
>2	60	75–85	60	10	70	50	35
On dialysis	>90	>90	75	50	N/A	N/A	N/A

CASE SCENARIO

A 28 years old G3P2L2 at 30 weeks of pog with SLE with BP well controlled on drugs, serum creatinine 1.2 mg% and proteinuria of 400 mg in 24 hours attends the antenatal OPD.

Q1. On what factors does a favorable outcome depend?

Best pregnancy outcomes in lupus nephritis are seen in:
- Women with quiescent lupus nephritis
- When SLE has been in remission for at least 1 year
- Normal or near normal renal function (serum creatinine ≤1.4 mg%)
- Proteinuria ≤500 mg/24 hours
- Hypertension controlled for at least 6 months before conception.

Q2. What points in history need to be stressed?

- Status of SLE at the time of conception (whether in a state of remission or exacerbation)
- Degree of renal involvement (risk is higher in women with renal involvement)
- Hypertension at conception
- Presence of antiphospholipid antibodies
- Presence of associated stigmata of SLE
- Treatment history—whether on steroids or immunosuppressive therapy.

Q3. What will be your management?

- The pregnancy should be booked in a tertiary care center under the guidance of a nephrologist, nutritionist, obstetrician and neonatologist. Good family support is essential to achieve best possible pregnancy outcome
- Baseline investigations at booking—KFT, liver function test (LFT), complete blood count (CBC), serum protein, serum cholesterol, creatinine clearance, serum electrolytes, anti-dsDNA complement titer, urine analysis for casts and culture, 24 hours urine estimation of proteins with protein-creatinine ratio
- Two weekly antenatal visits till 28–30 weeks and weekly thereafter
- Blood pressure, urine test for protein at each visit. If dipstick value is high then 24 hours urine protein
- Renal function tests every 4–6 weeks
- Mid-stream urine culture at 24, 28 and 32–34 weeks.
- Blood pressure should be maintained between 120/80 mm Hg and 140/90 mm Hg throughout pregnancy (preferably below 130/80 mm Hg). Suitable antihypertensives include alpha methyldopa, labetalol, nifedipine, hydralazine and beta blockers oxprenalol, metoprolol
- Anemia should be treated with hematinics/recombinant erythropoietin (frequent BP monitoring should be done in these patients)
- In the presence of gross edema as in nephrotic syndrome, low sodium diet, bed rest in left lateral position to increase GFR and careful addition of a loop diuretic
- Thromboprophylaxis with low dose aspirin and LMWH in the presence of proteinuria ≥1 g/24 hours.
- Uterine artery Doppler at 20–24 weeks may help in predicting preeclampsia and IUGR
- Serial biometry 3 weekly to assess fetal growth from 24 weeks onwards
- Fetal surveillance weekly from 30–32 weeks or earlier depending upon severity of disease
- Deliver at term with continous fetal heart rate monitoring. Avoid post-dates
- Intravenous glucocorticoid (hydrocortisone 100 mg 8 hourly 3 doses) during labor or cesarean in women who have received maintenance or steroid bursts during pregnancy
- Postnatally, monitor for exacerbation, restart maintenance therapy, check neonate for manifestations of SLE
- Nephrology review within first 4 weeks of delivery.

Q4. What is lupus flare?

- An acute exacerbation of SLE in pregnancy is termed lupus flare. It manifests as increasing proteinuria, presence of active urine sediments and rising serum creatinine. It is treated with 500 mg of methyl prednisolone IV daily for 3 days and increasing oral prednisolone to 60 mg daily. Azathioprine may also be used
- Though flares are more common in the postpartum period, increasing the dose of steroids prophylactically in the absence of signs of disease activity is not recommended
- Flares are more common in women who have had more than 3 flares before pregnancy, have antiphospholipid antibodies, C3 hypocomplementemia and hypertension
- Increased proteinuria in second and late third trimester may be sign of lupus flare or preeclampsia.
- Features favoring lupus flare are:
  - Increasing dsDNA
  - Fall in C3 and C4
  - Active urine sediments with hematuria and red blood cell casts
  - Extrarenal manifestations affecting skin and joints
  - Treatment is by increasing immunosuppression therapy.

Q5. What are the different stages of CKD?[8]

Table 4: Different stages of CKD

Stage	Description	Estimated GFR (mL/min/1.73m²)
1	Kidney damage with normal or raised GFR	>90
2	Kidney damage with mildly low GFR	60–89
3	Moderately low GFR	30–59
4	Severely low GFR	15–29
5	Kidney failure	<15 or dialysis

Abbreviation: GFR, glomerular filteration rate

Q6. What are the indications of early termination of pregnancy in CKD?

- Signs of impending intrauterine demise (IUD)
- Deteriorating renal function as shown by changes in serum creatinine or creatinine clearance of at least 25%
- Uncontrolled hypertension
- Eclampsia.

CASE SCENARIO

A 40 years old lady G3P2L2 with 26 weeks of gestation with CKD on dialysis.

Q1. What is the effect of dialysis on pregnancy?

- Increased risk of volume overload, exacerbation of hypertension, superimposed preeclampsia, polyhydramnios, increased fetal wastage[9]
- Only 60% pregnancies result in a live birth
- Limited prognosis raises doubts of advisability of pregnancy in these patients.

Q2. How will you manage such pregnancy?

- There is no superiority of hemodialysis over peritoneal dialysis and either modality can be used
- Lower concentration of sodium and bicarbonate should be used in dialysate so as to mimic physiological changes in pregnancy
- Increase total number of hours and number of sessions of hemodialysis per week (20–24 hours/weeks)
- Aim is to maintain predialysis BUN <50 mg/dL and serum creatinine <4.5 mg% and limit fluid removal to 400 mL/session
- Advise to take extra protein around 1.2 g/kg
- Anemia should be treated aggressively by IV/oral iron and erythropoietin
- Fetal monitoring after each dialysis session
- Consider delivery at 34–36 weeks.

CASE SCENARIO

A 35 years old nulliparous female who has undergone renal transplant 3 years back desires to conceive.

Q1. What prepregnancy counseling should she be offered?

According to guidelines issued by American Society of Transplantation Consensus Conference on Reproductive issues and transplantation, pregnancy is safe if:[10]

- Good general health for about 2 years post-transplantation
- Good stable allograft function (serum creatinine less than 2 mg/dL, preferably less than 1.5 mg/dL)
- No recent episode of acute rejection and no episode of ongoing rejection.
- Normal blood pressure or on minimal antihypertensive regimen
- Absent or minimal proteinuria (less than 0.5 g/day)
- Normal allograft ultrasound (absence of pelvicalyceal dilatation)
- Recommended immunosupression:
  - Prednisolone <15 mg/day, azathioprine <2 mg/kg/day, cyclosporine and tacrolimus at therapeutic level.

– Mycophenolate mofetil (MMF) and sirolimus are contraindicated in pregnancy and should be stopped 6 months prior to conception.

Q2. How will you monitor such pregnancy?

- Keep maintenance immunosuppression the same as before pregnancy
- Regular monitoring of renal function, electrolytes, plasma protein, calcium, phosphate levels 2 weekly
- Monitor allograft with monthly ultrasonography and technetium renal scan each trimester
- Aggressive treatment of hypertension and pre-eclampsia
- Anemia should be corrected
- Monthly urine cultures. Treat asymptomatic bacteriuria (ASB) for 2 weeks followed by suppressive therapy
- Maternal infection screening in each trimester
- Screening for impaired glucose tolerance due to prolonged steroid intake
- Close fetal surveillance to detect intrauterine growth restriction (IUGR)
- Careful watch for premature labor and preterm premature rupture of membrane (PPROM)
- Timing and mode of delivery depending upon fetal condition and pelvic adequacy.

Q3. What are the fetal and maternal risks in pregnancy after renal transplant?

Maternal Risks

Increased risk of gestational hypertension, preeclampsia, gestational diabetes, increased risk of infection.

Fetal Risks

Increased risk of preterm delivery, premature rupture of membrane, intrauterine growth restriction, defective organogenesis.

Q4. How will you manage acute graft rejection in pregnancy?

Graft rejection occurs in 5% of pregnant patients which is similar to nonpregnant population. It is diagnosed when ultrasonography shows alteration in renal parenchymal echogenicity, presence of indistinct corticomedullary boundary. Cyclosporin A should be used as treatment.

Q5. Is there any role of renal biopsy in pregnancy?

- Women less than 28 weeks pregnant with no preeclampsia and no history of renal disease showing sudden unexplained deterioration in renal function or new onset proteinuria >5 g/24 hours.
- Rapidly declining GFR with no obvious cause in a patient with renal transplant, so as to exclude acute rejection.
- Acute renal failure with active urine sediments before fetal viability is attained, where immunosuppression, plasma exchange or dialysis may be helpful.

REFERENCES

1. William DL. Renal disease in pregnancy. Obstet Gynaecol Reprod Med. 2007;17(5):147-53.
2. Smaill F. Antibiotics for asymptomatic bacteriuria in pregnancy. Cochrane database. Syst Rev. 2001;2:CD000490.
3. Lumbiganon P, Villar J, Laopaiboon M, et al. One-day compared with 7 day nitrofurantoin for asymptomatic bacteriuria in pregnancy. Obstet Gynecol. 2009;113:339-45.
4. Dwyer PL, O' Reilly M. Recurrent urinary tract infection in the female. Curr Opin Obstet Gynaecol. 2002;14:537-43.
5. Wing DA. Pyelonephritis in pregnancy. Treatment options for optimal outcomes. Drugs. 2001;61:2087-96.
6. Brady HR, Brenner BM. Acute renal failure. In: Braunwald E, Hauser SL, Fauci A, Longo DL, Kasper DL, Jameson JL (Eds): Harrison's Principles of Internal Medicine, 15th edition. McGraw Hill. United States of America; 2001. pp.1541-51.
7. Gilbert WM, Towner DR, Field NT, et al. The safety and utility of pulmonary artery catheterization in severe preeclampsia and eclampsia. Am J Obstet Gynecol. 2000;186:253-6.
8. Vidaeff AC, Yeomans ER, Ramin SM. Pregnancy in women with renal disease. Part II: Specific underlying renal conditions. Am J Perinatol. 2008;25:399-405.
9. Holley JL, Reddy SS. Pregnancy in dialysis patients: A review of outcomes, complications and management. Semin Dial. 2003;16:384-7.
10. McKay DB, Josephson MA. Reproduction and transplantation: Report on the AST Consensus Conference on Reproductive Issues and Transplantation. Am J Transplant. 2005;5:1592-9.

22

Liver Disorders in Pregnancy

Kashika Kathuria, Anjali Tempe

Liver diseases in pregnancy can cause significant maternal and fetal morbidity and mortality. Liver disorders related to pregnancy include conditions like ICP (0.5–1.5% prevalence), hyperemesis gravidarum (1 in 200 pregnancies), preeclampsia (10% prevalence in general population), HELLP syndrome (12% of pregnancies with preeclampsia); acute fatty liver of pregnancy (incidence—1 per 7270 to 16,000 deliveries). Management of these varies from simple supportive or medical measures to more aggressive measures including termination of pregnancy in some cases.

Liver Disorders in Pregnancy

Liver Disorders Caused By Pregnancy

Obstetric cholestasis, acute fatty liver of pregnancy (AFLP), liver damage due to severe preeclampsia and hemolysis, elevated liver enzymes and low platelet count (HELLP) syndrome, hyperemesis gravidarum-induced liver damage.

Liver Diseases Coincidental to Pregnancy

Acute viral hepatitis (Hepatitis A,B,C,D,E,G), drug-induced liver damage (isoniazid, rifampicin, phenothiazine); pre-hepatic causes: hemolysis, mismatched blood transfusion, malaria, severe septicemia; post-hepatic causes: common bile duct (CBD) stones, CBD strictures, biliary parasitosis.

Chronic Liver Diseases Preceding Pregnancy

Chronic hepatitis, liver cirrhosis, Budd-Chiari syndrome, congenital hyperbilirubinemia, autoimmune hepatitis, Wilson's disease, liver tumors, liver transplantation, Diseases of gallbladder (cholecystitis, cholelithiasis).

CASE SCENARIO

Intrahepatic cholestasis of pregnancy (ICP)

22 years old, primigravida with 37 weeks gestation comes to antenatal OPD with chief complaint of itching all over the body since 5 days. How will you manage this patient?

Relevant Findings in History and Examination

The patient had generalized itching, more severe in the night and on the palms and soles predominantly since 5 days. There was no history of skin lesions, yellowish discoloration of urine or skin, clay colored stools, fever or loss of appetite. She was admitted to the hospital as her liver function tests were abnormal. No history of drug intake, jaundice, blood transfusion or gall stones in the past. No history of jaundice or known liver disease in her family was present.

On Examination

Excoriated skin lesions (scratch marks) were present on the arms, legs and abdomen. No other rash or skin lesions seen. BP-120/80 mm Hg.

Q1. What is the differential diagnosis?

Viral hepatitis, cholelithiasis, AFLP, dermatitis (pruritic urticarial papules and plaques of pregnancy, pemphigoid gestations, atopic eruption of pregnancy), preeclampsia.

Q2. What is your provisional diagnosis and why?

It is most likely a case of intrahepatic cholestasis of pregnancy (ICP). It is also called icterus gravidarum, cholestatic hepatosis and recurrent jaundice of pregnancy.

Points which suggest the diagnosis: Pruritus which started and is more severe in the palms and soles; with its onset in the third trimester. It is worse at night, there is no rash and LFTs are deranged. Also scratch marks on the skin suggest the diagnosis. However, other causes of itching and liver dysfunction need to be excluded as ICP is a diagnosis of exclusion. Also postnatal resolution of pruritus and abnormal LFTs should be confirmed.

ICP is the second most common liver disorder in pregnancy (20% of all cases); second only to viral hepatitis.

Q3. What are the risk factors of ICP?

Risk factors of ICP are: Maternal age more than 35 years, personal or family history of ICP, multiple pregnancy, carriage of hepatitis C and gallstones.

Q4. What investigations are to be done in this case, apart from the routine antenatal investigations?

Liver function test, urine routine, PT/INR/aPTT, serum bile acids.

- *In ICP:* Hyperbilirubinemia (not exceeding 4–5 mg/dL) results from retention of conjugated pigment. Alkaline phosphatase is elevated even more than in normal pregnancy. Serum aminotransferases are normal to moderately elevated (seldom more than 250 U/L). There is rise in total serum bile acids >11 μmol/L. Increase in transaminases (ALT and AST) may occur weeks after onset of pruritus. In patients with persistent pruritus and normal biochemistry, LFT should be repeated 1–2 weekly.
- *Additional investigations to exclude other causes include:* HBs Ag, anti-HCV/HCV RNA, anti-HAV, anti-HEV; HSV, CMV and EBV screen; ultrasound of upper abdomen.
- *Tests for fetal well-being:* Daily fetal movement count (DFMC), nonstress test (NST), USG with biophysical score. A pregnant woman presenting with abnormal liver tests should undergo standard work up as for a non-pregnant individual.[1]

Q5. What are the physiological changes in hepatic functions during pregnancy?

There is no increase in liver size during pregnancy. Hepatic arterial and portal venous blood flow increase substantively.

For bilirubin, transaminases and gamma GT, upper limit of normal is 20% lower than the non-pregnant range. Total alkaline phosphatase activity almost doubles, much of it is attributable to heat stable placental alkaline phosphatase isoenzyme.[2] Total body albumin is increased, however, because of pregnancy associated increased plasma volume, the serum albumin concentration decreases. Serum globulin levels are higher.

Q6. Describe the pathophysiology of ICP.

It is a multifactorial disorder with environmental, genetic and hormonal contributions.

a. *Hormonal*: ICP tends to recur in subsequent pregnancies and may occur with OCPs as well. High circulating estrogen inhibits intraductal bile acid transport, hence causing cholestasis. Increased progesterone levels have also been implicated.
b. *Genetic*: Family history is present in half the cases; and increased risk in first degree relatives. Familial cases tend to be more severe. Mutations in certain genes have been implicated: ABCB4 gene which encodes MDR3 associated with progressive familial intrahepatic cholestasis,[3,4] ABCB11 which encodes bile salt export pump, ATP8B1 which encodes Farnesoid X receptor and transporting ATPase. These mutations predispose to increased sensitivity of bile ducts and hepatocytes to estrogens and progestogens.

As a result, bile acids are cleared incompletely and accumulate in plasma, leading to pruritus. Toxic bile acids can pass into fetal circulation, causing placental anoxia and fetal cardiac depression.

Liver biopsy shows mild cholestasis with bile plugs in hepatocytes and canaliculi of the centrilobular regions, but without inflammation or necrosis. Liver biopsy is usually not required for diagnosis. These changes disappear after delivery.

Q7. What are the risks of obstetric cholestasis?

a. *Meconium passage:* Risk increases with increase in total bile acid concentration. Meconium passage is more common in patients with severe cholestasis (defined as bile acids over 40 μmol/L) compared with mild cholestasis (bile acids less than 20 μmol/L);[5] bile acids stimulate fetal gut motility.
b. *Spontaneous preterm labour*: Bile acids increase expression and sensitivity of oxytocin receptors on the myometrium.
c. *Fetal arrhythmia*: Bile acids have been shown to be toxic to the fetal cardiomyocytes.

Table 1: Physiological changes in hepatic function in pregnancy			
Hepatic functions during pregnancy	Prepregnancy values	In pregnancy	Change during pregnancy
Bilirubin	<1 mg/dL or 0–17 μmol/L	<1 mg/dL or 3–14 μmol/L	No change
ALT (U/L)	0–40	6–32	No change or slight decrease
AST (U/L)	7–40	11–30	No change or slight decrease
GGT (U/L)	11–50	5–41	No change or slight decrease
Alkaline phosphatase(U/L)	30–130	130–418	Increased (almost double)
S. bile acids (cholic acid) μmol/L	0.4	0.41	No change
S. deoxycholic acid (μmol/L)	0.4	0.41	No change
S. chenodeoxycholic acid (μmol/L)	0.38–0.7	0.4–0.7	No change
S. albumin	4.3 g/dL	3 g/dL	Decrease

d. *Fetal asphyxia/still birth*: Bile acids cause vasoconstriction of placental chorionic veins leading to asphyxia. Fetal death is usually sudden and there is no evidence of placental insufficiency, fetal growth restriction or oligohydramnios.

There is increased incidence of *cesarean delivery and postpartum hemorrhage*.

Q8. How should patients of obstetric cholestasis be monitored?

LFT should be repeated weekly. Fetal well-being should be closely monitored owing to the inherent fetal risks; although no specific method of antenatal fetal monitoring has been recommended. Ultrasound and cardiotocography are not reliable methods for preventing fetal death in obstetric cholestasis. Continuous fetal monitoring in labor should be offered.[5]

Q9. What treatment should be offered to women with obstetric cholestasis?

There is no evidence that any specific treatment improves fetal or neonatal outcome.

Topical Emollients

Safe and provide temporary relief of pruritus. Their efficacy is unknown. Calamine lotion, aqueous cream with menthol can be used.

Systemic Treatment

- *Ursodeoxycholic acid (UDCA):* It improves pruritus, lowers bile acid and serum enzyme levels.[2] It may reduce fetal distress, preterm birth, asphyxial events;[6] certain neonatal complications, such as respiratory distress and NICU admissions. ACOG 2012a has concluded that UDCA relieves pruritus and improves fetal outcomes.[7] An ongoing trial named PITCHES is a phase III trial to evaluate the role of UDCA in improving perinatal outcome. The pilot study preceding this: PITCH (Pregnancy Intervention trial in cholestasis) found UDCA beneficial in improving perinatal outcome in patients with ICP. UDCA is the drug of choice; and is used in a dose of 300 mg 8–12 hourly. It is safe for the fetus with relatively low risk of adverse effects (Category B).
- *Mechanism of action:* UDCA (hydrophilic bile acid) displaces the more hydrophobic endogenous bile salts from the bile acid pool. This may protect the hepatocyte membrane from the damaging toxicity of the bile salts, enhance bile acid clearance across the placenta from the fetus and protect cardiomyocytes from damage by endogenous bile salts.
- *Antihistamines:* Chlorpheniramine 4 mg BD, fexofenadine 120 mg OD can relieve pruritus.
- *S-adenyl-methionine:* It inactivates estrogen metabolites, increases membrane fluidity, and alters bile acid metabolism.[8] There is insufficient evidence to show its effectiveness in improving outcomes; so it is not widely used.
- *Cholestyramine:* It is a bile acid chelating agent. It is effective but it causes further decreased absorption of fat soluble vitamins, enhancing vitamin K deficiency further. Fetal coagulopathy may develop and there are reports of intracranial hemorrhage and still birth. (Category C).[9]
- *Dexamethasone:* It is not a first line therapy. Studies have shown conflicting results and there are concerns about adverse fetal and neonatal neurological effects. It should be used only in the setting of a clinical trial.
- *Vitamin K:* It is given when the prothrombin time is prolonged. Water soluble vitamin K (menadiol sodium phosphate) 5-10 mg orally daily or vitamin K1 (phytonadione) 2.5–10 mg PO/SC once or twice daily. It reduces the risk of postpartum hemorrhage and fetal intracranial hemorrhage.

Obstetric cholestasis results in failure of excretion of bile acids into the gastrointestinal tract; hence, there is reduced micelle formation leading to reduced absorption of dietary fats and fat soluble vitamins. This leads to vitamin K deficiency which is required for manufacture of coagulation factors: II, VII, IX, X.

Q10. Should women with ICP be offered elective early delivery?

A discussion about induction of labor should take place at 37 weeks explaining the increased maternal and perinatal morbidity from early intervention versus the uncertain risk of still birth if pregnancy continues.[5] The case for intervention may be stronger in patients with more severe biochemical abnormalities (bile acids and transaminases).[5] Many recommend early delivery in ICP because of the associated fetal risks.[1] However, there is low level evidence to support this recommendation.

Q11. What follow-up should be provided to women who have pregnancy affected by obstetric cholestasis?

After delivery, resolution of LFTs and pruritus should be ensured. LFT should be repeated after a minimum of

10 days postnatally,⁵ usually at 6 weeks. The mother should be reassured about the lack of long-term sequelae for the mother and the baby. There should be a discussion about the high recurrence rate (45–90%) and increased incidence of obstetric cholestasis in family members. Contraceptive choices should be discussed especially avoiding estrogen-containing contraception. Maternal outcome is usually good and there is no permanent liver damage.

Q12. What are the other causes of pruritus in pregnancy?

Pruritus affects 20% of pregnant women.[10] Many cases of pruritus can be attributed to itchy dry skin, but may indicate a condition unique to pregnancy.

Pruritic Urticarial Papules and Plaques of Pregnancy (PUPPP)

Also called polymorphic eruption of pregnancy or prurigo of pregnancy. Lesions are urticarial papules that coalesce into plaques and spread from abdomen to thighs and buttocks. Microvesicles may overlie the striae gravidarum. Sparing of umbilicus, palms, soles and face is characteristic. Sparing of umbilicus helps to differentiate from pemphigoid gestationis (PG). It is self limiting illness with no serious consequences. Treatment is symptomatic with topical steroids and antihistamines.

Pemphigoid Gestationis (PG)

Self-limited autoimmune bullous disorder that presents after 20th week gestation or in the post partum period. Rash: pruritic, urticarial, erythematous papules, and plaques around umbilicus and extremities. Pregnancies with PG are at high risk of adverse fetal outcomes (preterm births and low birth weight).[11] Treatment: In mild pre-blistering state, topical corticosteroids with oral antihistamines may suffice. In all other cases: systemic steroids (prednisone 20–60 mg/day) are required.

Atopic Eruption of Pregnancy

Atopic eruption of pregnancy includes prurigo of pregnancy, Pruritic folliculitis of pregnancy and Eczema in pregnancy. These are benign pruritic conditions of pregnancy that include eczematous or papular lesions in patients with history of atopy.[12] Most women present with widespread eczematous changes affecting face, neck, chest and flexural surfaces of extremities. Treatment is with topical corticosteroids. In severe cases, systemic corticosteroids and antihistamines are used.

Diagnostic approach to *pruritus in pregnancy* is described in Figure 1.[13]

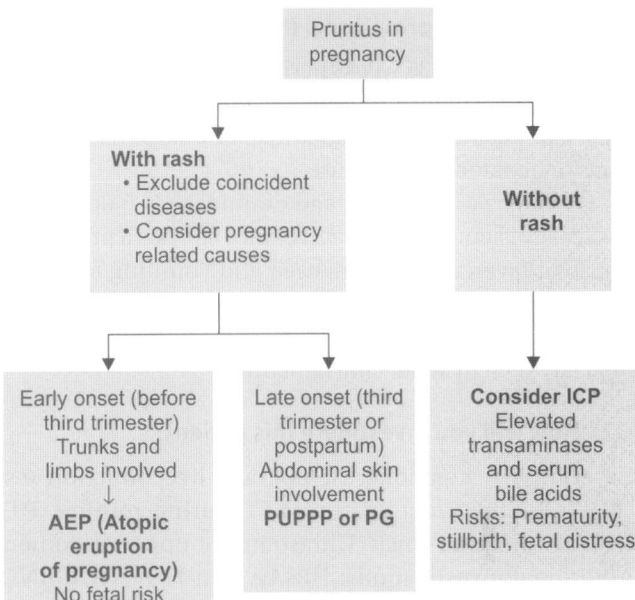

Fig. 1: Diagnostic approach to pruritus in pregnancy

Abbreviations: ICP, intrahepatic cholestasis of pregnancy; PUPPP, pruritic urticarial papules and plaques of pregnancy; PG, pemphigoid gestation

CASE SCENARIO

Acute viral hepatitis

28 years old, G2P1L1 with 35 weeks gestation came to gyne emergency with complaints of loss of appetite, nausea and vomiting for last 8 days, low-grade fever with mild chills which developed 8 days back and lasted for 5 days, yellowish discoloration of urine for last 7 days, yellowish discoloration of eyes and skin since 5 days, mild dull aching pain in right upper abdomen since 3 days. No history of itching, bleeding from any site, clay colored stools or drug intake [oral contraceptive pills (OCPs), rifampicin, isoniazid (INH)] and no disturbance in sleep pattern. No history of jaundice, blood transfusion, tattooing, acupuncture, high risk behavior in the past. She is nonalcoholic. No history of jaundice, HBV positivity or liver cancer in the family.

On Examination

Icterus seen, no pedal edema. No spider angioma or palmar erythema. No petechiae/purpura, no flapping tremors. Liver is enlarged 4 cm below the right costal margin, soft, tender, with regular margins, and smooth surface. There is no pulsation, rub or bruit. There is no splenomegaly, no free fluid, no dilated veins/caput medusa.

Q1. What is your provisional diagnosis and why?

Primigravida with 35 weeks period of gestation with single live fetus in cephalic presentation with jaundice and fever most likely acute viral hepatitis in icteric stage without any signs of hepatocellular failure.

On the basis of history and examination, it appears to be a case of acute viral hepatitis, since she has a prodromal phase of fever, anorexia, nausea and vomiting following which she developed jaundice (icteric phase). Also she has icterus with tender hepatomegaly. These findings are typically seen in acute viral hepatitis.

Q2. How will you investigate this patient?

Baseline investigations: Hemogram, liver function test (LFT), kidney function test (KFT), urine routine, PT/INR/aPTT, blood sugar. Ultrasound of upper abdomen. Additional investigations: HBsAg, anti-HCV/HCV RNA, anti-HAV, anti-HEV, CMV and EBV screen. Tests for fetal well-being.

Hemogram may reveal leucopenia/neutropenia and high ESR in the prodromal stage. LFT: S. bilirubin levels peak between 5–20 mg/dL. Aminotransferases vary from 400–4000 U/L.[9] Marked increase in ALT and AST is due to liver cell necrosis. Alkaline phosphatase is slightly increased (marked rise may occur in hepatitis A and E infection). Increase in prothrombin time (PT) indicates extensive hepatocellular necrosis and a worse prognosis. Blood glucose may be low due to vomiting, poor appetite and food intake and less hepatic glycogenolysis. USG of liver and biliary tract- helps in diagnosis of other causes of liver dysfunction, i.e. fatty liver, chronic liver disease and biliary tract disease.

Q3. What is the differential diagnosis?

Causes Unrelated to Pregnancy

Acute viral hepatitis (*Most common* cause of jaundice in pregnancy); acute fatty liver of pregnancy (AFLP); amoebic liver abscess; drug-induced hepatitis, alcoholic hepatitis, hemolytic jaundice; obstructive jaundice, acute malaria; congestive cardiac failure; chronic hepatitis (viral or autoimmune), cirrhosis of liver.

Pregnancy Related Causes

AFLP, HELLP syndrome, hyperemesis gravidarum, obstetric cholestasis

Q4. How will you differentiate this case from other causes of jaundice/liver disease in pregnancy?

Table 2: Features of various liver diseases in pregnancy

	Acute hepatitis	AFLP	ICP	Pre-eclampsia/ HELLP syndrome	Hyperemesis gravidarum
Onset in pregnancy	Any time/ variable	Late	Late	Mid to late	Early
Clinical features	Prodrome of fever, anorexia, nausea Jaundice in icteric phase	Moderate nausea and vomiting, jaundice, ±HTN, liver failure	Pruritus Jaundice in 10%	Hypertension, proteinuria, right upper quadrant pain, headache, epigastric sign of Chaussier	Severe nausea and vomiting
AST/ALT (U/L)	Very high (> 1000–2000)	Modestly high (200–800)	Upto 250	Mildly high (normal –300)	Normal –300
S. Bilirubin (mg/dl)	5–20	4–10	1–5	1–4	Normal–4
Ultrasound abdomen	Hepatomegaly, starry sky appearance, periportal edema and ↑ brightness of portal vein radical	Ascites and echogenic hepatic appearance (Swansea criteria)	Normal	Hyperechoic thickening of periportal area, ↓ liver echogenecity, Starry sky liver. Hyperechoic thickened Glisson's capsule	Normal
Hemolysis	No	+++	No	+++	No
Thrombocytopenia	+	++	No	++	No
PT	↑	↑↑	Normal	Normal	Normal

Contd...

Contd...

	Acute hepatitis	**AFLP**	**ICP**	**Preeclampsia/ HELLP syndrome**	**Hyperemesis gravidarum**
Other investigations	Hct↑, PT↑ Anti-HAV/HEV/HCV, HBsAg CMV/EBV	PS for hemolysis, LDH ↑, Hct↑↑↑, PT↑↑, fibrinogen↓↓↓, D dimer ↑, albumin ↓, creatinine ↑↑↑	S. Bile acids >11μmol/L(mild), S. Bile acids > 40 μmol/L (severe), Alkaline phosphatase↑↑↑ (5 to 10 fold)	PS for hemolysis, LDH↑, Hct↑, d–dimer↑, creatinine↑	Hct↑↑, creatinine↑, electrolyte imbalance
Etiopathogenesis	Viral infection, drug induced	AR mitochondrial abnormality of fatty acid oxidation (mutation of gene coding for LCHAD, MCHAD, CPT1)	Defective bile acid excretion: genetic and hormonal	Microangiopathic hemolysis	Strong association with hCG levels.
Liver pathology	Inflammatory cell infiltration of acini and portal tracts, hepatocyte swelling/ shrinkage/ necrosis	Small, soft, yellow and greasy liver. ↑microvesicular fat that crowds out normal hepatocyte function	Mild cholestasis with bile plugs in canaliculi of centrilobular regions, no inflammation or necrosis	Periportal hemorrhage and necrosis in liver periphery, hemorrhagic infarction, hepatic hematoma which may rupture	Minimal fatty changes
Effect on fetus	Vertical transmission of HBV and HCV infection. Fever, hypoglycemia, dehydration increase fetal morbidity.	Reduced uteroplacental perfusion due to hemoconcentration, maternal and fetal acidemia, fetal death	MSL, fetal distress, preterm labor, IUD	Perinatal mortality–7–20% due to prematurity, respiratory distress syndrome, intraventricular hemorrhage, necrotizing enterocolitis; FGR , abruption	↑incidence of SGA
Effect on mother	↑mortality in hepatitis A and E, fulminant hepatitis more common in hepatitis E	Mild to severe–disease: AKI, pulmonary edema, hypoglycemia, coagulopathy, liver failure/ encephalopthy	None	↑ morbidity due to renal/hepatic failure, pulmonary edema, eclampsia, stroke, coagulopathy. Mortality—1%	Dehydration leading to acute tubular necrosis. Excessive vomiting can cause Mallory weiss tear, splenic avulsion rarely. Wernicke's encephalopathy can occur due to thiamine deficiency.
Management	Supportive care (rest and nutrition)	Termination of pregnancy promptly	Emollients, UDCA Termination of pregnancy at 37 weeks	Termination of pregnancy	Hydration and antiemetics

Abbreviations: PT, prothrombin time; Hct, hematocrit; PS, peripheral smear; LDH, lactate dehydrogenase; AR, autosomal recessive; LCHAD, long chain 3 hydroxy acyl CoA dehydrogenase; MCHAD, medium chain dehydrogenase; CPT1, carnitine palmitoyl transferase 1; MSL, Meconium stained liquor; IUD, intrauterine death; AKI, acute kidney injury; FGR, fetal growth restriction; SGA, small for gestational age

Q5. What are the features of different types of hepatitis?

Table 3: Features of different types of viral hepatitis

	Hepatitis A	**Hepatitis B***	**Hepatitis C***	**Hepatitis E**
Transmission	Fecal-oral	Vertical, Parenteral, sexual	Parenteral (blood and body fluids), vertical, sexual	Fecal-oral
Incubation period (days)	15–45 (mean-30)	30–180 (mean = 8-12 weeks)	15–160 (mean = 7 weeks)	15–60
Severity	Usually mild; resolves in < 2 months	Asymptomatic in half, usually mild, Occasionally severe. Resolves in 3–4 months.	Acute infection: Usually asymptomatic or mild. Jaundice in 10–15%	Usually mild. More severe in pregnancy with frequent fulminant hepatitis

Contd...

Contd...

	Hepatitis A	Hepatitis B*	Hepatitis C*	Hepatitis E
Diagnosis	IgM Anti-HAV	Acute: HBs Ag, IgM Anti-HBc Chronic: HBs Ag	Anti-HCV, HCV RNA (gold standard)	IgM Anti-HEV, RT-PCR-HEV RNA
Mother to child transmission	Rare, if delivery occurs during incubation period (transmission due to viral shedding)	Not transplacental, occurs during delivery (10–20%)	4-7% in those with HCV positive, RNA positive. 1–3% in RNA negative	Can occur rarely
Effect of disease on pregnancy	↑preterm birth, neonatal cholestasis PROM, placental separation	Low risk of obstetric complications. Modest increase in preterm birth rates	Modest risk of low birth weight, NICU admission, preterm delivery/PROM and mechanical ventilation. Risk of gestational diabetes	Still birth, preterm delivery with high infant mortality rate upto 33%.[15]
Effect of pregnancy on disease	Not affected	Not affected	Not affected	Risk of fulminant disease and high maternal mortality- 20%[14]
Vaccination	Inactivated HAV vaccine (safe in pregnancy) After exposure in pregnancy: immunoglobulin 0.02 mL/kg	Recombinant HBV vaccine is safe	Not available	Recombinant HEV vaccine efficacious but not FDA approved. Available in China

Abbreviation: RTPCR, reverse transcriptase PCR; NICU, neonatal ICU; PROM, premature rupture of membranes.

*Note: Hepatitis B and C are known to cause chronic hepatitis and carrier state; more common with hepatitis C (80–90%) than hepatitis B (10%).

Hepatitis B virus (HBV) is a DNA virus, while others (Hepatitis A, C, E) are RNA viruses.

Hepatitis D: It is caused by delta (defective ss RNA) virus; causes hepatitis in patients infected with HBV. Transmission is by parenteral, sexual and rarely vertical routes. Chronic infection is common.

Hepatitis G: It is caused by a ss RNA virus- hepatitis G virus (HGV). Transmission is mainly through parenteral route (infected blood and blood products). Perinatal transmission is seen to occur in 75–80% cases.

Q6. On investigation, this patient was found to be Hepatitis E positive. How is hepatitis E infection different in pregnant women compared to non-pregnant women?

In non-pregnant individuals, Hepatitis E virus infection is usually mild to moderate in severity, with a mortality of 0.4–4%. Pregnant patients have a more severe illness with frequent fulminant hepatitis due to higher HEV viral loads, increased cytokine secretion and attenuated cellular immunity in pregnant women. The mortality rate rises with the term of pregnancy, with upto 20% mortality from acute infection in the third trimester.[14] Fetal or neonatal mortality and morbidity is high (still birth, preterm delivery, infant mortality rate of 33%).[15] The increased mortality may be attributed to associated complications like gestational hypertension, preeclampsia, proteinuria, edema and kidney disease. Management consists of supportive and symptomatic care. Patients with acute fulminant hepatitis may require liver transplantation.

CASE SCENARIO

Chronic hepatitis B carrier
30 years old primigravida was found to be HBs Ag positive on routine screening. She is asymptomatic and had an uneventful antenatal period so far.

Q1. How will you evaluate this patient?

For further evaluation: Detailed history, examination and relevant investigations are required.

Important points in *history and examination*: as for any case of liver disease (discussed in previous case).

Additional *investigations* in HBsAg + mother:

Liver function tests, HBe Ag, Anti-HBe, Anti-HBc IgM and IgG; HBV DNA levels; Tests to rule out other types of viral hepatitis; HBV testing of sexual partner and previous children; USG of upper abdomen.

The above mentioned case could be: (a) Chronic hepatitis B carrier or (b) Asymptomatic acute infection with hepatitis

B virus. This can be differentiated by the serological markers of HBV infection.

Interpretation of serological markers of HBV infection:

In acute infection, HBsAg (surface antigen) is the first to appear. Anti-HBc (IgM) appears thereafter, at the onset of symptoms and it indicates acute infection (<6 months). HBeAg appears during periods of active viral replication and indicates high infectivity. ALT and AST levels are high (1000-2000 IU/mL).

With the *resolution* of infection and *clearance of virus* from the body (convalescence): HBsAg and IgM anti-HBc disappear; Total (IgG) anti-HBc persists for life. Anti-HBs appears which indicates immunity from HBV infection. HBeAg disappears and anti-HBe antibody appears (a change known as "e"seroconversion), which is a predictor of long-term clearance of HBV.

In *Chronic HBV* infection: HBsAg persists; Total anti-HBc persists. High HBV DNA levels and HBeAg, if present, indicate high viral replication.

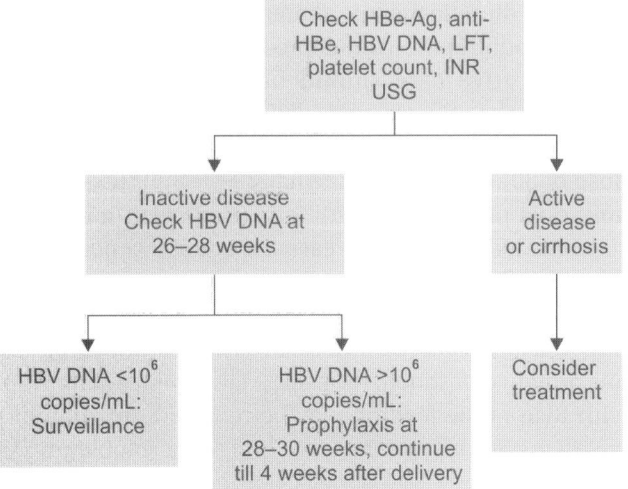

Fig. 2: Management of patient with HBV infection during pregnancy (HBsAg + ve)

If the mother is HBs Ag negative, and is also Anti-HBs and Anti-HBc negative; consider vaccination (recombinant HBV vaccine).

Q2. What is the clinical course of HBV infection?

Acute HBV infections are asymptomatic in 50% of the patients. Less commonly, acute fulminant hepatitis may occur. After acute hepatitis B infection; 2 outcomes are possible:
a. Clearance of virus with complete resolution of symptoms (within 3–4 months)—90%
b. Chronic carrier state >10%

After acute hepatitis B infection; risk of chronic carrier state is:
(a) 10% in adults, (b) 90% in infants, (c) 50% in young children

Patients with chronic infection are predisposed to develop chronic hepatitis, cirrhosis and hepatocellular carcinoma. Pregnancy does not affect course of disease or progression to chronic hepatitis. Acute hepatitis B infection in the third trimester is associated with higher risk of perinatal transmission.

Q3. How will you diagnose and manage a case of chronic hepatitis B?

Chronic HBV infection may be inactive or active. Inactive hepatitis B disease (chronic) is characterized by presence of HBsAg for more than 6 months, anti-HBc IgG and anti-HBe in serum. However, ALT and AST levels are normal; markers of infectivity such as HBeAg and HBV DNA are undetectable or at very low levels (<2000 IU mL). In these cases, laboratory evaluation every 3-4 months is recommended.

Chronic active hepatitis B disease is characterized by positive HBsAg and anti-HBc IgG, while HBeAg can be positive or negative. In HBeAg positive disease, there is mild to moderate elevation of aminotransferases (≤5 times the upper limit of normal); with ALT> AST. There are intermittent exacerbations of disease with elevations of ALT/AST, HBV DNA and hepatic dysfunction.

Management

Antepartum Care

Avoidance of alcohol and any potentially hepatotoxic drugs. They should be asked not to donate blood or share tooth brush/razor. Sexual partner should be counselled, informed and tested. Hepatologist/gastroenterologist consultation should be taken. Invasive procedures like amniocentesis/CVS/fetal scalp electrode should be avoided to decrease the risk of mother to child transmission (MTCT).

Indications for anti-viral drug treatment: Chronic active hepatitis or cirrhosis (for maternal health), HBV DNA> 10^6 log copies/ml (to reduce perinatal transmission).[1] Antiviral drugs like telbivudine, lamivudine and tenofovir appear to be safe in pregnancy[18] and should be offered to women with chronic HBV infection and high viral load to decrease risk of perinatal transmission (strong recommendation, low level of evidence).[1]

Intrapartum Care

Women with chronic hepatitis B who are HBsAg and HBeAg positive carry a 90% risk of transmitting the infection to the neonate as compared to a 10–20% risk in those who are only HBsAg positive.⁹ Infected neonates have a 90% risk of chronic infection, hence a high risk to develop chronic hepatitis B, cirrhosis and hepatocellular carcinoma. Therefore, all infants born to HBV-infected mothers are given active–passive immunoprophylaxis: HBIG (0.5 mL) is given soon after birth. This is accompanied by first of a three dose hepatitis B recombinant vaccine. When HBIG is given within the first 24 hours of birth, the risk of HBV infection can be reduced to 20%.[16,17] HBIG and vaccination are 85–95% effective in preventing HBV infection and chronic carrier state.

Cesarean section should not be performed electively in HBV-positive mothers to prevent fetal infection.

HBV infection is not a contraindication to breastfeeding (American Academy of Paediatrics). Although the virus is present in breast milk, the incidence of transmission is not lowered by formula feeding.

CDC recommends post vaccination serologic testing to assess response to vaccination at 9–12 months age. An anti-HBs titer>10 IU/L after 2–3 months is protective.

Q4. If the patient mentioned in case 3 is anti-HCV positive with positive HCV RNA; how will your management differ? Which patients should be screened for HCV infection in pregnancy?

All pregnant women with risk factors for HCV should be screened with anti-HCV antibody. Screening should not be performed in women without risk factors for HCV acquisition. Invasive procedures (e.g. amniocentesis, invasive fetal monitoring) should be minimized in infected mothers and their fetus to prevent vertical transmission of hepatitis C.

Cesarean section should not be performed electively in HCV-positive mothers to prevent fetal infection. Women chronically infected with HCV should be allowed to breastfeed as indicated for infant health. The treatment of chronic hepatitis C comprises pegylated interferon and ribavarin. However, these are contraindicated in pregnancy due to reports of decreased birth weight and increased fetal loss. US Food and Drug Administration (FDA) has labeled ribavarin as category X.[19,20] Therefore, hepatitis C therapy should not be offered to pregnant women to either treat HCV or decrease the risk for vertical transmission.[1]

CASE SCENARIO

Hepatic encephalopathy
28 years old primigravida presents at 30 weeks gestation with acute viral hepatitis and hepatic encephalopathy.

Q1. How will you manage this patient?

Admission to hospital is advised; Multidisciplinary care involving an obstetrician, hepatologist and intensive care specialist is required; Intensive care unit admission is preferable in patients with severe encephalopathy; other causes of altered mental function should be ruled out.

Airway, breathing and circulation should be secured; vitals should be assessed (Pulse rate, Blood pressure, temperature, respiratory rate). Wide bore intravenous access should be established.

Investigations should be sent: Hemogram, liver function tests, kidney function tests, blood sugar, serum electrolytes, serum protein, PT/INR, fibrinogen.

Cause of jaundice and hepatic dysfunction leading to encephalopathy should be determined. History of drug intake; anti-HAV, anti-HEV, anti-HCV, HBsAg, anti-HBc IgM; possibility of AFLP considered. Cause should be identified and treated.

Precipitating factors should be ascertained and corrected: constipation, GI bleeding, renal failure, infection, diuretic therapy, dietary protein overload, drugs like benzodiazepines, antidepressants and antipsychotics.

Supportive care should be given involving fluid balance, care of bowel and bladder. 5% dextrose infusion is given to prevent hypoglycemia. Lactulose is given in a dose of 30 ml once or twice daily as it inhibits intestinal ammonia production. Antibiotic (neomycin/ampicillin/rifaximin) is given to decrease the colonic concentration of ammoniagenic bacteria, hence decreasing ammonia production in the gut. Neomycin- 250 mg orally 2–4 times/day; Rifaximin: 400 mg thrice daily. High carbohydrate and low protein diet should be given. Maintenance of nutrition with Ryle's tube feeding may be required. Inj vitamin K 2.5–10 mg SC daily for 3 days or oral water soluble vitamin K is given.

Q2. How will you diagnose and manage a case of acute fatty liver of pregnancy (AFLP)?

AFLP is an uncommon but potentially life threatening condition unique to pregnancy. Women with multiple gestation, male fetus or nulliparous women are more likely to develop AFLP. It is characterized by microvesicular hepatic steatosis attributed to mitochondrial dysfunction in fatty acids oxidation.

Patients present with persistent nausea and vomiting, malaise, anorexia, epigastric pain and progressive jaundice. Half of the women also have hypertension, edema and proteinuria. Moderate to severe liver dysfunction is manifest by hypofibrinogenemia, hypoalbuminemia, hypocholesterolemia, and coagulopathy. Hypoglycemia and severe hemolysis may be seen. Fulminant hepatic failure with hepatic encephalopathy may occur in half the patients. In severe cases, there is profound endothelial cell activation with capillary leak causing hemoconcentration, acute kidney injury, ascites, and pulmonary edema. Hemoconcentration (leading to impaired uteroplacental circulation) along with maternal acidosis contribute to increased fetal compromise.

Infant morbidity may be increased due to risk of cardiomyopathy, neuropathy, myopathy, non-ketotic hypoglycemia and death.

Differential Diagnosis

Acetaminophen/drug-induced hepatotoxicity, viral hepatitis, preeclampsia-eclampsia, HELLP syndrome.

Investigations

- LFT: AST and ALT elevated, conjugated hyperbilirubinemia (S. bilirubin > 5 mg/dL)
- Blood glucose: decreased due to decreased gluconeogenesis
- Raised blood ammonia levels due to declining detoxification by liver.
- ↑PT, ↓fibrinogen and antithrombin: may suggest DIC (due to↓ production by liver)
- ↑ amylase, ↑ lipase (pancreatitis may be associated)
- ↑creatinine and uric acid—Metabolic acidosis (due to acute kidney injury).

Management

Obstetrical Management

Delivery of fetus, regardless of gestational age is the only treatment.

Perform urgent delivery when maternal condition is stabilized. Close fetal monitoring is essential because of risk of fetal acidemia, hypoxia and distress. Mode of delivery depends on the fetal status, period of gestation, maternal coagulation status and likelihood of success with induction of labor. Vaginal delivery is preferred. If delivery cannot be safely accomplished within 24 hours of diagnosis, cesarean is optimal. Replacement of coagulation factors and vitamin K administration is essential prior to delivery in patients with coagulopathy.

Supportive Care

Manage in intensive care unit/ high dependency care. Use multidisciplinary approach in liaison with hepatologist; 5% dextrose infusion to prevent and treat hypoglycemia; Careful monitoring of fluid balance is needed. Plasmapheresis has been shown to be beneficial in severe cases of AFLP with encephalopathy, ventilator support or liver/ renal insufficiency where conventional management has failed. Liver transplantation is being done in some centers in patients with liver failure. Maternal deaths are caused by sepsis, hemorrhage, GI bleeding, aspiration, renal failure and pancreatitis.

Postpartum Care

Intensive care management should be continued; Watch for wound hematoma, PPH and wound sepsis. Hepatic dysfunction usually resolves postpartum and long-term prognosis for the mother is good, if she survives the acute insult. Contraception should be encouraged.

Recurrence risk may be as high as 10–20%.

Screening the baby for Long chain 3-hydroxy acyl CoA dehydrogenase (LCHAD) deficiency can be considered. If previous baby is affected, prenatal diagnosis of LCHAD is possible by amniocentesis/CVS.

Q3. What are the challenges in dealing with liver cirrhosis in pregnancy?

Pregnancy is a rare event in patients with cirrhosis, since cirrhosis results in metabolic and hormonal derangements that lead to anovulation and amenorrhea. Improvements in the treatment of chronic liver disease have resulted in higher conception rates and more successful pregnancy outcomes.[21]

Maternal Risks during Pregnancy

Portal hypertension—increased risk of variceal hemorrhage especially during labor; hepatic encephalopathy; rupture of splenic aneurysm; hepatic decompensation; ascites and spontaneous bacterial peritonitis; postpartum hemorrhage; maternal mortality rate—10%

Fetal Complications

Spontaneous miscarriage in 30–40% cases; fetal growth restriction, prematurity; increased perinatal mortality rates.

Management

- *Preconceptional care:* Fetal and maternal risks should be explained. Liver function should be assessed. Upper GI endoscopy for any esophageal varices, which, if found can be subjected to band ligation or sclerotherapy. USG abdomen with Doppler should be done to look for splenic artery aneurysm.
- *Prenatal care:* Women with suspected portal hypertension should undergo screening with upper

GI endoscopy for esophageal varices in the second trimester. If they are found to have large esophageal varices, they should be treated with beta-blockers and/or band ligation. Acute variceal hemorrhage occurs more often in the second/third trimester due to increased intravascular volume and IVC compression. Treatment consists of endoscopic band ligation. If it fails, sclerotherapy may be done but is less preferred due to risks of chemical instillation. Octretide may be used but may have a risk of causing vasospasm. TIPS (Transjugular intrahepatic portosystemic shunt) is used if band ligation/sclerotherapy fail to control bleeding and benefit outweighs risk of radiation to the fetus.

- *Intrapartum management:* Second stage of labor should be cut short by using obstetric forceps due to risk of variceal hemorrhage because of raised intra-abdominal pressure during labor. Cesarean may be needed in patients with untreated large varices to prevent life threatening hemorrhage. Coagulopathy, if any should be corrected.

Q4. Describe your approach to a liver transplant recipient with respect to pregnancy?

Most experts advocate waiting at least 1 year, and some up to 2 years after liver transplantation before planning a pregnancy. Higher risk of acute cellular rejection and graft loss have been reported if pregnancy occurred within 6 months of liver transplantation. Preconceptional counseling and optimization of maternal health is essential prior to embarking on a pregnancy.

Management during pregnancy includes multidisciplinary care involving maternal–fetal medicine providers, hepatologist and the liver transplant center. In liver transplant recipients, there is a higher risk of prematurity, LBW, maternal hypertension, preeclampsia, and cesarean sections. Overall, pregnancy in liver transplant recipients is safe, with good outcomes provided careful management and monitoring is done. The key is to maintain liver graft function to support the mother's health and to maximize the chances of healthy pregnancy. The risks of immunosuppressive drugs in pregnancy should be balanced against the risk of graft rejection. Overall, risks of most drugs (cyclosporine, tacrolimus, AZA, sirolimus, everolimus, and corticosteroids) appear low compared with the risks of acute cellular rejection or graft loss with their discontinuation. Although a higher risk of prematurity and LBW have been reported, the risk of congenital malformation is not increased. However, mycophenolic acid should not be used in pregnancy because of emryo-fetal toxicity and risk of congenital malformations. Traditionally, breastfeeding has been opposed in such patients. However, recent studies have reported no adverse events in breastfed infants of transplant recipients.

Q5. What is the role of imaging in patients with liver disease?

- Ultrasonography with or without Doppler: Safe and preferred modality, helps to image the liver, hepatic vasculature and biliary system. It may identify calculi in the gallbladder and biliary tract. Liver echogenicity and size may suggest liver pathology.
- MRI without gadolinium can be used in the second and third trimester.
- CT scans: Carry a risk of teratogenesis and childhood hematologic malignancies but may be used judiciously with minimized radiation protocols (2-5 rads).
- Fibro scan/hepatic elastography: Indicated in patients with chronic liver disease. It can evaluate the liver hardness which will suggest the degree of hepatic fibrosis.

REFERENCES

1. Tran TT, Ahn J, Reau NS. ACG Clinical Guideline: liver disease and pregnancy. Am J Gastroenterol. 2 February 2016; doi: 10.1038/ajg.2015.430.
2. Cunningham FG, Leveno KJ, Bloom SL, et al. Williams Obstetrics. 24th edition. Mc Graw Hill education; 2014. p. 67.
3. Anzivino C, Odoardi MR, Meschiari E. et al. ABCB4 and ABCB11 mutations in intrahepatic cholestasis of pregnancy in an Italian population. Dig Liver Dis, 2013; 45(3): 226.
4. Dixon PH, Wadsworth CA, Chambers J. et al. A comprehensive analysis of common genetic variation around 6 candidate loci for intrahepatic cholestasis of pregnancy. Am J Gastroenterol. 2014;109:76
5. Green top guideline number 43. Royal College of Obstetricians and Gynecologists: Obstetric Cholestasis, 2011.
6. Gurung V, Middleton P, et al. Interventions for treating cholestasis in pregnancy. Cochrane Database Syst Rev. 2013;(6): CD000493. Doi10.1002/14651858.CD000493.pub2.
7. American College of Obstetricians and Gynecologists: Upper gastrointestinal tract, biliary and pancreatic disorders. Clinical Updates in Womens's Health Care. Vol. XI, No. 4,2012a
8. Frezza M, Pozzato G, Chiesa L. Reversal of intrahepatic cholestasis of pregnancy in women after high dose S-Adenosyl-Methionine administration. Hepatology. 1984;278-84.
9. Cunningham FG, Leveno KJ. Bloom SL, et al. Williams Obstetrics. 24th edition. McGraw Hill education; 2014. pp. 1084-97.

10. Wong RC, Ellis CN. Physiologic skin changes in pregnancy. J Am Acad Dermatol. 1984;10(6): 929-40.
11. Chi CC, Wang SH, Charles Holmes R, et al. Pemphigoid gestationis: early onset and blister formation are associated with adverse pregnancy outcomes. Br J Dermatol. 2009;160(6): 1222-8. Epub 2009 Mar 9.
12. Ambros Rudolph CM. Dermatoses of pregnancy- clues to diagnosis, fetal risk and therapy. Ann Dermatol. 2011; 23(3):265-75. Epub 2011 Aug 6.
13. Ambros Rudolph CM, Mullegger RR, Vaughan Jones SA, et al. The specific dermatoses of pregnancy revisited and reclassified: results of a retrospective two centre study on 505 pregnant patients. J Am Acad Dermatol. 2006; 54(3): 395-404.
14. Rein DB, Stevens GA, Theaker J, et al. The global burden of hepatitis E virus genotypes 1 and 2 in 2005.Hepatology. 2012; 55(4):988.
15. World Health Organization. Hepatitis E: fact sheet no. 280 (rev January 2005).
16. Hollinger FB, Liang TJ. Hepatitis B virus. In: Knipe DM, et al, (Eds). Fields Virology. 4th edition. Philadelphia, Pa: Lippincott Willams and Wilkins; 2001; 2971-3036.
17. Robinson WS. Hepatitis B virus and hepatitis D virus. In: Mandell GL, Benett JE, Dolin R, (Eds). Principles and Practice of Infectious Diseases. 4th edition. New York, NY:Churchill Livingstone;1995. 1406-39.
18. Brown RS Jr, MacMohan J, Lok AS, et al. Anti-viral therapy in chronic hepatitis B viral infection during pregnancy: A systematic review and meta-analysis. Hepatology. 2016.63 (1):319-33.
19. Boskovic R, Wide R, et al. The reproductive effects of beta interferon therapy in pregnancy: A longitudinal cohort. Neurology.2005.65(6):807-11.
20. Hiratsuka M, Minakami, et al. Administration of interferon-alpha during pregnancy: effects on fetus. J Perinat Med. 2000.28(5):372-6.
21. Russell MA, Craigo SD. Cirrhosis and portal hypertension in pregnancy. Semin Pernatol. 1988;22:156-65.

CHAPTER 23

Critically Ill Patients

Nilanchali Singh, Priyanka Khandey

We usually do not get critically ill patients as long cases in postgraduate examinations. However, simulated case scenarios or already managed postpartum or postoperative cases may be given during examinations. As a postgraduate, one needs to know how to tackle such emergency cases. Management of critically ill patients is very challenging and, if not managed timely, may lead to mortality; hence, early recognition, correct diagnosis, appropriate interventions and management are important to reduce maternal mortality. Although obstetric patients are young and healthy but the mortality rate is higher in those who need ICU admission, ranges 15-30% in developing countries.[1] Only few guidelines are available to identify critically ill patients in obstetrics, their diagnosis and treatment.[2-4] In this chapter, we will discuss about the critically ill patients in general, followed by some common causes of such illness in pregnancy.

Q1. How do you define a critically ill pregnant woman?

Any woman who is pregnant, laboring, postpartum or postabortal, who needs extensive medical or surgical management or urgent resuscitation or ICU admission is labeled as critically ill. Management of such patients needs multidisciplinary approach by involving obstetrician, anesthetist, pediatrician, hematologist, nephrologist, intensivist, clinical pharmacist, and senior nursing officers. Multidisciplinary team with protocol driven care have been demonstrated improved patient outcomes.[5]

Q2. How to identify women at risk of impending collapse or becoming critically ill?

Most of the patients have preexisting risk factors, but in some cases, maternal collapse occurs with no prior warning. An obstetric early warning score chart should be used routinely for all women, to allow early recognition of the woman who is becoming critically ill.[2]

Q3. What is the common scoring system/warning score used for obstetrics patient?

Modified early obstetrics warning score (MEOWS) measures physiological variables of the patients like temperature, systolic and diastolic blood pressure, heart rate, respiratory rate, level of consciousness and urine output (Table 1).

Use of these scoring systems also helps in early recognition of patients and their transfer to higher centers. A score ≥3 triggers the use of a 'call out cascade' providing specific instructions about level of monitoring, referral for advice, review, and immediate actions.[6]

Table 1: Modified early obstetric warning score chart							
Score	3	2	1	0	1	2	3
Temperature		<35°C		35–37.4°C			
Systolic BP	≤70	71–79	80–89	90–139	140–149	150–159	≥160
Diastolic BP			≤45	46–89	90–99	100–109	≥110
Pulse		≤ 40	40–50	51–100	101–110	111–129	≥ 130
Respiratory rate		≤ 8		9–14	15–20	21–29	≥30
AVPU				**A**lert	Responds to **V**oice	Responds to **P**ain	**U**nconscious
Urine output mL/hr	<10	<30		Not measured			

Q4. What are the various causes of maternal collapse?

The various causes of maternal collapse are mentioned in Table 2.

Table 2: Causes of maternal collapse

Pregnancy related conditions	Medical disorders worsen during pregnancy	Surgical/medical condition not related to pregnancy
Hemorrhage Sepsis Hypertensive disorders of pregnancy Amniotic fluid embolism Complex cardiac diseases Acute fatty liver Aspiration syndromes Infections Ovarian hyper-stimulation syndrome Tocolytic-induced pulmonary edema	Anemia Congenital heart diseases Rheumatic and non-rheumatic valvular diseases Pulmonary hypertension Renal failure Autoimmune diseases (e.g. SLE, myasthenia gravis), etc.	Trauma Asthma Diabetes Toxicity Anaphylaxis reactions Autoimmune diseases, etc.

Q5. What are the physiological and anatomical changes in pregnancy that affect resuscitation?

A pregnant woman undergoes many physiological changes, which affect her resuscitation and these factors need to be kept in mind before treating her (Table 3).

Table 3: Physiological and physical changes in pregnancy and their impact on resuscitation[2]

	Changes in pregnancy	Impact on resuscitation
Cardiovascular system		
Plasma volume	Increased by up to 50%	Dilutional anemia Reduced oxygen-carrying capacity
Heart rate	Increased by 15–20 bpm	Increased CPR circulation demands
Cardiac output	Increased by 40%	Increased CPR circulation demands
Uterine blood flow	10% of cardiac output at term	Potential for massive hemorrhage
Systemic vascular resistance	Decreased	Sequesters blood during CPR
Arterial blood pressure	Decreased by 10–15 mm Hg	Decreased reserve
Venous return	Decreased by pressure of gravid uterus on IVC	Increased CPR circulation demands
Respiratory system		
Respiratory rate	Increased	Decreased buffering capacity, acidosis more likely
Oxygen consumption	Increased by 20%	Hypoxia develops more quickly
Residual capacity	Decreased by 25%	Decreased buffering capacity, acidosis more likely
Arterial PCO_2	Decreased	Decreased buffering capacity, acidosis more likely
Laryngeal edema	Increased	Difficult intubation
Other changes		
Gastric motility	Decreased	Increased risk of aspiration
Lower esophageal sphincter	Relaxed	Increased risk of aspiration
Uterus	Enlarged	Diaphragmatic splinting reduces residual capacity and makes ventilation difficult Aortocaval compression causes supine hypotension, reduces venous return and significantly impairs CPR
Weight		Large breasts may interfere with intubation makes ventilation difficult

Q6. What are essential adaptations for the management of the collapsed pregnant woman because of the physiological and anatomical changes of pregnancy?

Following measures should be used for effective resuscitation of obstetric patients:[2]

- *A left lateral tilt:* The pressure of the gravid uterus must be relieved from the inferior vena cava and aorta, after 20 weeks of gestation. A left lateral tilt of 15° on a firm surface will relieve aortocaval compression and still allow effective chest compressions to be performed.
- *Airway:* It should be protected as soon as possible by intubation with a cuffed endotracheal tube.
- *Supplemental oxygen:* It should be administered as soon as possible. Bag and mask ventilation should be undertaken until intubation can be achieved.
- *Chest compression:* It should be commenced immediately in the absence of breathing despite a clear airway.
- *Circulation:* Two wide-bore cannulae should be inserted as soon as possible. There should be an aggressive approach to volume replacement.
- *Defibrillator:* The same defibrillation energy levels should be used as in the non-pregnant patient as there is no change in thoracic impedance.

CASE SCENARIO

History
A 28 years old lady, G3P2L2, was admitted in labor room at 39 weeks gestation in labor. She delivered vaginally with episiotomy, a female baby of weight 2.7 kg. Placenta delivered within 15 minutes and active management of third stage of labor was done. After two hours of delivery, she complained of bleeding per vaginum and passage of clots, which soaked her clothes and beddings. She also complained of pain abdomen, weakness and sudden dizziness.

Examination
Patient was very pale with cold and clammy extremities. Her pulse rate was 128 bpm, blood pressure was 70/54 mm Hg, and respiratory rate was 22/min. Abdominal palpation revealed the uterus, which was palpated just above the umbilicus, soft doughy like in consistency with mild tenderness. Per speculum examination revealed large clots of blood in the vagina. No active bleeding from the episiotomy site.

Q1. What is the diagnosis?

Hemorrhagic shock due to postpartum hemorrhage (PPH)

Q2. How do you define postpartum hemorrhage?

The terms mentioned in Table 4, are used to define PPH.[7,8]

Table 4: Definitions of PPH

Postpartum hemorrhage	Blood loss >500 mL (vaginal delivery); >1000 mL (in cesarean section)
Primary	Within 24 hours of delivery[5]
Secondary	After 24 hours postpartum[6]
Minor PPH	Blood loss = 500 mL – 1000 mL
Major PPH	Blood loss ≥1000 mL and/or unstable: • Moderate = 1000–2000 mL • Severe ≥ 2000 mL • Life-threatening ≥ 2500 mL

Q3. What are the risk factors for developing PPH?

Four Ts commonly predispose to PPH are tone, trauma, tissue and thrombin (Table 5).[9]

Table 5: Causes of PPH

Tone	Trauma	Thrombin	Tissue
Multiple gestation, good size baby, obesity, prolonged labor, placenta previa, previous history of PPH	Operative vaginal delivery, Episiotomy, cesarean section, local injury to cervix or vagina	Hypertensive disorder, pre-eclampsia and eclampsia, Abruption placentae	Retained placenta

Q4. How to manage a patient with major PPH?

Resuscitation, monitoring, investigation and treatment should occur simultaneously[10] (Flowchart 1)

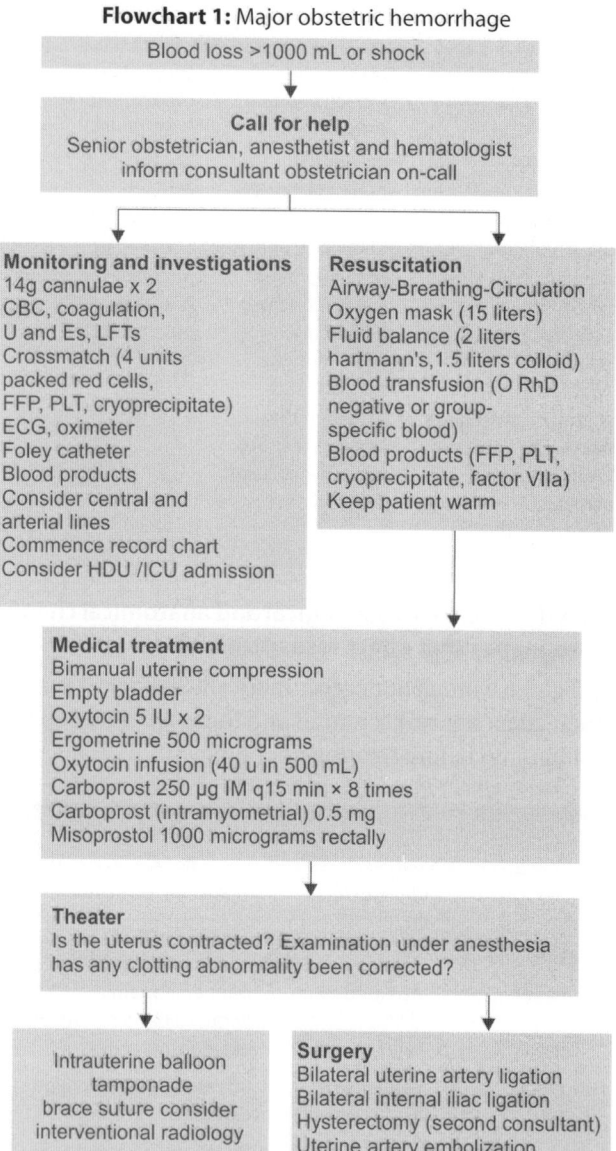

Flowchart 1: Major obstetric hemorrhage

Q5. How do you do fluid resuscitation in hemorrhagic shock?

In hemorrhagic shock there is depletion of ECF (extracellular fluid) compartment with an increase in intracellular water, so successful resuscitation depends on the prompt restoration of intravascular volume.[11]

- *Crystalloids:* The most commonly used crystalloid are 0.9% saline and lactated Ringer's solutions. Crystalloids distribute rapidly between the ICF and ECF. Equilibration within the extracellular space occurs within 20–30 minutes after infusion. In healthy non-pregnant adults, approximately 25% of the volume infused remains in the intravascular space after 1 hour as compared to less than 20% in critically ill obstetric patients.[12] Therefore, large amount of crystalloids, three to four times the amount of blood loss is needed.

- *Colloid solutions:* Colloids have large molecular weight so relatively impermeable to cell membranes. They increase COP (colloid osmotic pressure), resulting in the movement of fluid from the interstitial compartment to the intravascular compartment. They have prolonged duration of action due to their ability to remain in the intravascular space. They are costly as compared to crystalloids. Recent studies do not show any beneficial advantage of colloids over crystalloids in the management of critically ill patients.[13]
- **Total volume of 3.5 liters of clear fluids (up to 2 liters of warmed Hartmann's solution as rapidly as possible, followed by up to a further 1.5 liters of warmed colloid if blood still not available) comprises the maximum that should be infused while awaiting compatible blood.**[10]
- *Blood products:* Blood products are the best for volume replacement as they improve oxygen carrying capacity also. In emergency, group O Rh-D negative blood should be transfused to avoid risk of mismatch reaction. Cross-matched whole blood or packed RBCs are commonly used in clinical practice. ***During massive transfusion each packed cell transfusion should be accomplished by transfusion of platelet and fresh frozen plasma (FFP) in the ratio of 1:1:1 or 4:4:1, to restore coagulation factors.***[14]

The British Committee for Standards in Haematology summarizes the main therapeutic goals of management of massive blood loss is to maintain (Table 6).

Table 6: Main therapeutic goals of management of massive blood loss (The British Committee for Standards in Haematology)[15]

- Hemoglobin >8 g/dL
- Platelet count >75 x 10^9/L
- Prothrombin <1.5 x mean control
- Activated prothrombin times <1.5 x mean control
- Fibrinogen >1.0 g/L.

Q6. Is there any role of recombinant factor VIIa therapy?

The routine use of rFVIIa is not recommended but rFVIIa may be used as an adjuvant to standard management and should not delay or substitute the standard pharmacological and surgical treatment. It is used in a suggested dose is 90 micrograms/kg, which may be repeated within 15–30 minutes in the absence of clinical response. Before rFVIIa is given, fibrinogen should be above 1g/L and platelets greater than 20×10^9/L.[16]

Q7. Is there a use for antifibrinolytic drugs?

The fibrinolytic inhibitors (such as tranexamic acid) seldom, if ever, have a place in the management of obstetric haemorrhage. Tranexamic acid is used in a dose of 1 g intravenously and can be repeated after 30 minutes.[17]

Q8. What is the use of antishock garments?

They are lightweight, neoprene device resembles the bottom half of a wetsuit. It has five segments which wrapped around a mother's legs, pelvis, and abdomen, then tightened with Velcro straps. The garment, called "nonpneumatic" because it does not use air. It applies pressure to the lower part of the body, forcing blood to key organs, including the heart, lungs, and brain. It also increases resistivity index in internal iliac artery.[18]

CASE SCENARIO

History
A 27 years old lady, P1L1, with postpartum day 7 of cesarean section, had complaints of high-grade fever since two days, not associated with chills or rigor, no burning micturition and cough. She also complained of pain abdomen and abdominal distension.

Examination

On examination patient was febrile to touch; temperature was 39 degree Celsius; mild pallor was present; PR was 98 bpm; Blood pressure was 100/78 mm Hg; bilateral chest was clear; bilateral breasts were soft. On abdominal palpation, tenderness was present in lower abdomen with mild gaseous distension. Uterus was well contracted. Vaginal examination revealed foul smelling lochia.

Investigations

Hemoglobin was 9 g %, TLC of 18500/mm^3 and platelet count was 1.6 lac/mm^3. Urine microscopy and culture reports were normal. USG abdomen and pelvis showed bulky uterus with no retained products. A large collection of 10 × 12 cm seen at left side of lower abdomen. CT scan showed same collection at pelvis and lower abdomen suggestive of pyogenic foci.

Q1. What is the likely diagnosis?

Septic shock due to puerperal sepsis (pyoperitoneum).

Q2. How will you define septic shock?

Septic shock is sepsis with hypotension despite adequate fluid resuscitation combined with perfusion abnormalities that may include, but are not limited to, lactic acidosis, oliguria or an acute alteration in mental status. Patients who require inotropic or vasopressor support despite adequate fluid resuscitation are in septic shock. Septic shock is one of the forms of vasodilatory or distributive shock. It results from a marked reduction in systemic vascular resistance, often associated with an increase in cardiac output.[19]

Q3. Describe pathophysiology of septic shock.

Infection with a pathogenic organism results in cellular activation of monocytes, macrophages, and neutrophils and induction of a proinflammatory cascade. The pro-inflammatory mediators, in turn, induce a systemic response (characterized by tachycardia, tachypnea, and hypotension) and, if excessive or uncontrolled, can lead to end-organ dysfunction, including ARDS and acute renal failure. Endotoxin—a complex lipopolysaccharide (LPS) present in the cell wall of aerobic gram-negative bacteria, released at the time of the organism's death—appears to be a critical factor in inducing the pathophysiologic derangements associated with septic shock.[19]

Q4. How to diagnose septic shock?

There is no definitive diagnostic test, and a high index of clinical suspicion in the appropriate clinical setting is needed to confirm the diagnosis. A rapid and focused history and examination should be performed.

Q5. What are the various tests to be performed in such cases?

Laboratory evaluations include:[19]
- Complete blood count with differential count
- Basic biochemistry tests—LFT, KFT, serum electrolytes
- C- reactive protein
- Amylase and lipase (to diagnose pancreatitis)
- Coagulation profile, including fibrinogen and fibrin split products
- Lactate
- Arterial blood gases
- Toxicology screen (blood and urine)
- Chest radiograph
- Abdominal radiograph (to exclude intestinal obstruction)
- Electrocardiogram
- Urinalysis.

Search for infection, if indicated (including blood culture, urine culture, CXR, lumbar puncture).

Blood cultures should be obtained prior to antibiotic administration; however, antibiotic treatment should be started without waiting for microbiology results.

Serum lactate should be measured within 6 hours of the suspicion of severe sepsis to guide management. Serum lactate ≥ 4 mmol/L is indicative of tissue hypoperfusion.[20]

Q6. How will you manage this patient?

Fluid replacement: Aggressive volume replacement to improve the functional circulating intravascular volume and to treat hypotension as evidenced by meeting the targeted hemodynamic goals:[21]
- CVP 8 – 12 mm Hg,
- MAP ≥ 65 mm Hg,
- SvO_2 > 70%, and
- Urine output ≥ 0.5 mL/kg/hour.

Airway: Establishment and maintenance of an adequate airway to facilitate management of respiratory failure.

Oxygenation: To assurance adequate tissue perfusion and as evidenced by normalization of mixed venous oxygenation, arterial lactate levels, and acid – base status.

Diagnostic evaluation: Initiation of diagnostic evaluations to determine the septic focus and remove it, if possible (abscesses should be drained and extensive soft-tissue infections should be debrided or amputated).

Antimicrobial therapy: Institution of empiric antimicrobial therapy to eradicate the most likely pathogens.
- Administration of intravenous broad-spectrum antibiotics within one hour of suspicion of severe sepsis, with or without septic shock, is recommended as part of the surviving sepsis resuscitation care bundle
- If genital tract sepsis is suspected, prompt early treatment with a combination of high-dose broad-spectrum intravenous antibiotics may be lifesaving
- A combination of either piperacillin/tazobactam or a carbapenem plus clindamycin provides one of the broadest ranges of treatment for severe sepsis.
- MRSA may be resistant to clindamycin, hence if the woman is highly likely to be MRSA-positive, a glycopeptide, such as vancomycin or teicoplanin may be added until sensitivity is known.

Q7. What is the role of laparotomy in this patient?

This patient has intra-abdominal collection suggestive of pyoperitoneum, so laparotomy should be undertaken. Postpartum hysterectomy indicated if microabscess formation is identified within myometrial tissues or if there is clinical evidence of deterioration in the patient's condition despite appropriate antibiotic therapy.

Q8. What are the features of sepsis in the puerperium that should prompt hospital admission?

Following 'red flag' signs and symptoms, prompt urgent hospital admission:[20]
- Pyrexia more than 38°C
- Sustained tachycardia more than 90 beats/minute
- Breathlessness (respiratory rate more than 20 breaths/minute; a serious symptom)
- Abdominal or chest pain
- Diarrhea and/or vomiting
- Uterine or renal angle pain and tenderness
- Woman is generally unwell or seems unduly anxious or distressed.

Q9. What are the common organisms causing sepsis in the puerperium?

The major pathogens causing sepsis in the puerperium are:[20]
- GAS, also known as *Streptococcus pyogenes*
- *Escherichia coli*
- Staphylococcus *aureus*
- *Streptococcus pneumoniae*
- Methicillin-resistant *S. aureus* (MRSA), *Clostridium septicum* and *Morganella morganii*.

Q10. What are the indications for admission to the intensive care unit (ICU)?

The presence of shock or other organ dysfunction in the woman is an indication for admission to the ICU[22] (Table 7).

Table 7: Indications for admission to the ICU

System	Indication
Cardiovascular	Hypotension or raised serum lactate persisting despite fluid resuscitation suggesting the need for inotropic support
Respiratory	• Pulmonary edema • Mechanical ventilation • Airway protection
Renal	Renal dialysis
Neurological	Significantly decreased conscious level
Miscellaneous	• Multiorgan failure • Uncorrected acidosis • Hypothermia

Q11. What is the role of intravenous immunoglobulin (IVIG)?

- IVIG is recommended for severe invasive streptococcal or staphylococcal infection if other therapies have failed. IVIG has an immunomodulatory effect and in staphylococcal and streptococcal sepsis also neutralizes the superantigen effect of exotoxins and inhibits production of tumor necrosis factor and interleukins
- It is effective in exotoxic shock (i.e. toxic shock attributable to streptococci and staphylococci), but there is little evidence of benefit in gram-negative (endotoxin-related) sepsis.[23] The main contraindication to IVIG use is a congenital deficiency of immunoglobulin A.

Q12. Is there any role of steroid in the treatment of severe sepsis or septic shock?

- Use of high-dose corticosteroid is a controversial modality which has theoretical benefit of stabilization of lysosomal membranes, inhibition of complement-induced inflammatory changes, and attenuation of the effects of cytokines and other inflammatory mediators.
- Potential role of steroid is to treat refractory shock or multiorgan failure with adrenal insufficiency.

CASE SCENARIO

History

A 29 years old lady, G3P1L1A1 at 37 weeks of gestation came to gynecology casualty with complaints of bleeding per vaginum and pain lower abdomen for four hours. She was diagnosed as gestational hypertension at sixth month amenorrhea and started on tab labetolol 100 mg BD, on which her BP was controlled.

Examination

She was pale; pulse rate was 120 bpm; systolic BP was 80 mm Hg; respiratory rate was 18/min and bilateral chest was clear. On abdominal examination fundal height corresponded to term pregnancy, with tenderness, mild contractions and increased tone. A note was made of single fetus in longitudinal lie and cephalic presentation and heart rate of 156 bpm. Speculum examination revealed bleeding through os.

Investigations

Her investigation showed hemoglobin of 7.8 g%, platelet count was 76000/mm^3, peripheral smear showed signs of hemolysis, PT was 28 sec (C-10.1) and aPTT was 58 sec (C-22), FDP was increased to 42 µg/dL and D dimer was 26 mg/dL.

Q1. What is the most probable diagnosis?

Abruptio placentae leading to disseminated intravascular coagulation (DIC)

Q2. Define disseminated intravascular coagulation (DIC).

DIC is defined as a systemic thrombohemorrhagic disorder found in association with well-defined clinical situation and laboratory evidence of procoagulant activation, fibrinolytic activation, inhibitor consumption and biochemical evidence of end-organ damage or failure.[24]

Q3. Describe pathophysiology of DIC in brief.

DIC is mostly secondary to another underlying condition that provokes clotting within vascular compartment. In cases of placental abruption there is release of thromboplastin from placental and decidual tissues into the maternal circulation. Damage to endothelial exposes the underlying collagen to plasma and procoagulants, which provokes coagulation cascades. Red cells and platelets injury may occur as in incompatible blood transfusion reaction which leads to release of phospholipids and initiation of coagulation system (Flowchart 2).

Hemostasis is a complex and dynamic balance between coagulation and fibrinolytic system. In DIC, there is excessive and widespread coagulation and depletion of coagulation factors resulting in hemorrhage.

In response, fibrinolytic system get activated. Plasminogen is converted to plasmin, which breaks fibrin into fibrin degraded products (FDP). FDP also have anticoagulant activity. It inhibits platelets function and thrombin action, which further aggravates coagulopathy. Extensive microvascular thrombosis also occurs which leads to organ ischemia and infarction.

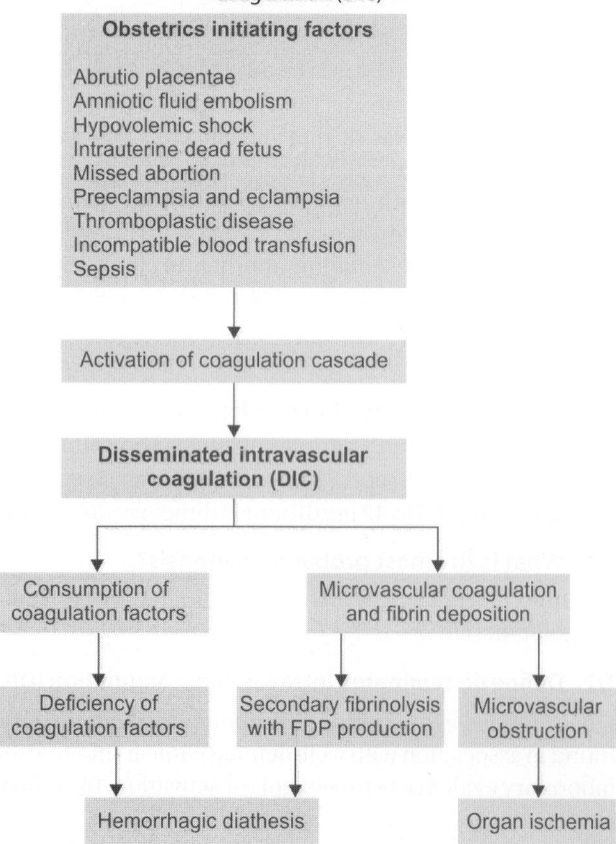

Flowchart 2: Pathophysiology of disseminated intravascular coagulation (DIC)[25]

Q4. What is the clinical presentation of DIC?

It has wide spectrum of presentation from no clinical manifestation with only hematological changes to torrential bleeding and collapse. In subtle cases, bruising, epistaxis, purpuric rash and oozing from venopuncture sites seen.

Q5. How to diagnose DIC?

Diagnosis is mainly supported by hematological investigations and coagulation profile.
- Platelet count (falling or low)
- PT and APTT (usually prolonged)
- Thrombin time (prolonged)
- Fibrinogen level (increases; 400–650 mg/dL)
- D-dimer (level increases but not very reliable test).

Q6. How to manage a patient of DIC?

- Treatment of underlying cause like delivery of fetus in intrauterine fetal demise, abruption placentae, correction of coagulopathy and hematological changes in preeclampsia, HELLP syndrome
- Maintenance of circulation by crystalloids, colloids and blood products. It clears FDP from circulation
- Maintenance of ventilation, oxygen administration and intubation if needed.

Q7. How will you replace of procoagulants?

- If available, fresh whole blood is to be administered.
- Fresh frozen plasma (FFP): Administer one unit of platelet and one unit of FFP for each unit of packed cell transfusion in case of massive hemorrhage.
- Cryoprecipitate: It is rich in fibrinogen, vWF and factor VIII and XIII. It should be given if fibrinogen level falls below 100 mg/dL.
- Platelets transfusion in cases with severe thrombocytopenia (count <30,000/mm^3)
- Antithrombin if available.
- Recombinant activated factor VII (Novo 7): It combines with local tissue factor at sites of hemorrhage to enhance thrombin generation and stabilize fibrin formation. Recommended dose is 90 μg/kg, and can be repeated within 15–30 minutes in absence of clinical response in cases of life threatening PPH.[26] Before administration fibrinogen should be above 1 g/L and platelet > 20 × 10^9/L.

CASE SCENARIO

History

A 28 years old lady, G4P2L2A1 underwent LSCS for fetal distress at 38 weeks POG. Antepartum period and intracesarean events were uneventful. Uterus was well contracted and estimated blood loss was around 600 mL.

In immediate postpartum period patient was complaining of sudden onset breathlessness. She was a booked case with no history of high BP records and deranged sugar test. She had intake of hematinics through out pregnancy and received 2 doses of tetanus toxoid. She had previous 2 normal vaginal deliveries followed by one spontaneous abortion 4 years back.

Examination

Patient was conscious but drowsy. Her pulse was 128 bpm; blood pressure was 80/50 mm Hg; respiratory rate was 18/min. On auscultation, bilateral clear chest with normal heart sounds. Abdominal palpation revealed well-contracted uterus, below umbilicus and no active bleeding per vaginum.

Investigations

Her hemoglobin was 10.4 g%, platelet count was 1.8 lac/mm³, and normal coagulation profile.

Q1. What is the most probable diagnosis?

Amniotic fluid embolism

Q2. What is amniotic fluid embolism?

Amniotic fluid embolism (AFE) is a rare but life-threatening condition with high mortality rates. It commonly occur during late pregnancy, labor or immediately postpartum period. Amniotic fluid may gain access into the maternal circulation due to breach in the physiological barrier between maternal and fetal circulation. Risks factors are abruptio placentae, intrauterine fetal demise, amnioinfusion and operative deliveries.

Q3. Define pathophysiology of amniotic fluid embolism.

Amniotic fluid emboli containing fetal epithelial cells, fat, lanugo hairs and meconium lead to activation of inflammatory cascades which resemble anaphylactic reaction, so also called as *anaphylactoid syndrome of pregnancy*. The initial transient phase is pulmonary and systemic hypertension, followed by left ventricular failure leading to profound hypotension and shock. Damage to pulmonary capillary endothelium and alveoli due to inflammatory reaction along with vasoconstriction leads to ventilation perfusion imbalance, result in severe hypoxia, cyanosis, convulsion and coma.[27] DIC may also occur due to release of thromboplastin from placenta or decidual tissue into maternal circulation. Because of severe hypoxia, those who survive may develop neurological impairment.

Q4. How to diagnose a case of amniotic fluid embolism?

Diagnosis is made by exclusion as no specific diagnostic tests are available yet. Clinical presentations are variable but help in diagnosis. A woman in late stage of labor or immediate postpartum, develops gasping, breathlessness, seizure or cardiorespiratory arrest followed by consumptive coagulopathy, massive hemorrhage and death leads toward the diagnosis of AFE.

Q5. Criteria to diagnose AFE[28]

In the absence of any other clear cause, acute maternal collapse with one or more of the following features:
- Acute fetal compromise
- Cardiac arrhythmias or arrest
- Coagulopathy
- Convulsion
- Hypotension
- Maternal hemorrhage
- Premonitory symptoms, e.g. restlessness, numbness, agitation, tingling
- Shortness of breath

Excluding woman with maternal hemorrhage as the first presenting feature in whom there was no evidence of early coagulopathy or cardiorespiratory compromise.

Postmortem finding of amniotic fluid content (fetal squames or hair) in pulmonary vessel confirm the diagnosis of AFE.

Q6. What is the differential diagnosis of amniotic fluid embolism?

Cardiac causes	Myocardial infarction, cardiomyopathy, heart failure, vulvular disease
Pulmonary causes	Pulmonary edema, acute asthma, pulmonary embolism
Infection	Severe sepsis, chorioamnionitis, endocarditis
Pregnancy related	Preeclampsia, eclampsia, HELLP syndrome, APH, PPH
Others	Anaphylaxis, air embolism, anesthetic toxicity

Q7. How to manage a patient suspecting of AFE?

- Treatment is mainly supportive. Immediate administration of oxygen and intravenous fluid are most important step. Blood component therapy should be started timely
- Early effective CPR should be initiated, if CPR is not effective within 5 minutes then delivery of fetus and placenta is to be performed.
- Intubation and ventilation with inotropic support if needed and correction of coagulopathy is to be performed
- Recently, plasma exchange and hemofiltration have been used in selected cases with some benefit possibly

by clearing or washing out the inflammatory effect of amniotic fluid in circulation.[29]

CASE SCENARIO

History
Mrs X, 28 years old lady, delivered her third baby vaginally at labor room at 39 weeks 4 days POG. Placenta was delivered by controlled cord traction after 10 minutes of delivery. Uterotonic was given. Patient suddenly collapsed, not responding and gasping.

Examination

She was unconscious, PR was 128 bpm and systolic BP was 80 mm Hg, RR -18/min and bilateral chest were clear. On palpation, uterus not felt per abdominally. A large boggy mass seen at introitus.

Q1. What is the most probable diagnosis?

Acute uterine inversion.

Q2. What is acute uterine inversion?

Acute uterine inversion is rare life-threatening complication of third stage of labor. Incidence varies between 1 in 2000 and 1 in 50000 deliveries.

Q3. What are the types of inversion?

Acute uterine inversion	Within 24 hours of delivery
Subacute inversion	Between 24 hours and 4 weeks of delivery
Chronic inversion	Nonpregnant woman or after 4 weeks of delivery
Incomplete inversion	When fundus of uterus has turned inside out but not descended through cervix
Complete inversion	When inverted uterine fundus has passed completely through cervix and lie within vagina or outside introitus
1 degree	Incomplete inversion
2 degree	Complete inversion but fundus lies in vagina
3 degree	Fundus lies outside in the introitus

Q4. What are the predisposing factors for uterine inversion?

Predisposing Factors[30]
- Relaxed uterus with fundal insertion of placenta is an important risk factor
- Mismanagement of 3rd stage of labor involving fundal pressure and/or cord traction before placental separation when uterus is still relaxed
- Rarely, abnormally short umbilical cord or functionally shortened by being wrapped around the fetus may cause pulling of fundus inside out while delivery
- Sudden increase in intra-abdominal pressure due to maternal coughing or vomiting
- Morbidly adherent placenta with fundal insertion
- Manual removal of placenta may also ends in inversion
- Connective tissue disorder, such as Marfan syndrome may predispose to acute uterine inversion.

Q5. What are the clinical signs and symptoms?

Clinical Presentation[31]

- Most obvious and least common presentation is appearance of large boggy mass at introitus
- Patient complaints of severe sustainable hypogastric pain in 3rd stage of labor
- Shock out of proportion of apparent blood loss, due to pulling of infundibulopelvic and round ligament, ovaries and associated nerves, which produces vasovagal stimulation. Woman becomes pale, sweaty, develops sudden bradycardia, profound hypotension and rarely cardiac arrest
- Uterus not palpated per abdominally and mass felt at introitus in complete inversion, whereas a dimple felt abdominally in incomplete inversion.

Q6. How to manage a patient with uterine inversion?

- Acute inversion can be fatal if not managed as soon as it occurs. Immediate manual reposition of uterus under anaesthesia is recommended (Flowchart 3).
- Use of tocolytics to relax cervicouterine junction ensures rapid replacement of uterus.
- If manual reposition failed then hydrostatic replacement by O'Sullivan method can be remarkably effective. Principle of this technique is to instill 3–5 L of warm normal saline into upper vagina, thus distending the fornices, which pulls open the cervical ring and facilitate replacement of uterine fundus[32]
- In rare cases when manual and hydrostatic repositioning failed then surgical replacement with laparotomy has to undertaken. In Huntington's operation, Allis forceps are used to grasp the myometrium just inside the dimple of the inverted fundus. Cervical ring may be stretched either by fingers or by opening forceps and by using forceps on both sides, the inverted fundus is withdrawn to correct inversion
- Abdominal procedures:[33] In few cases when the cervical ring is too tight then incision over posterior cervical ring (Haultain's operation) or over anterior cervical ring (Ocejo procedure).

Flowchart 3: Managing acute uterine inversion

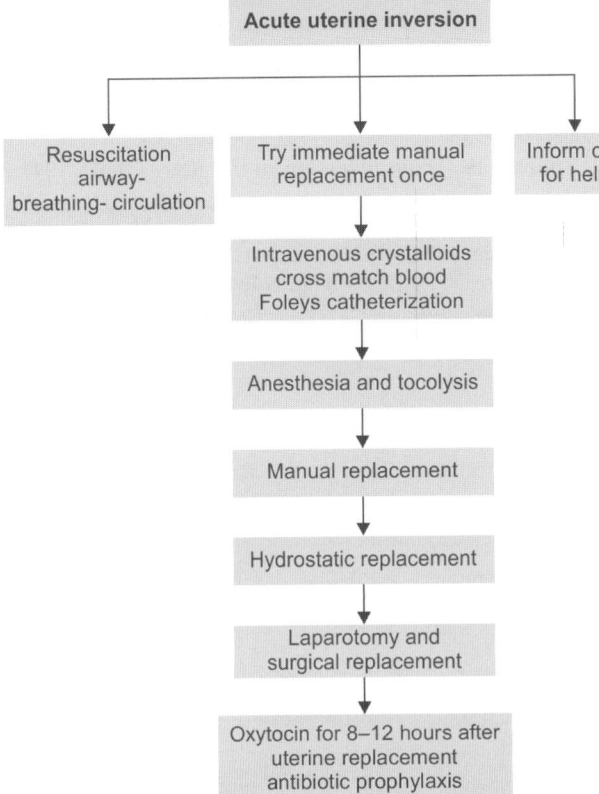

- Vaginal procedures: Spinelli—The cervical ring and the lower part of uterus are divided anteriorly and the inversion is replaced. Kustner—Involves division of the cervical ring posteriorly.

REFERENCES

1. Boerma JT. Maternal mortality in sub-Saharan Africa: Levels, causes and interventions. Ann IFORD. 1988;12:49-68.
2. Royal College of Obstetricians and Gynaecologists. Maternal Collapse in Pregnancy and the Puerperium, Green-top Guideline No. 56: London: RCOG; Jan 2011.
3. American College of Obstetricians and Gynecologists: Critical care in pregnancy. Practice Bulletin No. 100, February 2009, Reaffirmed 2011a.
4. Maternal Near Miss Review Operational Guideline. Ministry of Health & Family Welfare. Government of India. December 2014.
5. Wall RJ ,Dittus RS , Ely EW . Protocol - driven care in the intensive care unit: a tool for quality. Critical Care 2001 ; 5 (6): 283 – 5.
6. Daisy Nirmal. Clinical Guideline for: The use of the Modified Early Obstetric Warning Score (MEOWS). Maternity Guidelines Committee. 2016
7. Mousa HA, Blum J, Abou El Senoun G, Shakur H, Alfirevic Z. Treatment for primary postpartum haemorrhage. Cochrane Database Syst Rev 2014;(2):CD003249.
8. Alexander J, Thomas PW, Sanghera J. Treatments for secondary postpartum haemorrhage. Cochrane Database Syst Rev 2002;(1): CD002867.
9. Oyelese Y, Ananth CV. Postpartum hemorrhage: epidemiology, risk factors, and causes. Clin Obstet Gynecol 2010;53:147–56
10. Royal College of Obstetricians and Gynaecologists. Prevention and Management of Postpartum Haemorrhage Green-top Guideline No. 52 December 2016
11. Scorza WE, Scardella A. Fluid and Electrolyte Balance. In Belfort MA, Saade GR, Foley MR, et al (eds): Critical Care Obstetrics, 5th ed. Wiley-Blackwell, 2010, p70.
12. Hauser CJ , Shoemaker WC , Turpin I et al. Oxygen transportresponses to colloids and crystalloids in critically ill surgical patients.SurgGynecolObstet1980; 150:811-6.9.
13. Perel P, Roberts I, Ker K. Colloids versus crystalloids for fluid resuscitation in critically ill patients. Cochrane Database Syst Rev. 2013 Feb 28;(2):CD000567.
14. Borgman MAQ, Spinella PC, Perkins JG, et al. The ratio of blood products transfused affects mortality in patients receiving massive transfusion at a combat support hospital. J Trauma. 2007;63(4):805-13.
15. Stainsby D, MacLennan S, Thomas D, Isaac J, Hamilton PJ. Guidelines on the management of massive blood loss. Br JHaematol2006;135:634–41.
16. Sobieszczyk S, Breborowicz G. Management recommendations for postpartum hemorrhage. Arch Perinat Med. 2004;10:1–4
17. Ducloy-Bouthors AS, Jude B, Duhamel A, Broisin F, Huissoud C, Keita-Meyer H, et al.; The EXADELI Study Group. High-dose tranexamic acid reduces blood loss in postpartum haemorrhage. Crit Care 2011;15: R117.
18. Magwali T, Butrick E, Mambo V, El Ayadi A, Lippman S, Bergel E, et al. Non-pneumatic anti-shock garment (NASG) for obstetric hemorrhage: Haraze, Zimbabwe. Int J Gynecol Obstet. 2010;119:S410.
19. Norwitz ER, Lee HJ. Septic Shock. In Belfort MA, Saade GR, Foley MR, et al (eds): Critical Care Obstetrics, 5th ed. Wiley-Blackwell. 2010; p571-2.
20. Royal College of Obstetricians and Gynaecologists. Bacterial sepsis following pregnancy. Green-top Guideline No. 64b. April 2012.
21. Rivers E , Nguyen B , Havstad S , et al. Early goal - directed therapy in the treatment of severe sepsis and septic shock. N Engl J Med. 2001; 345: 1368-77.
22. Plaat F, Wray S. Role of the anaesthetist in obstetric critical care. Best Pract Res Clin Obstet Gynaecol. 2008;22:917-35.
23. Darenberg J, Ihendyane N, Sjölin J, Aufwerber E, Haidl S, Follin P, et al.; Streptlg Study Group. Intravenous immunoglobulin G therapy in streptococcal toxic shock syndrome: a European randomized, double-blind, placebo-controlled trial. Clin Infect Dis. 2003;37:333-40.
24. Bick RL. Disseminated intravascular coagulation: a review of etiology, pathophysiology, diagnosis, and management: guideline for care. Clin Appl Thromb Hemost. 2002;8:1-31.
25. Basket TF. Dessiminated intravascular coagulation. In: Essential management of obstetric emergencies. 4th ed. Bristol : Clinical Press Ltd; 2004.p.242-5.

26. Zupanic SS, Sokolic V, Viskovic T, Sanjug J, Simic M, Kastelan M. Successful use of recombinant factor VIIa for massive bleeding after caesarian section due to HELLP syndrome. Acta Haematol. 2002;108:162-3.
27. Clark Sl. New concepts of amniotic fluid embolism: a review. Obstet Gynecol Surv. 1990;45:360-8.
28. Knight M, Tuffnell D, Brocklehurst P, Spark P, Kurinczuk JJ, on behalf of the UK Obstetric Surveillance System. Incidence and risk factors for amniotic fluid embolism. Obstet Gynecol. 2010;115:910-7.
29. Kancho Y, Ogihara T, Tajima H, Mochimaru F. Continuous hemofiltration and shock due to amniotic fluid embolism:report of a dramatic response. Intern Med 2001;40:945-7.
30. Basket TF. Acute uterine inversion. A review of 40 cases. J Obstet Gynecol Can. 2002;24:953-6.
31. Achama S, Mohamed Z, Krishnan M. Puerperal uterine inversion: a report of four cases. J Obstet Gynecol Res. 2006;32:341-5.
32. O'Sullivan JV. Acute inversion of the uterus. BMJ. 1945;2: 282-4.
33. Stafford I, Belfort MA, Dildy GA. Etiology and Management of Hemorrhage. In Belfort MA, Saade GR, Foley MR, et al. (eds): Critical Care Obstetrics, 5th ed. Wiley-Blackwell; 2010; p312.

CHAPTER 24

Postnatal and Postoperative Ward Round

Pallavi Sharma, Pushpa Mishra

CASE SCENARIO

Mrs. X, P2L2 day 1 of normal vaginal delivery (4 hours postpartum) shifted to postnatal ward two hours back: She does not have any complaints

On Examination

- She looks conscious, comfortable and oriented to time, place and person.
- General condition is good
- Hydration adequate
- No pallor/icterus/pedal edema
- Pulse rate 82/minute
- Afebrile on touch
- BP 110/78 mm Hg
- Chest/CVS unremarkable.
- B/L Breasts soft and lactating.
- P/A: Uterus well contracted
- Palpable just below the umbilicus.
- Local examination: Episiotomy present over right medio-lateral aspect, stitch line healthy
- Bleeding per vaginum is within normal limits
- Baby is with the mother and had been breastfed.
- Patient has passed urine.

Course in the Hospital

27 years old Mrs. X G2P1L1 came to the casualty at 39 weeks gestation with the complaint of leaking per vaginum since 2 hours. She was a booked case of the hospital with no high risk factors. Her present pregnancy was uneventful till date. Labor augmentation was done and she delivered normally. Labor course was uneventful.

Patient was observed for some time in the postnatal room with vital monitoring and was transferred to the ward after she passed urine. Baby was breastfed on demand.

Q1. What are the common important clinical features you look for immediately postpartum?

- Immediately after delivery ask for general wellbeing of the patient
- Vitals such as temperature, blood pressure and pulse rate should be taken routinely during the first 24 hours starting from the first hour after birth
- Look for any pallor
- Chest and CVS examination should be done
- Fundal height and contractility of the uterus along with vaginal bleeding should be checked
- In case of suspected abnormal blood loss timely oxytocics, gentle messsage should be given
- Bladder should be assessed since it interferes with the contraction of the uterus, and patient should be encouraged to pass urine as early as possible. Voiding should be documented within six hours[1]
- Status of newborn should be seen at every visit
- Initiation of breastfeeding should be enquired and encouraged.

Q2. What are the important features to be seen on the second postnatal day?

At each subsequent visit, patient should be assessed for her general wellbeing and following:

- Micturition and urinary incontinence
- Bowel function
- Episiotomy healing
- Headache, fatigue, back pain
- Perineal pain and perineal hygiene
- Breast pain and breastfeeding progress
- Uterine tenderness and lochia
- Dietary intake.

Apart from all these, women should be asked about their emotional wellbeing, their family and social support and their usual coping strategies for dealing with day-to-day matters.

Any changes in mood, emotional state or behavior pattern that are outside of the woman's normal pattern should be noticed and taken care off.[1]

Q3. When should the woman be mobilized after delivery?

- All women should be encouraged to mobilize as soon as possible following the birth. She should be encouraged to pass urine as soon as possible (**within first 6 hours of delivery**)
- WHO recommends gentle exercise and rest during the postnatal period.[1]

Q4. What is the rationale for routine episiotomy in normal delivery?

- ACOG does not recommend routine episiotomy and clinical judgment remains the best guide for giving it[2]
- ACOG further states that there has been a decline in the use of routine episiotomy since 2000 and it does not offer any decrease in perineal lacerations, pelvic floor dysfunction, or pelvic organ prolapse compared with restrictive episiotomy
- Episiotomy has been associated with increased risk of postpartum anal incontinence, dyspareunia and increased chances of wound infection, requiring additional treatment at times.

Q5. What is the recommendation on antibiotics after uneventful normal delivery?

Routine use of antibiotics is not recommended in uneventful vaginal or instrumental delivery or even in a delivery with meconium stained liquor.

As per WHO, the antibiotics should be given:
- In manual removal of placenta
- There are third or fourth degree perineal tears for prevention of wound complications.[1]

Q6. When should breastfeeding be started after a normal delivery?

WHO recommends that mothers should initiate breastfeeding within one hour of birth. Babies should be placed in skin-to-skin contact with their mothers immediately after birth for at least an hour. Mothers should be encouraged to recognize when their babies are ready to breastfeed, help should be provided if required.[1]

Q7. Elaborate on kangaroo mother care.

- WHO emphasizes on close bonding between mother and baby through **kangaroo mother care**
- Here preterm infants are carried skin-to-skin touch with the mother. It is a powerful, easy-to-use method to promote the health and wellbeing of infants born preterm as well as full-term.

Its key features are:
- Early, continuous and prolonged skin-to-skin contact between the mother and the baby
- Exclusive breastfeeding (ideally).

It is initiated in hospital and can be continued at home. It is quite beneficial as:
- Small babies can be discharged early
- Mothers at home require adequate support and follow-up
- It is a gentle, effective method that avoids the agitation routinely experienced in a busy ward with preterm infants.[3]

Q8. When can a patient be discharged after a normal delivery?

After an uncomplicated vaginal birth in a health facility, healthy mothers and newborns can be discharged after 24 hours of observation.[1]

Q9. What important dietary advice should be given to the woman at the time of discharge?

- Stress should be made on the importance of a balanced diet along with iron and folic acid supplementation for three months postpartum.[1]
- An additional of 500 calories is recommended for breastfeeding women. The calories intake can be further increased if the mother is underweight or she is feeding two babies or doing vigorous exercises.

Q10. What postnatal precautions are advised to the patient on discharge?

WHO recommends that women should be discharged after explaining the physiological changes expected during puerperium and other warning signs and symptoms suggestive of:

- **Postpartum hemorrhage** (heavy vaginal bleeding, fainting attacks, dizziness, palpitations and tachycardia).
- **Preeclampsia/eclampsia** (headaches, visual disturbances, nausea, vomiting, epigastric or hypochondrial pain, feeling faint, convulsions)
- **Infection** (fever, shivering, abdominal pain and/or offensive vaginal loss)
- **Thromboembolism** (unilateral calf pain, redness or swelling of calves, shortness of breath or chest pain)

- Counseling should be given on nutrition, hygiene and importance of regular hand washing.[1]

NICE guidelines also recommend that on any subsequent visit enquiry should be made about the perineal health, if any complaints are found then local examination needs to be done:
- Signs and symptoms of infection should be evaluated
- Ask about any dyspareunia
- Headaches
- Undue fatigue
- Domestic abuse should be looked for
- Hemoglobin levels should be done if pallor is clinically evident
- Backache, hemorrhoids, urinary and fecal incontinence, urinary retention
- Immunization in case of Rh negative mothers.

At the end of 6–8 weeks postpartum the overall assessment of her physical, social and emotional wellbeing should be done.

Q11. What counseling should be given on contraception?

- Women should be counseled on birth spacing and family planning. The earliest known time for ovulation after delivery is 27 days so no conception can occur before 21 days
- Immediately after birth and for up to 6 months following a birth, a woman who is exclusively breastfeeding can use the lactational amenorrhea method (LAM)
- The criteria to be met for LAM include amenorrhea, baby is fed for at least 4 hourly in the day and six hourly in the night and baby is less than six months old. If a mother chooses LAM, she should switch from LAM to another modern contraceptive method by the time the infant reaches 6 months of age, or sooner[1]
- The effectiveness depends on the user, if used correctly less than 1 pregnancy per 100 women using LAM is seen in first six months after childbirth
- In addition to IUCD and sterilization, progestogen-only pills can be initiated immediately following birth. For **non-breastfeeding women**, combined pills can be initiated starting at 3 weeks after birth
- All **breastfeeding** women can use progestogen-only methods; can be initiated at 6 weeks following birth, as per WHO MEC
- Progestogen-only pills
- Injections
- Implant.

The POP should be taken at a specific time only and a gap of more than 3 hours can make it ineffective and lead to spotting.

Cerazette is a POP containing desogestrel and can be used with a gap of 12 hrs if the woman forgets to take it.

- All women, breastfeeding or not, can initiate use of condoms immediately after birth, emergency contraception after 4 weeks, and the diaphragm or cervical cap after 6 weeks
- A copper-bearing intrauterine contraceptive device (IUCD) can be inserted immediately or up to 48 hours after birth, or any time after 4 weeks postpartum
- A female sterilization procedure or tubal occlusion (TO) can be performed immediately or up to 4 days after birth, or any time after 6 weeks postpartum.

Q12. Elaborate on Janani Suraksha Yojana (JSY) and Janani Shishu Suraksha Karyakaram (JSSK).

Janani Suraksha Yojana (JSY) is a safe motherhood intervention under the National Rural Health Mission (NHM).

JSY is 100% Central Government sponsored program to promote the institutional delivery among the poor pregnant mothers by integrating cash assistance to reduce MMR, perinatal mortality and IMR in poor families.

The Yojana has identified ASHA, the accredited social health activist as an effective link between the Government and the poor pregnant women in 10 low performing states, namely the 8 EAG states and Assam and J and K and the remaining NE states. The scheme focuses on the poor pregnant woman with special dispensation for states having low institutional delivery rates, namely the states of Uttar Pradesh, Uttaranchal, Bihar, Jharkhand, Madhya Pradesh, Chhattisgarh, Assam, Rajasthan, Orissa and Jammu and Kashmir. Low performing states (LPS) and the remaining states have been named as high performing states (HPS)[4]

- Eligibility for cash assistance in HPS
- Schedule caste
- Scheduled tribe
- BPL mothers
- However all mothers are given assistance in LPS.

Cash assistance to mothers		
Areas	LPS	HPS
Rural	Rs 1400/-	700/-
Urban	Rs 700/-	600/-

All the details of the mother are documented antenataly and money is transferred to the accounts of mothers directly within 7 days of delivery.

Janani Shishu Suraksha Karyakaram: This programme was launched on June 1, 2011 by the Ministry of Health and Family Welfare to ensure better facilities to the mother and the newborn. It is an initiative to provide free and cashless services to pregnant woman in government institutions. The free entitlements under JSSK include:
- Free and cashless delivery
- Free c-section
- Free treatment of sick-new-born up to 30 days
- Exemption from user charges, free drugs and consumables
- Free diagnostics
- Free diet during stay in the health institutions for 3 days in case of normal delivery and 7 days in case of caesarean section
- Free provision of blood
- Free transport from home to health institutions
- Free transport between facilities in case of referral and also drop back from institutions to home after 48 hrs stay
- Free entitlements for sick newborns till 30 days after birth similarly include free treatment, free drugs and consumables, free diagnostics, free provision of blood, exemption from user charges, free transport from home to health institutions, free transport between facilities in case of referral and free drop back from institutions to home.[4]

Q13. What is care around birth program (CAB)?

- United States Agency for International Development (USAID) in association with the Ministry of Health and Family Welfare, Government of India has taken an initiative to scale up RMNCH +A (Reproductive, Maternal, Newborn Child and Adolescent Health) strategy
- This project started with the aim of reducing preventable maternal and child deaths in 2012. It supports six Indian states which are Delhi, Haryana, Himachal Pradesh, Jharkhand, Punjab and Uttarakhand and 30 high priority districts (HPDs)
- This is a comprehensive approach which focuses on the quality of care around the time of birth. This is because by improving services and practices during intrapartum and immediate postpartum period has the maximum potential to save maximum maternal and newborn lives. It aims at improved behavior and practices, and strengthened service delivery mechanisms. It involves an approach which brings together
  - Technical interventions
  - Health system strengthening efforts
  - Quality improvement methodology
  - Respectful maternity care.

This strategy is currently being implemented across 141 high case load facilities accounting for close to 2,00,000 annual deliveries across 26 high priority districts of India. The care around birth package also includes strengthening of:
- Postpartum family planning (PPFP) services
- Improved management of diarrhea and pneumonia through ensuring availability of ORS/Zinc and antibiotics
- Strengthening of adolescent-friendly health clinics (AFHC).

The technical intervention package to strengthen 'care around birth' has been designed in two phases
- The first phase, technical intervention package-1 (**TIP-1**), lays emphasis on strengthening the universal interventions for mothers and newborns
- The second phase **TIP-2** focuses on the management of complications.[5]

CASE SCENARIO

Mrs X P2L2 is day one of forceps delivery; delivered 5 hours back was examined in the postnatal ward.
- She looks conscious and oriented to time, place and person.
- Afebrile on touch, vitals are normal.
- No pallor or edema.
- Well hydrated
- Chest/CVS unremarkable.
- B/L breasts soft and lactating.
- P/A: Uterus well contracted just below the umbilicus.
- Local examination: Episiotomy seen over the right mediolateral aspect, stitch line healthy.
- Bleeding per vaginum is within normal limits.
- Baby is with the mother and had been breastfed.
- Patient has passed urine.

Course in Hospital

Patient came to casualty as G2P1L1 with 39 weeks POG with labor pains. She progressed well into the second stage, however forceps application was done in view of poor maternal bearing down effort with fetal distress.

- The forceps was applied by a skilled obstetrician in the presence of a neonatologist
- Baby was handed over immediately to neonatologist for examination
- Vaginal and cervical exploration was done for any tear or laceration after delivery of the placenta
- Episiotomy was sutured in layers
- Patient was observed for some time in the labor room and she was shifted out with normal vitals and after passing urine to the ward
- Breastfeeding was initiated after the baby was examined.

Q1. What should be looked after the delivery in case of forceps application?

- Do a detailed pelvic and rectal examination to detect any injuries and lacerations. Cervical exploration should be done. If any actively bleeding tears are seen, suture them properly. Severe and painful edema of the vulvovaginal area is common in these patients
- Look for any periurethral tears. Along with other injuries, these are very painful and make spontaneous voiding difficult, in which case an indwelling catheter should be placed
- Proper postoperative pain control is essential
- These patients are at increased risk for hemorrhage, and a postoperative hemogram should be obtained and the condition corrected as needed
- The newborn should be carefully examined for any injury. Common injuries associated with forceps application are facial injuries, facial palsy, bruising and swelling in the eyes and head and skull fracture.

Q2. What are the recommendations on antibiotics after instrumental delivery?

- There are insufficient data to justify the use of prophylactic antibiotics in operative vaginal delivery. Good standards of hygiene and aseptic techniques are recommended.[6]
- WHO does not recommend use of routine antibiotics in cases of uncomplicated instrumental deliveries.[1]

Q3. What analgesia should be offered to the mother in the postnatal period?

Regular paracetamol and diclofenac should be offered after an operative vaginal delivery in the absence of contraindications [6.]

Q4. What precautions should be taken for bladder care after delivery?

- The timing and volume of the first void urine should be monitored and documented. A post-void residual should be measured if retention is suspected
- Women who have had a spinal anesthesia or an epidural that has been topped up for a trial may be at increased risk of retention and should be recommended to have an indwelling catheter in place for at least 12 hours post-delivery to prevent asymptomatic bladder overfilling.[6]

Q5. When can a patient be discharged after forceps delivery?

- If patient is not having any complaints she can be discharged on the second day of delivery. A thorough pelvic and rectal examination must be done before discharge.[6]

Q6. When should the patient be called after forceps delivery?

- In the absence of specific forceps-related complications, a follow-up postpartum examination within 4–6 weeks, with a thorough pelvic examination, usually is sufficient.

Q7. What advice should be given for future deliveries?

- Women should be encouraged to aim for a spontaneous vaginal delivery in a subsequent pregnancy as there is a high probability of success.
- Care should be individualized for women who have sustained a third or fourth-degree perineal tear.[6]

CASE SCENARIO

Mrs X day 1 of LSCS was examined in the postnatal ward (done in view of previous 2 cesarean sections). The LSCS was done under spinal anesthesia 3 hours back. Blood loss was average. Baby was shifted to the mother side.
- On examination she was oriented to:
- Time, place and person
- Lying in the bed, looks comfortable.
- On examination her, pulse rate is 80/min and BP 110/70 mm Hg.
- There was no pallor or pedal edema. The chest and CVS examination was unremarkable.
- Per abdomen examination: Uterus was contracted just below the level of umbilicus.
- Dressing was applied in the lower abdomen and it was dry.
- Local examination: Vulval pad kept was superficially soaked with no active bleeding.
- Bladder was catheterized and there was total output of around 400 cc since the LSCS.

Course in the Hospital

Mrs X came to the casualty at G3P2L2 with 38 weeks gestation with previous 2 LSCS with the complaint of pain abdomen since 2 hours, there was no history of leaking or bleeding per vaginum. She was a booked patient of the hospital with no associated co morbidities. She was taken up for LSCS immediately in view of previous 2 LSCS with labor pains.

Q1. What signs are to be looked for, on the first postoperative day of cesarean section?

- After CS, women should be observed on a one-to-one basis by a properly trained member of staff until they have regained airway control and cardiorespiratory stability and are able to communicate
- After recovery from anesthesia, vital should be seen after every half hour for the initial 2 hours and then hourly provided that the vitals are stable. If any abnormality is seen, more frequent observations and medical review are recommended.[7]

Q2. What is the recommendation on antibiotics after LSCS?

- Women should be given prophylactic antibiotics at CS before skin incision. This reduces the risk of maternal infection more than when given after skin incision, with no effects on the baby
- Prophylactic antibiotics at CS reduce the risk of postoperative infections. Antibiotics chosen should be effective against endometritis, urinary tract and wound infections, which occur in about 8% of women who have had a CS.[7]

Q3. What analgesia can be offered?

Women who have a CS should be prescribed and encouraged to take regular analgesia for postoperative pain; in case of severe pain, paracetamol and codeine combination with added ibuprofen for moderate pain paracetamol and codeine combination and only paracetamol for mild pain.[7]

Q4. When can the woman be orally allowed after a cesarean section?

Women who are recovering well after CS with regional anesthesia and who do not have complications can eat and drink when they feel hungry or thirsty.[7] If the cesarean section is done under general anesthesia then orals can be allowed after 6 hours.

Q5. When should breast feeding be initiated after CS?

Women who have had a CS should be offered additional support to help them to start breastfeeding as soon as possible. This is because women who have had a CS are less likely to start breastfeeding in the first few hours after the birth, but when breastfeeding is established, they are as likely to continue as women who have a vaginal birth.[7]

Q6. What are the recommendations on wound care?

- The dressing should be removed 24 hours after the CS, look for signs of infection (such as increasing pain, redness or discharge), separation or dehiscence gently cleaning and drying the wound daily
- Advise her to wear loose, comfortable clothes and cotton underwear[7]
- Sutures can be planned for removal after 7–10 days.

Q7. What is the recommendation on catheter care and removal after LSCS?

Removal of the urinary bladder catheter should be carried out once a woman is mobile after a regional anesthetic and no sooner than 12 hours after the last epidural 'topup' dose.[7]

Q8. When should the patient be discharged?

- NICE guidelines advocate that length of hospital stay is likely to be longer after a CS with an average of 3–4 days
- However, women who are recovering well are afebrile and do not have complications following CS should be offered early discharge even after 24 hours.[7]

Q9. What is the recommendation on thromboprophylaxis?

- Routine thromboprophylaxis is not recommended in low risk women. Women should be encouraged early mobilization
- Risk assessment should be performed in each woman at least once following delivery and before discharge and arrangements made for LMWH prescription and administration (usually by the woman herself)
- Thromboprophylaxis should be continued for 6 weeks in high-risk women and for 10 days in intermediate-risk women
- In women who have additional persistent (lasting more than 10 days postpartum) risk factors, such as prolonged admission, wound infection or surgery in the puerperium, thromboprophylaxis should be extended for up to 6 weeks or until the additional risk factor/s is/are no longer present.[8]
- Other methods of preventing VTE can be use of graduated stockings, hydration, and early mobilization.[7]

Q10. What is the importance of exercises after delivery?

- Depending on the mode of delivery exercises can be started soon after the delivery.
- It has been stated that initiation of perineal exercises after delivery reduces the risk of future urinary incontinence.
- Women who have had cesarean delivery may slowly increase their aerobic and strength training, depending

on their level of discomfort and other complicating factors, such as anemia or wound infection[5]
- Kegel exercises reduces the chances of future pelvic organ and anal prolapse and strengthens the pelvic floor musculature.

CASE SCENARIO

A 26 years old P1L1, presented to us on day 12 of an uneventful normal vaginal delivery with abnormal behavior. Her vitals were stable. General and systemic examination was normal. She was discharged in a satisfactory condition from the hospital after delivery.

Her husband stated that she showed the following signs:
- Abnormal behavior and disinterest in life
- Not attending the baby properly
- Thoughts of harming the baby
- Poor sleep and personal hygiene
- Feeling of being a horrible mother
- Hearing voices, commanding her to throw away her baby.

These hallucinations terrified her and became stronger after she returned home from the hospital. The husband immediately brought her to the casualty. This is a **typical case of postpartum psychosis**. Patient was managed in association with psychiatry team. She received sessions of psychotherapy along with drug therapy and improved with time. Her husband and one other relative throughout this period observed her baby, so that she does not cause any harm to it.

Q1. What are the common psychiatric disorders witnessed in the postpartum period?

Many mental disorders can be seen in the postpartum period. The important ones include:
- Postpartum blues (25–80%)
- Postpartum depression (10–15%),
- Postpartum post-traumatic stress disorder (1.5–6%).
- Postpartum psychosis (0.1–0.2%).

Q2. What are the risk factors associated with postpartum mental disorders?

All psychiatric events generally manifest within 2–4 weeks postpartum. The risk factors include:
- Previous history of any psychiatric illness
- Poor socioeconomic status
- Psychological disturbances during pregnancy
- Lack of proper antenatal care
- Previous stressful life events
- Disturbed marriages
- Coexisting medical disorders
- Family history.

Q3. What is the treatment of acute psychiatric events in the postpartum period?

- Reassurance, love and care plays a vital role in managing these events. Patient should be managed in association with psychiatric team
- Majority of these can be settled with behavioral therapy
- Antidepressants and mood stabilizers can be prescribed in some cases for some time
- Electroconvulsive therapy has to be prescribed in acute cases only.

Q4. Elaborate on the various medications used for psychiatric disorders and their effect on breast-feeding?

Breastfeeding has an important role in the development of an infant. The treatment of such mothers raises several dilemmas, including the risk of drug exposure to the infant through the breast milk.

Most of the newer antidepressants produce very low to undetectable concentrations in infant's blood. Drugs should not be stopped in such mothers, since it can lead to adverse maternal outcomes.

WHO Recommendation for drugs during lactation[9]

Drug	Compatibility	Side effects
Amitriptyline	Compatible with breastfeeding in doses up to 150 mg/day	
Carbamazepine	Compatible with breastfeeding	Monitor infant for side-effects (jaundice, drowsiness, poor suckling, vomiting and poor weight gain)
Lithium carbonate	Avoid if possible	Monitor the infant for side-effects (Restlessness or weakness). Monitor lithium levels in mother's blood
Valproic acid	Compatible with breastfeeding	Monitor infant for side-effects (jaundice)
Chlorpromazine fluphenazine haloperidol	Avoid if possible	Monitor the infant for drowsiness

Q5. How can we prevent postpartum psychiatric events?

- The importance of mutual love and family support is very important
- Nutritious and balanced diet should be explained. Counsel to restrict alcohol intake, smoking, tobacco and substance abuse

- Spend quality time with loved ones, shopping and other routine work. Engaging in a hobby and recreational classes is one good suggestion
- Exercise under supervision and a sound and regular sleep is immensely helpful
- Practice the concept that good babies come from healthy mothers.[10]

REFERENCES

1. WHO recommendations on Postnatal care of the mother and newborn OCTOBER 2013.
2. ACOG: New Recommendations on Obstetric Lacerations-Medscape-Jun 24, 2016.
3. Who kangaroo mother care a practical guide 2003.
4. Website Mohfw.nic.in.
5. Web source: Rmncha.in
6. RCOG Green-top Guideline No. 269of 19© Royal College of Obstetricians and Gynecologists.
7. NICE Guideline on Cesarean Section. Clinical guideline [CG132]
8. RCOG Green-Top Guideline No. 37A
9. Breastfeeding and Maternal Medication Recommendations for Drugs in the Eleventh WHO Model List of Essential Drugs.
10. Sharma P, Singh N, Tempe A, et al. Psychiatric disorders during pregnancy and postpartum. J Preg Child Health. 2017; 4:317.

25
CHAPTER

Neonatal Resuscitation for an Obstetrician

Ashish Jain

CASE SCENARIO

A 33 weeks male preterm baby is born to a primigravida mother vaginally. The liqour was clear. The baby is LMP and has no breathing efforts. The Neonatologist is busy attending another delivery in emergency OT. The nursing staff calls upon the attending obstetrician for newborn resuscitation.

Q1. Why is neonatal resuscitation important?

Spontaneous breathing after birth is not a problem for most babies, however 10% of neonates require assistance at birth to breathe and about 25% of all neonatal deaths are attributed to birth asphyxia. Hence, learning the knowledge and skill in the neonatal resuscitation may prevent many neonatal deaths and the long-term neurological impairment associated with perinatal asphyxia. As 50% of the babies who need resuscitation are born un-anticipated without any high-risk antenatal factors, the attending obstetricians may often face a situation when pediatrician is not available and the baby is born. Knowing the physiology of the normal transition of the neonate immediately after birth will also generate a thorough understanding among obstetricians and generate a very good perinatal team along with the attending Neonatologist. In hospitals with high delivery rates, the preparation for the neonatal resuscitation before the baby is born is also organized by the obstetrician and the birthing place staff. Obstetrician also plays a very important role in the perinatal interventions like, delayed cord clamping, immediate skin-to-skin contact after birth and early initiation of breastfeeding, which are an integral part of the routine care of the baby at birth. The early monitoring of the baby who had successful resuscitation is also very often assisted by the delivery team. Considering above, acquiring the knowledge and skills of neonatal resuscitation is very important for the obstetricians and birthing staff.

Q2. What are the different aspects of neonatal resuscitation an obstetrician should know?

An obstetrician should know the following aspects of neonatal resuscitation:
- Preparedness for newborn resuscitation
- Assessing a newborn at birth
- Determine if a newborn needs resuscitation
- Perform resuscitation of a newborn using standard guidelines, if required
- Anticipate the aftercare that will be given to the baby following successful resuscitation
- Forming a team with the Neonatologist during resuscitation.

Q3. What are the risks factors associated with the need for resuscitation at birth?

Antenatal Risk Factors

Maternal hypertension, antepartum bleed, diabetes in mother, maternal infections, polyhydramnios, oligohydramnios, multiple gestation, premature rupture of membrane, malformation in fetus, etc.

Intrapartum Risk Factors

Abnormal heart rate, meconium stained amniotic fluid, abnormal presentation, prolonged labor, chorioamnionitis, etc.

An increased risk of breathing problems may occur in babies who are preterm, born after traumatic labor and born to mothers who received sedation during late stage of labor. However, it should be kept in mind that any baby may have breathing difficulty at birth (50% of the time problem is unanticipated). Therefore, it is important to be prepared for resuscitation in all deliveries.

Q4. How does one prepare for resuscitation before the delivery?

The obstetricians and the healthcare providers present at the time of birth must be skilled at resuscitation and know how to recognize babies at risk. They should learn to work in coordination with the pediatric team attending the delivery. When the baby is sick and being resuscitated often multiple (up to 4 people) may be required within a very short time, hence all healthcare providers should be aware of the basic knowledge and skills of neonatal resuscitation. One should prepare oneself by observing all the universal precautions while resuscitating the baby. Preparations should include having warm place to perform the resuscitation (Radiant warmer that is switched on in a manual mode at least 20 minutes prior to delivery), all other equipment and supplies that may be needed starting from the first step to the last step of resuscitation (Articles required is enclosed as annexure). Each of these articles should be checked for the sterility, efficacy and the safety prior to every delivery. One should use disposables wherever required. The medications, e.g. Adrenaline, should be prepared in the required dilution (1:100000) and kept ready prior to delivery of the baby. One should also, keep the neonatal case record and the other logistics required by the institution (e.g. Identity bands) ready before resuscitation.

Q5. What are the guidelines on Neonatal Resuscitation Program (NRP) that should be followed while resuscitation of a baby?

Since 1985, the NRP algorithm is revised every 5 years and updated based on the accumulating evidence by the international Liaison Committee on Resuscitation (ILCOR). Many countries are a part of this committee. The latest guidelines available have been published in 2015. Different countries also have a country-specific guideline based on these guidelines. The "NRP India" are the guidelines developed by the National Neonatology Forum of India (NNFI) for the Indian context. Similarly, the AAP/AHA American Association of Pediatrics/American Heart Association NRP is developed for the USA. Hence, one can follow any of these latest guidelines. The tertiary referral hospitals should follow the international ILCOR/AAP guidelines as they are evidence based and not context specific recommendations for resource restraint situations.

Q6. How does one determine the need of resuscitation in the newborn?

At birth, the time of birth is noted and the newly born baby is received in clean, dry and warm linen. While the baby is received he/she is assessed for breathing or crying (some normal babies may have good breathing efforts but not cry). If the baby is breathing or crying, then the baby needs only "routine care". The babies who do not cry at birth will be needing additional resuscitation. These steps are to be followed in sequence from initial steps to medications. (refer the NRP Algorithm).

Q7. What are the steps of routine care for babies who do not need resuscitation?

The steps of routine care are to dry the baby on mother's abdomen, provide warmth by skin-to-skin contact, cut cord in 1–2 minutes (delayed cord clamping) and evaluate respiration and heart rate of the baby. The secretions in the oral cavity if any can be cleared by a clean gauze piece. The breastfeeds are initiated immediately on the mother's abdomen itself (Fig. 1).

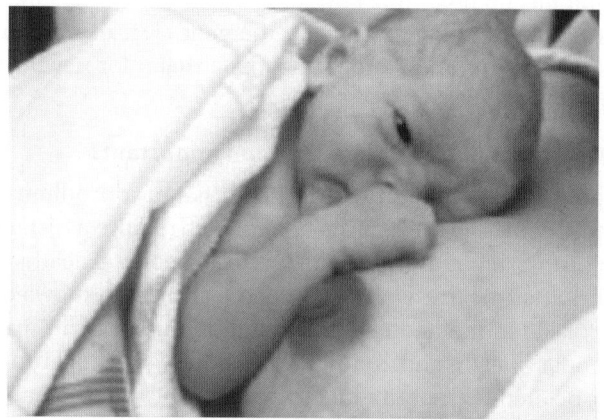

Fig. 1: Skin-to-Skin contact soon after birth

Q8. What is the first step of resuscitation for a baby who does not cry at birth?

The first steps performed in resuscitation when the baby does not cry or breathe are the "initial steps", they consist of;

Provision of Warmth

The cord of the baby needing the initial steps should be cut (without delay) and the baby should be placed under the radiant warmer with direction of baby's head towards the resuscitator. In all deliveries, the warmer should be pre-warmed prior to the delivery for at least 20–30 minutes in the manual mode. In this way, the resuscitation team will have access to the baby and the heat loss is prevented by the radiant warmer. At this stage, full visualization of the baby is needed and the baby should not be covered. In case of suspicion of birth asphyxia, due care should be taken not to overheat the baby (Fig. 2).

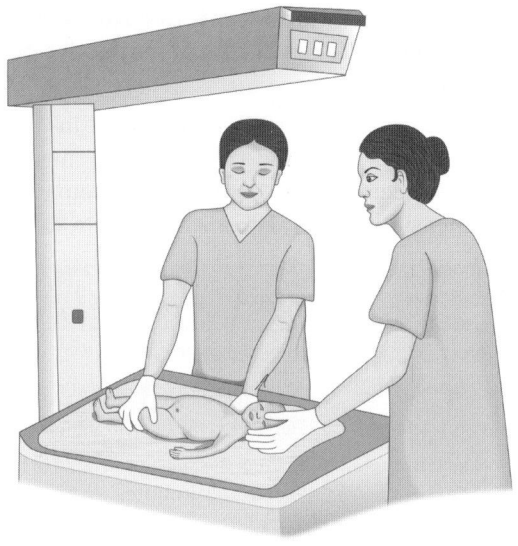

Fig. 2: Provision of warm and positioning the baby

Positioning the Baby

The baby should be positioned on the back with the neck slightly extended in the "sniffing" position. To attain a correct posture, a rolled piece of cloth/gauze piece (shoulder roll) may be placed under the shoulder of the baby. This is particularly useful when there is a large occiput (back of head) resulting from molding or edema. An appropriate position as described facilitates an unrestricted air entry, by bringing the posterior pharynx, larynx and trachea in line.

Clearing the Airway

After the baby is positioned well, the presence of secretions may prevent the entry of air into the lungs. Hence, the clearing of the airway if required should immediately follow once the newborn has been positioned. However, suction should not be done as a 'routine ritual' in all cases. Secretions may be removed from the airway by wiping the nose and mouth with a towel or by suctioning with a mucus extractor or suction catheter attached to mechanical suction device. The turning of the head to one side will allow the secretions to collect in the cheek where they can be removed easily. This is important when there are copious secretions. When using suction from the wall or from an electric suction machine, the suction pressure should be set so that when the suction tubing is blocked, the negative pressure (vacuum) reads approximately 100 mm Hg or less. The mouth (M) is suctioned before the nose (N) to ensure that there is nothing for the newborn to aspirate if he/she should gasp when the nose is suctioned.

Drying

The baby is then dried with and warm and dry cloth. It is important to dry all the parts of the baby including the back. The wet linen should be immediately removed and the baby cared always on a dry and warm linen.

Tactile Stimulation

Drying and suctioning stimulate a baby to breathe. For many newborns, these are sufficient to initiate respiration. If a baby does not have vigorous breathing, additional tactile stimulation may be briefly provided by:

1. Gently flicking or slapping the soles
2. Gently rubbing of the back, trunk and the extremities of the baby

If a baby is in primary apnea, any form of stimulation will initiate breathing.

Q9. How do you evaluate the baby during resuscitation?

The evaluation of the baby is done after each of the steps Viz Initial Steps (30 Sec), positive pressure ventilation (30 Sec), Chest compression (45–60 Sec) and the medications (ongoing evaluation every 45 sec to 1 minutes). The effectiveness of a step and the decision for progressing to next step depends on the results of this quick evaluation. The method of evaluation is the same after all the steps. The respiration is evaluated by looking at the chest and the abdomen movements. The heart rate is estimated by the auscultation of the chest with a stethoscope and counting for 6 seconds. This is multiplied by 10 to determine the heart rate. The oxygenation is estimated by applying the pulse oximeter probe to the right upper hand (Preductal). Saturation targets for a normal baby at 1 minute are 60–65% and gradually increase to 85–90% at 10 minutes.

Q10. What are the indication to start the positive pressure ventilation (PPV) after the initial steps?

After the initial steps, an evaluation is done on the baby as described above. The PPV is started if, on evaluation the baby is apneic or gasping, or the heart rate is less than 100 bpm even with breathing, and/or has persistent central cyanosis or low oxygen saturation, despite free flow oxygen increased to 100%.

Q11. What are the equipment that can be used to deliver positive pressure ventilation in the newborn? How is the PPV given to the neonate?

Equipment available for PPV in newborns are the self-inflating bag (Fig. 3), flow inflating bag and T piece resuscitator. Select appropriate size mask (0- pre-term and 1 for term baby) to cover the tip of chin, mouth, and the nose but not the eyes (Fig. 4). Ventilate newborn at a rate of 40 breaths per minute until the baby starts crying or breathing using room air. If heart rate of the baby is does not increase even after 5 inflations, look for chest rise. If the baby's chest is NOT rising, then probably the PPV given is ineffective. The corrective measures should be taken to optimize the PPV. If the chest is rising and the heart rate is increasing, the PPV is effective it is continued at a rate of 40/minutes. This rate is achieved by vocalizing and generating a rhythm as (breathe-two-three) → (breathe-two-three) and so on.

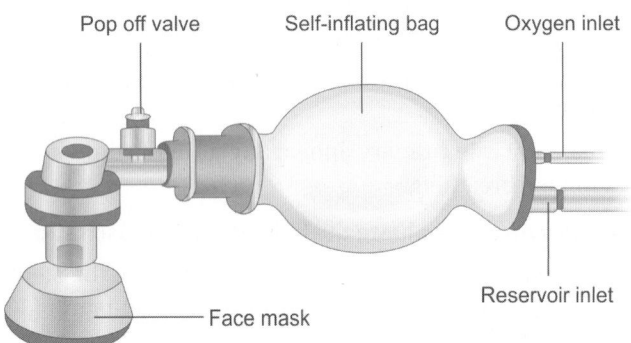

Fig. 3: Different parts of a self-inflating bag

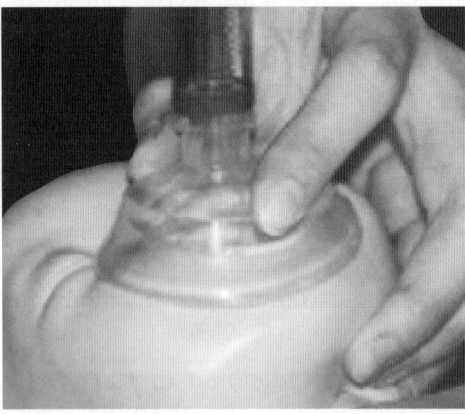

Fig. 4: Application of Face Mask

Q12. What is the concentration of oxygen that should be used during resuscitation?

Oxygen is a drug and should be used judiciously. It has been shown that the normal saturations of the baby are 60–85% in the first 5 minutes after birth and 90% only at 10 minutes of life. Hence, one should always keep in mind these targets and accordingly titrate the use of oxygen (Acceptable targets at 2 minutes, 3 minutes, 4 minutes, 5 minutes and 10 minutes after birth are 60%, 70%, 80%, 85% and 90% respectively). In all term babies, the resuscitation can be started with room air and in preterm babies at 30%. After this, a close watch is kept on the oxygen targets and the use of oxygen titrated to achieve the target.

Q13. What are the important problems and the corrective measures taken in case of ineffective positive pressure ventilation?

One should suspect that the PPV is ineffective in case of no increase in the heart rate and/or absence of chest rise on inspection of the chest. The common problems and the corrective measures to be taken are detailed in Table 1.

Table 1: Problem and the corrective measures (MRSOPA) taken for ineffective PPV

	Problem	Remedial steps
M	Inadequate seal	Mask adjusted to ensure airtight seal
R	Inappropriate position	Reposition the head in sniffing position
SO	Blocked airway	Suction the airway and open baby's mouth and ventilate
P	Inadequate pressure	Inadequate pressure increase pressure by squeezing the bag till a chest rise is visible
T	No improvement with above steps	Consider endotracheal intubation

Q14. When do you stop the positive pressure ventilation?

Provide uninterrupted effective ventilation for 30 seconds and assess for spontaneous breathing, heart rate and oxygen saturation. If spontaneous breathing present (baby breathing regularly at >30 breaths per minute), heart rate is 100 or more, and no 'in-drawing' of the chest wall then gradually discontinue PPV. In case of baby having chest in-drawing, continue with continuous positive airway pressure (CPAP) or free flow of oxygen.

Q15. What is the important precaution to be taken when the PPV is prolonged?

If PPV is prolonged over several minutes place an orogastric tube (8F) to prevent distention of stomach with air which may interfere with ventilation. Endotracheal intubation can be considered any time during the resuscitation.

Q16. What are the indications of chest compressions?

Despite 30 seconds of initial steps and 30 seconds of effective PPV, if there is progressive fall in the heart rate and the estimated heart rate is less than 60 on evaluation, then the chest compressions are promptly initiated with the PPV continued at 30/min.

Q17. How is the chest compression performed?

The chest compression can be done either by the "2-Thumb Method" or by the "2-Finger Method". The 2-Thumb Method is seen to be more effective and less tiring. However, when the umbilical venous line is inserted from the foot end of the baby for the medications, this may be difficult and the 2-finger method must be used. The chest compressions should be done on just above the xiphoid, midway between the xiphoid and the nipple line on the sternum. The compression should be deep enough to compress 1/3rd of the anteroposterior diameter of the neonate's chest. The rate and the rhythm should be 3 compressions for every breath (Hence in minute 90 compressions and 30 breaths are given). Each compression is a cycle of downward stroke and a release. Ventilation is more important during resuscitation than any other step—hence it should be continued even while administering chest compressions. It is recommended to intubate the baby and increase the oxygen to 100% during chest compression to ensure effective ventilation. This might require at least two persons with the necessary skills. The 2 persons should coordinate. The person compressing should call the counting sequence of "One and Two and Three and Breathe and". The person ventilating squeezes the bag during "Breathe and" and releases during "one and". Chest compressions are used to temporarily increase circulation and oxygen delivery. After 45 seconds to 1 minute of coordinated PPV and chest compressions, the baby's heart rate should be re-assessed. If heart rate is still less than 60 per minute, chest compressions should be continued (after administering injection adrenaline); if heart rate is >60/min, stop chest compressions.

Q18. What is the indication of administering drugs during new-born resuscitation?

Extensive resuscitation with need for medications is seen in only 1% of the cases. Medications are administered during resuscitation when despite adequate ventilation and cardiac compression, together for more than 45 seconds to 1 minute, the heart rate remains <60/min and is not improving. Epinephrine at a dose of 0.1 mL to 0.3 mL of 1:100000 per kg body weight administered through umbilical vein or any peripheral vein or 0.5 mL to 1 mL per kg body weight into the endotracheal tube if the IV access is not possible. The intravascular administration is always better than the endotracheal route, as the absorption from trachea is variable. In cases where there is no improvement and a history of blood loss is evident, volume expanders (saline, ringer lactate) at dose of 10 mL/kg are infused over 10–15 minutes through the umbilical venous line.

Q19. When do you need to intubate the baby during the neonatal resuscitation?

The endotracheal intubation is not synonymous with ventilation. A baby may be ventilated effectively without any intubation. Hence, the intubation should be performed only when it is indicated. Endotracheal intubation may be performed at various stages of resuscitation for different purposes. It may be used as soon as the baby is born in very preterm babies to administer surfactant. The babies with condition like diaphragmatic hernias also should be ventilated only after intubation. It is used during the PPV, if one cannot achieve the effective ventilation even after all the corrective measures are taken (See "A" in MR SO PA). The babies who are given chest compressions should be intubated and ventilated with 100% oxygen, as the effective and sustained ventilation is very important during this stage. Finally, the intubation may be also done for administration of the medications, if the venous line is fails.

Q20. What is the follow-on care after successful resuscitation?

Follow on care after successful resuscitation is of two types:

Observational Care

Observational care is given to those babies who have required PPV for less than 1 minute should be provided, which includes providing warmth, initiating breastfeeding and monitoring newborn (temperature, heart rate, breathing, and color every 30 minutes for 2 hours).

Postresuscitation Care

Postresuscitation care is provided to those babies who have received PPV for more than 1 minute or more extensive resuscitation like intubation, chest compression is at high risk of further deterioration. These babies should be managed in neonatal intensive care unit (NICU).

Q21. What should be discussed before the baby is discharged?

Record what has happened as soon as possible after the baby is stable. The information is important if a baby needs to be referred or becomes sick in the next few days. Also, one should discuss and de-brief about the resuscitation followed on the baby. This will help understand the gaps and improve the resuscitation and team coordination next time.

Clinical Obstetrics: A Case-based Approach

Flowchart 1: Newborn resuscitation program in India

```
Birth
 │
 ▼
Note the time
Receive baby in dry, warm linen
 │
 ▼
◇ Is baby breathing/crying? ──Yes, place with mother──▶ Routine care
 │                                                      • Dry baby on mother's abdomen
 │ No                                                   • Provide warmth (skin to skin care)
 ▼                                                      • Assure open airway if needed
• Cut cord immediately and place                        • Cut cord in 1-2 min
  under radiant warmer                                  • Ongoing evaluation of neonate.
• Provide initial steps (Dry,                                        ▲
  position, clear airway, tactile                                    │ No
  Stimulus)*                                                         │
 │
30 sec
 ▼
◇ Gasping, apnea or HR <100 bpm? ──No──▶ ◇ Labored breathing or persistent cyanosis?
 │ Yes                                          │ Yes
60 sec                                          ▼
 ▼                                     Ensure Open airway
Initiate PPV using room air*           Consider SPO₂ monitoring
 │                                     Consider CPAP (in preterm);
 ▼                                     (If not possible start supplemental
◇ Heart rate after 5 inflations:       oxygen) and shift to NICU
   <100 bpm? ──No──▶ Baby breathing well and
 │ Yes                  heart rate >100 bpm
 ▼                            │                       Observational
Look for Chest Rise; if Not   ▼                       care with Mother
• Ensure open airway      ◇ PPV <1 min ──Yes──▶       • Warmth (skin to
• Reduce leaks                │                         skin care)
• Consider increasing         │ No                    • Initiate breast
  pressure *                  │                         feeding
 │                            ▼                       • Monitor neonate
 ▼                     Baby breathing well and          (Temperature,
If Heart rate <60 bpm     heart rate >100 bpm           heart rate,
and chest rising              │                         breathing and
• Continue PPV, add 100%      ▼                         color every
  oxygen*                 Post resuscitation            30 min for 2 hr)
• Start chest compressions   care in NICU
  3 compression to 1 breath
 │
 ▼
If heart rate not detectable or <60 bpm
Administer epinephrine (1:10000),
0.1-0.3 mL/kg IV; If endotracheal
route give 0.5-1.0 mL/kg
```

Assessment

A

Evaluation

B

Evaluation

C

Evaluation

D

* Critical points when endotracheal intubation to be considered

Annexure 1

Box 1 shows the articles required for neonatal resuscitation.

Box 1: Articles required for neonatal resuscitation

- A draught free, warm room with temperature >25°C
- A clean, dry and warm delivery surface
- A radiant warmer
- A clock with seconds hand
- Warmed linen
- Shoulder roll (1/2 to 1 inch thickness)
- Oxygen with flow meter and tubing
- Stethoscope
- Mucus extractor, suction devices and catheters, No. 12 FG, 14 FG (oral suction), 5 or 6 F for preterm and 8 F for term baby for ET suction
- Positive pressure device: Self-inflating bag (250–750 mL) with oxygen reservoir
- Face masks, term (1) and preterm (0) sizes
- Laryngoscope with straight blades with an extra set of batteries and bulbs, blade 1 (term infant), 0 (preterm newborn) and 00 (extremely preterm infants)
- Endotracheal tubes of 2.5, 3.0, 3.5 and 4.0 mm
- Scissors and adhesive tape
- Umbilical catheter 3.5, 5 F
- Three way stopcock
- Syringes 1, 2, 5, 10, 20 mL
- Sterile gloves
- 8 F feeding tube
- Medications: Epinephrine, normal saline, ringer lactate

26 CHAPTER

Postpartum Contraception

Rachna Sharma, Anubhuti Rana

Postpartum Contraception

Family planning interventions is the key to achieve India's commitment for reducing maternal and child mortality. It is important that the high unmet need during postpartum period be reduced by expanding the scope of family planning services. Aside from socioeconomic benefits, these services will provide significant health benefit. The postpartum contraception counseling should begin in antenatal period. According to NICE guidelines, contraception should be discussed within the first week of delivery.[1]

In this chapter, the various methods of family planning with respect to specific situation of postpartum women are elaborated.

CASE SCENARIO

A 23 years old woman who is six weeks postpartum and also breastfeeding comes to OPD and asks how she can prevent another pregnancy for minimum 2 years. She knows about some oral preparations but she is not sure if these medicines will be safe for the baby also or not.

Q1. What are the oral preparations available for use?

The oral hormonal preparations that can be used are:
- Progesterone-only pills (POPs), also called as mini pills
- Combined oral contraceptive pills (COCs).

Q2. What is the mechanism of action of POPs?

They contain very low doses of a synthetic hormone progestin in the form of levonorgestrel or desogestrel. The mechanism of action is:
- Endometrium involutes and becomes hostile to implantation
- Cervical mucus becomes thick and impermeable
- Tubal physiology may also be affected.

Q3. How should she take the pill?

One pill should be taken every day at the same time. The new pack should be started on the next day at the same time.[2]

Q4. What is the medical eligibility criteria (MEC) for the use of POPs in postpartum women and when can they be started?

The MEC categories for POP are described in Table 1.[3]

Table 1: Medical eligibility criteria for POP

Postpartum (breastfeeding)	MEC category
<6 weeks	2
> 6 weeks but <6 months	1
> 6 months	1
Postpartum (not breastfeeding)	*MEC category*
<21 days	1
>21 days	1

Q5. What are the common side effects of POPs?

The common side effects and their management are described in Table 2.[2]

Table 2: Common side effects and their management

Side effects	Management

Irregular and unexpected bleeding	• Reassurance
	• Check compliance
	• To reduce irregular bleeding:
	  – Take a pill each day and at the same time.
	  – For short-term relief, Tranexamic acid can be used. If irregular bleeding continues or starts after several months of normal or no monthly bleeding, some other conditions unrelated to method use is suspected and further evaluation is required

Contd...

Contd...

Side effects	Management
No monthly bleeding	• Reassurance • Check compliance
Ordinary headaches (non-migrainous)	• Ibuprofen (200–400 mg), paracetamol (500–1000 mg) or other pain relievers can be used • If it gets worse, further evaluation is required
Breast tenderness	• A supportive inner wear to be worn • Ibuprofen (200–400 mg), paracetamol (500–1000 mg) or other pain reliever can be used
Mood changes or changes in libido	• Counseling and support

Q6. What should be done if the woman misses her POPs?

The management of missed pill is suggested in Table 3.[2]

Table 3: Management of missed pills

Missed pill	Management
3 or more hours late taking a pill or misses one pill	• A pill should be taken as soon as possible. • Keep taking pills as usual, one each day (she may take 2 pills at the same time or on the same day)
If she has severe vomiting or diarrhea	• If she vomits within 2 hours after taking a pill, she should take another pill from the pack as soon as possible and continue with the schedule pill as usual • If her vomiting or diarrhea continues, follow the instructions for making up for missed pills above

Q7. What are the contraindications for POPs?

Contraindications
- Absolute: Breast cancer current or past
- Relative
  - Active viral hepatitis
  - Severe cirrhosis, liver tumor (benign or malignant)
  - H/O breast cancer with no evidence of disease for at least 5 years
  - Medications that induce liver enzymes
  - Unexplained abnormal vaginal bleeding.

Q8. What preparations of COCs are available for use in government supply?

The available COC pills supplied free of cost through government health centers and hospitals Mala-N which contains levonorgestrel (0.15 mg) + Ethinyl estradiol (30μg). Each strip of Mala-N contains 21 hormonal tablets and 7 nonhormonal (iron) tablets. One pill should be taken at a fixed time every day. When one pack is finished, it is very important to start the first pill from the next pack on the very next day, irrespective of bleeding.[2]

Q9. What is the medical eligibility criteria (MEC) for the use of COCs in postpartum women and when can they be started?

The MEC categories for COC shown in Table 4.[3]

Table 4: MEC categories for COC

Postpartum (breastfeeding)	MEC category
< 6 weeks	4
>6 weeks but < 6 months	3
> 6 months	2
Postpartum (not breastfeeding)	**MEC category**
a. <21 days	
i. Without other risk factors for VTE	3
ii. With other risk factors for VTE	4
b. >21 days to 42 days	
i. Without other risk factors for VTE	2
ii. With other risk factors for VTE	3
c. >42 days	1

Q10. What is ormeloxifene and how can it used in postpartum women?

The nonhormonal preparation that can be used is Centchroman (ormeloxifene). It is a nonsteroidal, nonhormonal once a week oral contraceptive pill. It acts as selective estrogen receptor modulator (SERM). For initiation of Centchroman, the first pill is to be taken on the first day of period and the second pill three days later for the first three months. After that, the pill is to be taken once a week on the first pill day and should be continued on the weekly schedule regardless of the menstrual cycle.[2]

Medical Eligibility Criteria for Centchroman (Ormeloxifene)

Women with following conditions **should not use** Centchroman (ormeloxifene): polycystic ovarian disease, cervical hyperplasia, recent history of clinical evidence of jaundice or live disease and several allergic states, chronic illnesses, such as tuberculosis, renal disease. **It can be safely used by lactating mothers.**[2]

Side Effects

It causes delayed periods in around 8% of users, usually in the first three months.

Management of Missed Pill

- A pill should be taken as soon as possible after it is missed[2]
- If pill is missed by 1 or 2 days but lesser than 7 days, the normal schedule should be continued and she needs to

use a backup method (e.g. condoms) till the next period starts[2]
- If pill is missed by more than 7 days, she needs to start taking it like a new user that is twice a week for 3 months and then once a week.[2]

Q11. What is the effectiveness of the various oral contraceptive methods described above?

The effectiveness of oral contraceptive pills is described in Table 5.[2]

Table 5: Effectiveness of OCPs

	With perfect use	With typical use
Combined oral contraceptive pills	0.3 pregnancy per 100 women	8 pregnancy per 100 women
Progestin-only pills	• Breastfeeding women: 0.3 • Pregnancy per 100 women • Non-breastfeeding: 0.9 pregnancy per 100 women	• Breastfeeding women • Pregnancy per 100 women • Non-breastfeeding: 3–10 pregnancies per 100 women
Centchroman	1–2 pregnancy per 100 women	No documented failure rate with typical use available

CASE SCENARIO

A 23 years old mother of an 18 months old girl has been taking COCs for 3 months. She has noticed nausea on the first day of starting a new pack. She wants to switch to another method which does not involve daily administration, till she plans to become pregnant again after about 1–2 years.

Q1. What are the types of injectable contraceptives?

The main types of injectable contraceptives are:
- DMPA-IM (150 mg of DMPA given intramuscularly, 3 monthly)
- DMPA-SC (104 mg of DMPA given subcutaneously, 3 monthly)[5]
- NET-EN (200 mg of NET-EN given intramuscularly, 2 monthly) (not available in India).

Q2. What is the mechanism of action of DMPA?

It acts in the following way:
- Inhibiting ovulation—by suppressing mid cycle peaks of LH and FSH
- Thickening of cervical mucus due to depletion of estrogen. The thick mucus prevents sperm penetration into the upper reproductive tract
- Thinning of endometrial lining due to high progesterone and depleted estrogen, making it unfavorable for implantation of fertilized ovum.

Q3. What is the effectiveness of DMPA?

The effectiveness is 99.7% when the drug is used correctly; the perfect use failure rate of 0.3%.[4]

Q4. What are the advantages of DMPA?

The advantages are:
- Safe, effective
- Does not cause any significant changes in blood pressure or on the coagulation or the fibrinolytic system
- Convenient and easy to use (does not require daily routine or additional supplies)
- Acts for 3 months with a grace period of 4 weeks
- Completely reversible: 7–10 months from date of last injection (average 4–6 months after 3months effectivity of last injection is over)
- A private and confidential method
- Does not interfere with sexual intercourse/pleasure
- Pelvic examination not required prior to use
- Suitable for women who are not eligible to use an estrogen containing contraceptive
- Suitable for breastfeeding women (after 6 weeks postpartum) as it does not affect quantity, quality and composition of breast milk
- Provides immediate postpartum (in non-breastfeeding women) and post-abortion contraception
- May be used by women at any age or parity, if they are at risk of pregnancy.

Q5. What are the MEC categories for DMPA?

The MEC categories described in Table 6.[3]

Table 6: MEC categories for DMPA

Postpartum (breastfeeding)	MEC category
<6 weeks	3
>6 weeks but <6 months	1
>6 months	1
Postpartum (not breastfeeding)	**MEC category**
<21 days	1
>21 days	1

Q6. What is the preferred site for injection DMPA?

The injection site for DMPA is the upper arm (deltoid muscle), the buttocks (gluteal muscle, upper outer portion) or thigh (outer anterior).[4]

Q7. What are the common side effects with DMPA?

Irregular bleeding, prolonged/heavy bleeding (bleeding longer than 8 days or twice than usual) amenorrhea, weight gain and headache.[4]

Q8. What are the types of implants available for postpartum period?

Progestogen-only implants are a type of long-acting, reversible contraception. The various types of implants that are considered here are the following:
- Levonorgestrel (LNG): The LNG-containing implants are Norplant®, Jadelle® and Sino-implant (II)®.
    - Norplant® is a 6-rod implant, each rod containing 36 mg of LNG (no longer in production).
    - Jadelle® is a 2-rod implant, each rod containing 75 mg of LNG
    - Sino-implant (II) R is a 2-rod implant, each rod containing 75 mg of LNG
- Etonogestrel (ETG): The ETG-containing implants are Implanon® and Nexplanon®. Both consist of a single-rod implant containing 68 mg of ETG.[3]

The MEC category for the implants is described in Table 7.[3]

Table 7: MEC category for the implant	
Postpartum (breastfeeding)	MEC category
<6 weeks	2
>6 weeks but <6 months	1
>6 months	1
Postpartum (not breastfeeding)	MEC category
< 21 days	1
>21 days	1

CASE SCENARIO

A 35 years old woman, G3 P2 L2 with 36 weeks period of gestation wishes to use Cu-T as contraceptive in postpartum period. How will you counsel her about the same regarding timing of insertion, advantages, disadvantages, effectiveness, contraindications, side effects and follow-up care?

Q1. What is the timing of insertion of PPIUCD?

The CuT-380A is approved for postpartum insertion as a method of contraception. The PPIUCD can be inserted at the following timings:

Immediate Postpartum
- *Postplacental:* After vaginal delivery it can be done within 10 minutes after expulsion of the placenta on the same delivery table.[6]
- *Intracesarean:* After removal of the placenta and before closure of the uterine incision.
- *Within 48 hours after delivery:* It can be done within 48 hours of delivery and prior to discharge from the postnatal ward.[6]

Extended Postpartum/Interval

It can be done any time after 6 weeks postpartum. The IUCD should not be inserted from 48 hours to 6 weeks following delivery because there is an increased risk of infection and expulsion.[6]

Q2. What is the mechanism of action of IUCD?

The IUCD interferes with the capacity of sperm to survive and to reach the fallopian tubes where fertilization occurs. It alters sperm migration, ovum transport and fertilization. It also stimulates a sterile foreign body reaction in endometrium potentiated by copper.[6]

Q3. What is the effectiveness of IUCD?

The CuT-380A is a highly effective (>99%). There are 0.6–0.8 pregnancies per 100 women in first year of use. The CuT-380A is effective for 10 years of continuous use.[6]

Q4. What are the advantages of using an IUCD in postpartum period?

The advantages of an IUCD inserted in the immediate postpartum period include:
- It is convenient as it saves time and an additional visit
- It is safe because it is certain that she is not pregnant at the time of insertion
- Less perception of initial side effects (bleeding and cramping)
- Less chances of heavy bleeding, especially when lactating
- No effect on amount or quality of breast milk.

Q5. What are the disadvantages of using an IUCD in postpartum period?

The disadvantage of insertion of an IUCD in the immediate postpartum period is the increased risk of spontaneous expulsion. The chances of expulsion can be reduced by inserting IUCD within 10 minutes and placing the IUCD high enough at uterine fundus by using PPIUCD insertion forceps.[6]

Q6. What are the MEC categories for IUCD?

The MEC categories are:
- *Category 1:* Immediate post-placental, immediate postpartum <48 hours or during cesarean section or more than 4 weeks postpartum.[3]

- *Category 2:* No conditions.[3]
- *Category 3:* Between 48 hours and 4 weeks postpartum, chorioamnionitis, prolonged rupture of membranes >18 hours.[3]
- *Category 4:* Puerperal sepsis, unresolved postpartum hemorrhage.[3]

Q7. How is IUCD inserted in postpartum period and what are the precautions to be followed?

Postplacental (Vaginal Delivery)

- The IUCD is held in a long forceps without a lock (e.g. long placental forceps)
- The instrument is inserted up to the fundus of the uterus, and the IUCD is released
- Insertion of a post-placental IUCD should not interfere with the active management of third stage of labor.[6]

Postplacental (Cesarean)

- The IUCD is inserted through the uterine incision and placed at the uterine fundus
- This is done manually or using a regular ring forceps
- It is important to *not* attempt to pass the strings of the IUCD through the cervical os before closure of the uterus to prevent infection by contamination of the uterine cavity with vaginal flora, and to prevent displacement of the IUCD from the fundus of the uterus.[6]

Q8. What are the side effects of insertion of postpartum IUCD?

The side effects are slight discomfort related to insertion of IUCD, changes in menstrual pattern, mild cramping pain in first few weeks and infection (<1%).[6]

Q9. How will you counsel the woman after insertion of IUCD in postpartum period?

- Reassure IUCD does not affect breastfeeding and to continue exclusive breastfeeding[6]
- To follow up after six weeks for checkup and then whenever necessary[6]
- To report any time if she has any warning sign (heavy vaginal bleeding, severe lower abdominal discomfort, fever and unusual vaginal discharge) or if IUCD is expelled.[6]

Q10. What is the management of missing strings of PPIUCD?

After the involution of uterus, the PPIUCD strings usually come down. If the strings are not seen through the cervical os after involution (6 weeks after delivery), the following needs to be done:[6]

- History of expulsion of IUCD
- If she is not sure whether it has fallen out or not, an ultrasound should be done to locate the IUCD
- If IUCD is not seen on ultrasound, the woman should be counselled to replace the IUCD
- If IUCD is seen on ultrasound, then a follow up at 12 weeks is required. If again at 12 weeks the strings are not visible, the above protocol is repeated. If the strings are still not seen then either IUCD can be removed and replaced or reassurance and follow-up is advised.

CASE SCENARIO

A 34 years old woman, P4 L4, after delivery wants a permanent method of contraception. How will you counsel the woman about the same?

Q1. What is the criteria for case selection for female sterilization?

The criteria are:
- She should be married (including ever-married)[7]
- The range of is below 49 years and above 22 years[7]
- The couple should have at least one child whose age is above one year[7]
- She or her spouse/partner must not have undergone sterilization in the past[7]
- She must be in a sound state of mind so as to understand the full implications of sterilization.[7]

Q2. How will you counsel the woman and explain the consequences of the procedure?

The following features should be explained to her:
- It is a permanent procedure
- There are possibilities of complications, including failure
- It does not affect sexual pleasure or ability
- It will not affect her ability to perform daily activities
- It does not protect against STIs, or HIV/AIDS
- The consent of the spouse is not required for sterilization.[7]

Q3. What is the timing of sterilization?

The timing of surgical procedure are as follows:
- *Interval sterilization:* After 42 days of delivery or anytime in nonpregnant state. It should be done within 7 days of the menses[7]
- *Postpartum sterilization (minilaparotomy):* After 24 hours up to 7 days of delivery. **Laparoscopic tubal ligation should not be done in postpartum period**[7]
- *Sterilization with medical termination of pregnancy (MTP)* but **laparoscopic tubal ligation should not be done with second-trimester abortion**[7]
- *Sterilization following spontaneous abortion* can be done if MEC fulfiiled.[7]

Q4. What is the surgical technique used in sterilization?

- *Minilaparotomy (interval, post-abortal, or postpartum)* is done with a transverse or longitudinal incision.
  - In postpartum patient uterus should be palpated and a midline vertical (3–4 cm) incision should be given at the level of the fundus.
  - Modified Pomeroy's procedure is done for tubal liagtion[7]
  - In the Pomeroy's method, after bringing out the tube through the incision, a loop is made by holding the tube by Babcock's forceps
  - A needle with catgut no. 1 is passed through an avascular part in the mesosalpinx and the base of the loop is then tied while keeping 2 cm of the loop above the tie
  - The loop is cut and about 1.5 cm of the tube is removed
  - The stumps of the tubal ends are inspected carefully to make sure that the tube is cut completely and that there is no bleeding from the stump
  - The tubal segment removed is sent for histopathology. The same procedure is done for the other side.
- *Laparoscopic ligation* is done with Falope's rings. The fallopian tube should be identified up to the fimbrial end and the site of the occlusion of the fallopian tube must always be within 2–3 cm from the uterine cornu in the isthmus portion.[7]

Q5. What are the possible intraoperative complications?

Intraoperative complications can be nausea, vomiting, vasovagal attack, respiratory depression, cardiorespiratory arrest, uterine perforation, bleeding from the mesosalpinx, injury to urinary bladder, injury to intra-abdominal viscera, injury to blood vessels, convulsions and toxic reaction to local anesthesia.[7]

Q6. What are the postoperative complications of sterilization procedure?

Postoperative complications can be wound sepsis, hematoma in the abdominal wall, intestinal obstruction, paralytic ileus, peritonitis, incisional hernia and failure of procedure.[7]

Q7. What are the MEC categories for sterilization procedure?

There are no absolute contraindications for performing a sterilization operation. However, there are certain relative contraindications where the criteria of "C", "D", and "S" given below have to be applied which are elaborated in Tables 8 and 9.[3]

Table 8: Various MEC categories

Category		Explanation
A	Accept	No medical reason to deny the procedure
C	Caution	Procedure requires extrapreparation and precautions
D	Delay	Delay the procedure till the condition is evaluated
S	Special	The procedure should be done in a setting with an experienced surgeon and staff, the equipment needed for providing general anesthesia, and other back-up medical support

Table 9: MEC categories for sterilization in various conditions

Conditions	MEC category
Breastfeeding	A
Sterilization concurrent with cesarean section	A
<7 days postpartum	A
>7 days but <42 days postpartum	D
>42 days postpartum	A
Mild preeclampsia	D
Severe preeclampsia/eclampsia	D
Prolonged rupture of membranes (>24 hours)	D
Puerperal sepsis, intrapartum or puerperal fever	D
Severe antepartum or postpartum hemorrhage	D
Severe trauma to the genital tract	D
Uterine rupture or perforation	S
Uncomplicated	A
Post-abortal sepsis or fever	D
Severe post-abortal hemorrhage	D

REFERENCES

1. National Collaborating Centre for Primary Care. Postnatal Care: Routine Postnatal Care of Women and Their Babies (Report No. 37). 2006. http://www.nice.org.uk/nicemedia/pdf/CG037fullguideline.pdf
2. Reference Manual for Oral Contraceptive Pills. Family Planning Divison, Ministry of Health and Family Welfare, Government of India; 2016.
3. World Health Organization. Medical Eligibility Criteria for Contraceptive Use. Geneva: WHO Press; 2015.
4. Reference Manual for Injectable Contraceptive (DMPA). Family Planning Divison, Ministry of Health and Family Welfare, Government of India; 2016.
5. Supplement for Medroxy Progesterone Acetate-Subcutaneous Injectable Contraceptive (MPA-SC). Family Planning Divison, Ministry of Health and Family Welfare, Government of India; 2016.
6. IUCD Reference Manual for Medical Officers and Nursing Personnel. Family Planning Division, Ministry of Health and Family Welfare, Government of India; 2013.
7. Standards for Female and Male Sterilization services. Research Studies and Standards Division, Ministry of Health and Family Welfare, Government of India; 2014.

27
CHAPTER

Surgeries in Obstetrics

Pushpa Mishra, Aparna Setia

FIRST AND SECOND TRIMESTER ABORTIONS

Abortions can be:
- Spontaneous
- Induced (MTP).

SPONTANEOUS ABORTION

Pregnancy loss without any outside intervention before 20 weeks of gestation.

Classification

- *Complete abortion:* All products of conception have passed without the need for any surgical or medical intervention
- *Incomplete abortion:* Some of the POC's have passed while few products are still retained inside the uterine cavity
- *Inevitable abortion:* Herein the cervix has dilated but the POC's have not been expelled
- *Missed abortion:* A pregnancy wherein there has been a fetal demise but the POC's have not been expelled and the os is closed (diagnosed incidentally on USG or when signs of pregnancy start regressing)[1]
- *Recurrent spontaneous abortion:* ≥3 consecutive pregnancy losses
- *Septic abortion:* A spontaneous abortion which is complicated by intrauterine infection
- *Threatened abortion:* A confirmed viable pregnancy complicated by bleeding before 20 weeks of gestation.

Incidence

Twenty percent of pregnant women experience some bleeding before 20 weeks GA, and roughly half of them end in spontaneous abortion.[1]

Etiology and Risk Factors[2]

- Chromosomal abnormalities (most common)
- Advanced maternal age
- Drugs like misoprostol, methotrexate, retinoids or anesthetic agents
- Substance abuse, i.e. smoking, alcohol, cocaine, caffeine
- Chronic maternal diseases like poorly controlled DM, autoimmune diseases (e.g. APLA)
- Conception within 3 to 6 months after delivery
- Pregnancy with IUCD in situ
- Maternal infections like TORCH bacterial vaginosis, chlamydia, etc.
- Exposure to toxins like arsenic, lead, heavy metals
- Uterine anomalies like adhesions, cervical incompetence, etc.

Presurgery Work Up

- History—to establish gestational age and if any other symptoms (bleeding, pain, any medical history)
- Per abdominal and per vaginal examination
- Complete blood count to rule out anemia and infection
- Blood typing and Rh testing (in case of RH negative pregnancy anti D has to be administered post-abortion or any blood requirement)
- USG to intrauterine pregnancy and gestational age.

Treatment

Lines of Management

- Expectant
- Medical
- Surgical (treatment of choice in unstable patients)

Management

- *Complete abortion:* No further treatment required.

- *Incomplete abortion:* Expectant management (82–96% success rate)[6-8] till 2 weeks followed by surgical evacuation if required.
- *Inevitable abortion:* Expectant followed by surgical evacuation.
- *Missed abortion:* Medical therapy with intravaginal misoprostol (80% success rate).

Surgical Treatment

- Manual vacuum aspiration (MVA)
- Dilatation and curettage (D and C)
- Dilatation and evacuation (D and E)

INDUCED ABORTIONS

They can be first trimester (up to 12 weeks of gestation from LMP) or second trimester abortions (12–20 weeks).

Incidence

- About 16.5% of all abortions in the United States are managed medically and 25.2% of all abortions <9 weeks of gestation.
- Mifepristone, combined with misoprostol, is the most commonly used medical abortion regimen worldwide.

Surgical Abortion

A surgical procedure is carried out for termination of pregnancy.

Indications

- If on follow up of medical abortion a gestational sac is present or the pregnancy is continuing with or without cardiac activity (failed medical management)
- Patient wants immediate termination
- Patient is bleeding excessively
- MTP with ligation or IUCD.

Medical Abortion versus Surgical Abortion[10]

Medical Abortion

Advantages

- Avoid invasive procedure
- Avoid anesthesia
- Good success rate (approximately 95%)

Disadvantages

- Takes days to weeks to complete
- Requires follow-up
- Side effects of drugs used (e.g. nausea, vomiting, diarrhea, headache, dizziness, and fever)[11,12]
- Causes pain and cramps needing NSAIDs
- Can cause excessive bleeding which warrants immediate surgical intervention, rarely blood transfusion.
- About 5% cases require surgical evacuation.

Surgical Abortion

Advantages

- Completed in a predefined period of time
- High success rate (99%)
- Does not require follow-up
- Patient compliance not required
- Less blood loss
- Patient can be discharged same day.

Disadvantages

- Invasive procedure
- Needs anesthesia/sedation/analgesics
- Risk of surgical trauma
- Asherman syndrome can be there in few cases.

SURGICAL ABORTION

First-trimester Surgical Abortion

- Preoperative preparation of the cervix with misoprostol to overcome any stenosis or scarring of the cervix if present.
- Local anesthesia given
- Painting and draping done
- Sims speculum is inserted and cervix is held with sponge holder.
- Cervical dilatation is done with serial hegar dilators if required followed by:
  - MVA wherein with the help of vacuum aspirator, we remove the POC's, done up to 63 days of pregnancy.
  - *Suction and evacuation:* Cervix (internal os) is dilated according to gestational age (8 mm for 8 weeks pregnancy) and then products are sucked with appropriate number of suction cannula. Cannula size is matched with the GA and the pressure generated is 60–70 mm Hg
  - Curettage is done either as a last step of suction evacuation or for the incomplete abortion or for retained POC's. It is done with the blunt end of the curette (blunt and sharp curette).
- The instrument is placed 1–2 cm short of the fundus and is gently rotated and withdrawn till internal os.
- Completion of the procedure is confirmed when a gritty sensation is appreciated or when the uterine

walls adhere to the suction tip or when no more tissue is evacuated from the uterus.

Second Trimester Abortion
- Labor induction with the help of misoprostol/dinoprost/mechanical methods.
- Digital evacuation with ring forceps to be done in retained bits of placenta or POCs.
- Very rarely hysterotomy too required if patient fails to progress and leads to complications.

Post-procedure Care
- Observation for 24 hours if excessive blood loss occurred during procedure
- Volume replacement and blood transfusion if required
- If signs of infection seen, IV antibiotics are given.

MANUAL REMOVAL OF PLACENTA (MRP)

Introduction
Among the causes of postpartum hemorrhage (PPH), retained placenta which occurs in 0.6–3.3% of normal deliveries, has a case fatality rate of 10% in rural areas.[3,4]

Definition
Placenta not expelled within 30 minutes after delivery of the baby is known as a retained placenta.

Indications for MRP
- Partial separation of placenta
- Retained placental bits

Pathogenesis
Due to retained placenta, the uterus is unable to contract and the sinusoidal arteries keep bleeding from the placental bed leading to PPH.

Treatment
Removal of the placenta and/or retained placental tissue and membranes.

Timing to do MRP
- In the absence of hemorrhage-Conservative management:
  - Observe for a further 30 minutes as spontaneous expulsion of the placenta can still occur.
  - Intraumbilical vein injection of oxytocin with saline can be given.[5]
  - Active management of the third stage of labor (AMTSL) to be done.
- In the presence of hemorrhage and failure of conservative management—MRP is the definitive treatment.

Steps
1. Under aseptic condition, give a single dose of prophylactic intravenous antibiotics[5] and adequate analgesia.
2. Place your non-dominant hand over the abdomen and stabilize the uterus.
3. Make a cone with your dominant hand and enter the uterus.

1. Retained Placenta
- Trace the umbilical cord and identify the edge of the placenta.
- Strip off the membranes from the margins of the placenta with your fingers directed towards the placenta to prevent uterine rupture.
- Go between the placenta and the uterine wall.
- With an up and down motion establish a cleavage plane thus separating the placenta from the wall of the uterus.
- After complete separation of the placenta, draw it out gently through the cervix.
- Examine the placenta and membranes for completeness.
- Reinsert your hand to remove any tissue if left behind.

2. Retained Placental Bits
- Identify and remove the clots and tissue bits by same sweeping motion.
- If any placental tissue fails to separate then likelihood of abnormal placentation should be thought for and USG should be done to plan further management.

Post-procedure Care
- Observation till bleeding controlled.
- Volume replacement and blood transfusion as per need.
- Monitor the vitals every 30 minutes for 6 hours or until patient is stable.
- Regular P/A examination to pick up uterine atony.

PERINEAL INJURIES

Anatomy[7]

Perineum is the region between mons pubis to anus and inferior to uro-genital diaphragm. The structures which form it are the muscles of the anus, sphincter and urogenital region, medial part of the levator ani muscles with fascia over them and the subcutaneous tissue and skin. These structures aid in supporting the pelvic organs and maintaining fecal continence.

Definition

A perineal tear is an injury involving some or all of these structures which form the perineum.[8]

Rcog Classification of Perineal Tears[9,10]

- *First-degree tear:* Injury to skin and/or vaginal mucosa
- *Second-degree tear:* 1st degree + Injury to perineal muscles
- *Third-degree tear:* 2nd degree + Injury to anal sphincter complex:
  - Grade 3a tear: <50% of external anal sphincter (EAS) thickness torn
  - Grade 3b tear: >50% of EAS thickness torn
  - Grade 3c tear: Both EAS and internal anal sphincter (IAS) torn
- Fourth-degree tear: 3rd + Injury to anorectal mucosa.

*Obstetric anal sphincter injuries (OASIS) = 3rd and 4th degree perineal tears.

Risk Factors[11,12]

- Birth weight >4 kg
- Median episiotomy
- Nulliparous
- Shoulder dystocia
- Kristeller's maneuver/fundal pressure
- Instrumental delivery
- Prolonged second stage of labor
- Family risk of similar tear in first degree relatives
- Occipitoposterior position.

Prevalance

- Over 85% of women having a vaginal delivery sustain perineal trauma, and 60–70% require suturing.[13]
- An increasing incidence of higher grade perineal tears in the past few decades has been reported mainly due to an improved rate of detection.[14]

Diagnosis

By careful inspection of the perineum after vaginal delivery.

Treatment

- Adequate general or regional anesthesia to provide a maximal sphincter relaxation and a sufficient pain relief
- Preoperative prophylactic antibiotic (e.g. with 2nd generation cephalosporin) should be administered[15]
- Proper aseptic precautions.

Steps

1. Identify and classify the tear by inspection and via speculum and digital rectal examination (DRE).
2. In case of doubt, it is advisable to classify to the higher degree.
3. Repair of the cervical and high vaginal tears should be done first.
4. In case of 3rd and 4th degree tear, repair should be done in OT under good analgesia and light:
   - First repair the anorectal epithelium with atraumatic, 3-0, end-to-end sutures.
   - Then identify the edges of the torn internal anal sphincter and repair with atraumatic interrupted mattress sutures, preferably 3-0.
   - Thirdly, suture the external anal sphincter muscle with atraumatic sutures—preferably 2-0.
   - Per rectal examination should be done after the repair.

Complications

- Fecal incontinence
- Fecal urgency
- Chronic perineal pain
- Dyspareunia
- Residual defects.

*First and second-degree tears rarely cause long-term problems except dyspareunia occasionally.

Postoperative Care

1st and 2nd Degree Tear
- *Antibiotics:* No evidence of benefit seen after repair.
- Perineal care and hygiene is all needed the postoperative care.

3rd Degree Tear
- Antibiotics (broad spectrum) should be started before repair in OASIS.
- Nil per oral for 24 hours followed by oral liquid diet followed by soft diet for initial 72 hours.
- *Laxatives:* Given to reduce the mechanical stress on the sutures.
- *Physiotherapy:* To strengthen the pelvic floor musculature.
- *Timely follow-up:* After 6 weeks followed by after 3 months.

Look for:
- Symptoms of anal incontinence—if present patient requires further investigations and surgical assistance.
- Residual dehiscence or defects.
- Counsel regarding subsequent pregnancies and births (5% risk of renewed injuries with vaginal birth) and hence a cesarean section should be offered to women with history of 3rd/4th degree perineal tears and its complications.

EPISIOTOMY (FIG. 1)

Definition
An episiotomy is a surgical procedure where we incise the perineum to enlarge the vaginal opening to improve fetal and maternal outcomes (ACOG, 2006; Downe, 2009).

Indications
- *Large size baby:* EFW >4 kg
- Suspected shoulder dystocia
- Preterm or SGA baby

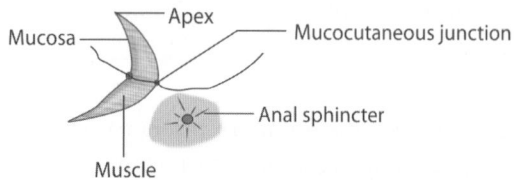

Fig. 1: Episiotomy incision

- Malposition and malpresentation
- A thick and rigid perineum
- Prior to instrumental delivery
- To quicken the second stage of labor.

Types
There are four types of episiotomy:[14]

Mediolateral
The incision is made downward and outward from the midpoint of the fourchette either to the right or left midway between the anus and the ischial tuberosity.

Advantage
Less risk of anal tears.

Disadvantages
- Increased blood loss
- Severe pain
- Difficult repair
- Higher risk of long-term discomfort and dyspareunia.

Median
The incision commences from the center of the fourchette and extends on the posterior side along the midline.

Advantages
- Less blood loss
- Less pain
- Easier to perform
- Easier to repair
- Better cosmetically.

Disadvantage
More risk of anal tears.

Lateral
The incision starts from about 1 cm away from the fourchette and extends laterally.

Disadvantages
High chance of injury to the Bartholin's duct (strongly discouraged).

J-shaped
The incision begins in the center of the fourchette and is directed posteriorly along the midline for about 1.5 cm and

then directed downwards and outwards along the 5 or 7 o'clock position to prevent the internal and external anal sphincter (not widely practiced).

Epidemiology

- Episiotomies were done routinely in the past but no benefit was reported.[17]
- In 2009, a Cochrane meta-analysis concluded that: "Restrictive episiotomy is more beneficial than routine episiotomy".
- ACOG (2016) concluded that mediolateral episiotomy is better than midline episiotomy when clinically indicated.

Procedure

- Consent is taken
- Local anesthesia (M/C lignocaine 0.5%) is given
- The incision is given at the time of crowning (If given too early, increased bleeding may occur and if too late there will not be any protective effect and tears already might have taken place).

Precaution

While incising, insert two fingers into the vagina to prevent injury to fetal presenting part.

- Controlled birth of the presenting part is done to prevent any extension of the episiotomy. If it is taking time, compress the incision in between contractions to prevent PPH.
- After completion of the third stage, thoroughly examine the vagina and perineum for any injuries.

Repair of episiotomy:
- We first repair the vaginal mucosa by continuous suturing technique with rapid vicryl using a round body needle and starting above the apex of the cut or tear to include the retracted vessels.
- Secondly, muscles are sutured with interrupted stitches.
- Thirdly, skin closed by mattress stitches, starting from the apex to the fourchette for a good apposition.
- Gentle examination is done for any missed tears or inappropriate apposition of anatomy to correct it.
- Finally put a finger in the rectum and check that no sutures have passed through into the rectal mucosa and that the sphincter is intact. If sutures are felt, remove them and re-suture.

Complications

- Excessive blood loss.
- Extension of the wound causing anal incontinence.
- Perineal infections can occur rarely (necrotizing fasciitis is a rare but potentially fatal complication).
- Postpartum perineal pain (if excessive it may be a sign of perineal hematoma).
- Wound dehiscence.
- Dyspareunia.

Advice on Discharge

- Analgesics and anti-inflammatory drugs (Acetaminophen or paracetamol is the safest choice, since it can be taken even while breastfeeding)
- Cold sponging for soothing
- Perineal hygiene
- Avoiding pressure on the stitches (use laxatives)
- Pelvic floor exercises (advantage: strengthening the pelvic floor musculature and increasing the blood circulation leading to early healing).

BROAD LIGAMENT HEMATOMA (Fig. 2)

Anatomy[18,19]

The broad ligaments consist of anterior and posterior leaflets of peritoneum covering the lateral uterine corpus and upper cervix.

Boundaries

- *Superior:* Round ligament
- *Inferior:* Cardinal and uterosacral ligaments
- *Lateral:* Infundibulopelvic ligament and lateral pelvic wall
- *Medial:* Lateral boundary of uterus.

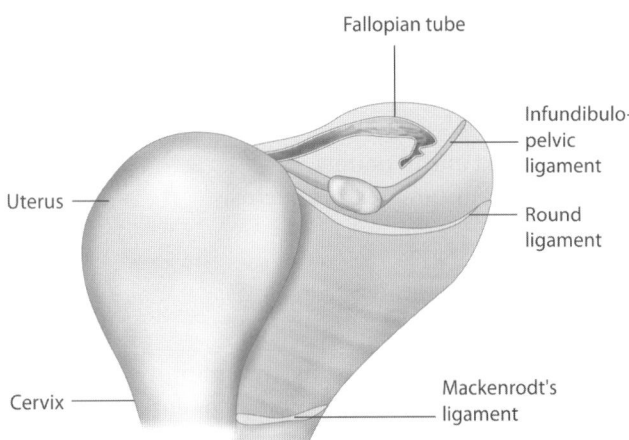

Fig. 2: Anatomy of broad ligament

Contents
- The fallopian tubes, ovaries and round ligaments
- Blood supply to the uterus:
  - *Arterial:* Uterine and ovarian arteries which anastomose near the upper lateral aspect of the uterus.
  - *Venous:* The uterine wall is occupied by many venous sinuses which come together within the broad ligament to form the large pampiniform plexus.

Incidence
Broad ligament hematoma is a rare but dangerous complication with the incidence from 1 in 20,000 to 1 in 35,000 deliveries.[20]

Predisposing Factors
- Tears in cervix or upper vagina or uterus that extends to uterine or vaginal arteries:
  - During dilatation during D and C or D and E procedures (most common)
  - Spontaneous vaginal deliveries (very rare complication)[21]
  - Difficult traumatic and instrumental deliveries
  - Prolonged second stage of labor
  - Precipitate labor
  - Intrauterine instrumentation.
- Post-cesarean section (trauma to the broad ligament or extension of the uterine incision into the broad ligament)
- Pelvic fractures
- During or following tubal ligation (hematoma within mesosalpinx)
- Coagulopathy.

Classification
- Early onset due to trauma
- Late onset due to pressure necrosis.

Source
- *Venous:* Typically results in slow expansion and may appear dark red or bluish in color.
- *Arterial:* Typically results in a rapidly expanding hematoma and may appear bright or dark red.
- Both.

Symptoms
- Asymptomatic
- Persistent postpartum localized pelvic pain, fullness or discomfort
- Abdominal distension
- Back pain
- Fullness or pressure in the recto-anal area
- Dizziness, syncopal attacks.

Examination
Signs
- Tachycardia
- Tachypnea
- Hypotension
- Pallor
- Prolonged capillary refill time
- Trembling, sweating, anxiety and collapse.

Per Abdominal Examination
- Tenderness
- Unilateral fluctuating mass
- Elevated and deviated uterine fundus.

Pervaginal Examination
- Vaginal or cervical tear
- Adnexal mass
- Cervical motion tenderness.

Per Rectal Examination
- Tenderness
- Mass.

Investigations
Ultrasound is Diagnostic
- Hemogram
- Coagulation profile
- Blood grouping and cross matching
- CT scan or MRI.[22]
- USG guided paracentesis from the mass.

Patient hemodynamically stable and small hematoma, diagnosed on USG, can be managed conservatively with:
- Strict pulse, temperature, respiratory rate
- Antibiotics
- Serial USGs.

Patient Hemodynamically Unstable

- Resuscitation
- Volume replacement with crystalloids
- Blood transfusion
- Blood products if indicated
- Laparotomy is required in large and progressive hematomas
  - Hematoma is drained by incising anterior leaf of the broad ligament.
  - If any active bleeder, it should be ligated.
  - For generalized ooze, uterine, internal iliac or branches of ovarian artery can be ligated on ipsilateral side.
  - Repair of tears present in broad ligament, lateral vaginal fornices or uterus should be done.
  - Care should be taken not to include ureter in the stiches or traumatize it.
  - Feeding vessel embolization can be done if facilities are there.
- Routine postoperative care.[23]

CERVICAL TEARS

Introduction[24]

Cervical tears are the commonest form of traumatic postpartum hemorrhage.

Classification

- *First degree:* Up to 2 cm
- *Second degree:* More than 2 cm but limited to the cervix
- *Third degree:* Extending into the vaginal fornices
- Rarely, cervical avulsion with colporrhexis with or without extension to involve the LUS and uterine artery and its major branches.

Risk Factors

- Delivery through an undilated cervix whether spontaneously or by forceps or vaccum.
- Precipitate labor.
- Rigid cervix due to previous operations like the LEEP procedure, conisation, or cervical amputation.
- Very vascular cervix as in case of a low level placenta previa.
- Trauma due to the after coming head of breech.

Diagnosis

By visual inspection of cervix, by using right angle vaginal retractors and grasping the patulous cervix with a ring forceps, under proper light. It is done if:

- Clinical suspicion present in a case of vaginal bleeding after childbirth despite a well-contracted uterus with no injury to the vagina and perineum
- In case risk factors are present

*Most common site: The lateral angle at 3 o'clock and the nine o'clock positions, between the anterior and posterior lips of the cervix.

Treatment

Aim: Control of bleeding

- Minor lacerations not actively bleeding should not be stiched.
- Major cervical lacerations or tears need stat repair, under anesthesia and good light.
- Treatment varies with the extent of the lesion:
  - If limited to the cervix—suture the cervix followed by the repair the vaginal lacerations.
  - Cervical tear that has extended deep beyond the vaginal vault—arterial embolization or laparotomy may be required to repair it.

Technique

- Apply antiseptic solution to the vagina and cervix
- Anesthesia may be required for cervical tears that are high and extensive
- Ask an assistant to massage the uterus and provide fundal pressure
- Proper cervical inspection is done with sponge forceps.
- Close the cervical tears under direct vision with continuous chromic catgut suture starting at the apex (upper edge of tear)
- If a long section of the rim of the cervix is tattered, under-run it with continuous chromic catgut suture.

PERIURETHRAL TEARS

Definition

Vaginal tears that occur at the region around the urethra.

Cause

Normally, at the time of delivery the head is born by extension. If a sudden extension occurs, it will cause a sudden pressure on upper vaginal area resulting in a periurethral tear.

Precaution

Press gently on the fetal head at the time of delivery and guide it to a slow and gradual extension at the time of birth.

Treatment

Periurethral tears need to be stitched carefully under proper light and with bladder catheter in situ. Minute tears with no bleeding does not require any repair.

Postpartum Care

- Prevention of infections
- Analgesics and anti-inflammatory
- Cold packing to prevent retention of urine due to inflammation.

CESAREAN SECTION (FIG. 3)

Definition

Delivery of a fetus through surgical incisions made through the abdominal wall (laparotomy) and the uterine wall (hysterotomy).

Incidence

- In 2014, the rate of CS delivery in the United States was 32.2%.[25]
- According to the NFHS 2015-16, rate of cesarean section (CS) in some states of India is as high as 87.1%.
- WHO norms prescribe CS deliveries to be at 10–15% of the total number of deliveries in the country and to be resorted for medical reasons alone.
- A rapid increase in cesarean rates from 1996 to 2014 without evidence of concomitant decrease in maternal or neonatal morbidity or mortality raises a concern that CS delivery is overused.

Causes for Increase CS Rates[26]

- Previous cesarean delivery
- Multifetal gestations
- Increase in the intrapartum electronic fetal monitoring
- Increased parental and social expectations of pregnancy outcome
- Maternal autonomy in decision making regarding mode of delivery
- Lack of adherence to standard guidelines
- Use of ART/IVF.

ACOG/SMFM guidelines for prevention of primary cesarean delivery:[27,28]

- Promote prolonged latent (early)-phase labor.
- The start of active-phase labor can be defined as cervical dilation of 6 cm, rather than 4 cm.
- In the active phase, more time should be permitted for labor to progress.
- Increase use of instrumental deliveries should be encouraged.
- Increase in delivery of primi breech, vaginally.
- Trial of labor in women with twin gestations if the first twin is cephalic.

Classification

1. **RCOG classification according to urgency (Table 1):**
   - *Category 1:* Emergency CS
   - *Category 2:* Urgent CS
   - *Category 3:* Scheduled CS
   - *Category 4:* Elective CS

Table 1: A classification relating the degree of urgency to the presence or absence of material or fetal compromise

Urgency	Definition	Category
Maternal or fetal compromise	Immediate threat to life of woman or fetus	1
	No immediate threat to life of woman or fetus	2
	Requires early delivery	3
No maternal or fetal compromise	At a time to suit the woman and maternity services	4

Proposed by "Lucas et al" April 2010

2. **According to gestational age:**
   - Before the age of viability—hysterotomy
   - After the age of viability—cesarean section
3. **According to the incision:**
   - *Lower segment cesarean section (LSCS):* Incision is made on the lower part of the abdomen and uterus to deliver the baby (M/C).
   - *Classical cesarean section:* A midline vertical incision on the abdomen and the uterus is made to deliver the baby.

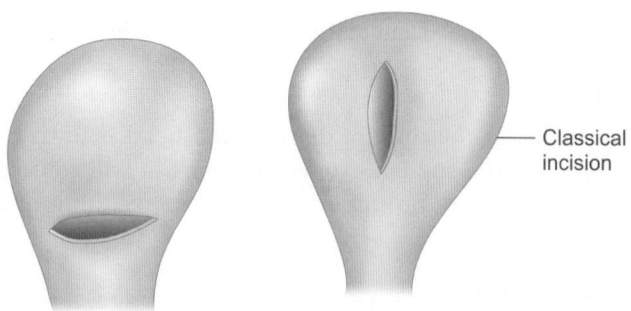

Fig. 3: Uterine incisions

- *Cesarean hysterectomy:* It is a life-saving procedure in which the uterus is removed after delivering the baby.

CONTRAINDICATIONS

- Dead fetus: Except in extreme degree of pelvic contraction, neglected shoulder or severe accidental hemorrhage
- Disseminated intravascular coagulation (DIC)
- Extensive scar or pyogenic infection in the abdominal wall.

LOWER SEGMENT CESAREAN SECTION

Definition

A surgery in which the incision is made in the lower segment of the uterus. The incision could be transverse (Kerr incision) (M/C) or low vertical (Kronig) in case of:
- Presence of lateral varicosities
- Constriction ring to cut through it
- Deeply engaged head.

Indications

85% cases of CS are due to:[29]
- Previous cesarean delivery
- Breech presentation
- Dystocia
- Fetal distress.

Maternal Factors

- Prior classical C-section or transmural myomectomy
- Active genital herpes infection
- Cervical carcinoma
- Maternal trauma.

Fetal and Maternal Factors

- Cephalopelvic disproportion
- Placenta previa
- Placenta abruption
- Failed operative vaginal delivery
- Post-term pregnancy.

Fetal Factors

- Fetal malposition
- Fetal distress
- Cord compression
- Erythroblastosis fetalis.

Emergency

- Fetal distress
- Meconium stained liquor
- Cord prolapse
- Maternal distress (like excess bleeding or surge of blood pressure)
- Mechanical impedance to the progress of labor (due to passage, passenger, power).

Elective CS

- Previous CS
- Previous classical cesarean section
- Placenta previa grade 4
- Malposition
- Pelvic tumors or large ovarian cysts
- Genital herpes in the mother
- Medical problems in the mother like high blood pressure or diabetes
- Multifetal gestation
- IVF/ICSI pregnancies
- HIV infection in the mother
- Macrosomia >4 kg
- Uterine deformity like a bicornuate uterus.

Advantages of LSCS over Classical CS

- Peritoneum is loosely attached to the uterus at LUS
- Less damage to the vascularized areas of uterus
- Easier to repair
- Sutures remain intact (less problem with suture loosening)
- Less blood loss
- Healing is more efficient
- Less chance of scar rupture
- Cosmetically more acceptable.

Investigations Needed before Doing CS

Blood Tests

- Hemoglobin, hematocrit
- Blood sugar
- Blood grouping and cross matching
- Viral markers (HIV, HBsAG, anti-HCV) and VDRL

Ultrasonography

To know the lie, position, placental localization, estimated fetal weight, etc.

Operative Procedure—LSCS

- Adequate nil per oral status (at least six hours prior to the surgery)
- Adequate hydration
- Prophylactic antibiotics an hour before surgery (preferred first generation cephalosporin)
- Urinary catheterization
- Monitoring of the mother (pulse, BP and ECG) and the baby (FHR)
- Inform the pediatrician
- Give anesthesia: Level-up to T4
  The anesthesia can be of the following types:
  - Spinal anesthesia (most common)
    - Easy to administer
    - Safe for the mother and the baby
    - Early return to normal activities including breastfeeding
  - Epidural anesthesia if it is already in place (labor analgesics) or in maternal heart disease
  - General anesthesia if:
    - There are bleeding or clotting problems in the woman
    - Fetal distress
    - Eclampsia or severe PE
- Paint and drape the patient
- A transverse (Pfannenstiel) incision is given 2 to 3 cm above the symphysis pubis cutting the skin and subcutaneous tissue.
- The rectus sheath is incised transversely and the rectus muscles is separated in the midline followed by opening of the parietal peritoneum.
- The loose UV fold of peritoneum over the lower uterine segment is held and incised transversely in a semilunar fashion and the bladder is pushed downward.
- Then the uterine incision is given over LUS and liquor is drained out.
- The presenting part is delivered followed by the rest of the body.
- Then umbilical cord is clamped and cut and the placenta is delivered out.
- The uterus is then explored to remove any remaining membranes or placental tissue.
- The uterine massage and oxytocics are given to promote uterine contractions.
- Uterine incision is closed in 2 layers.[30]
- Lastly, abdomen is closed in layers and aseptic dressing applied followed by a vaginal toileting.

Complications

In Mother

Intraoperative Complications

- Injury to the nearby structures like—ureters, urinary bladder, intestines
- Perforation of the uterus
- Aspiration of the contents of the stomach into the lungs during anesthesia
- Amniotic fluid embolism (very rare). It cannot be prevented
- Shock due to excess bleeding due to uterine atony (normal expected blood loss—1000 mL)
- Uterine rupture (0.5–1% risk in previous transverse or low vertical incision).

Postoperative Late Complications

Approximately 2-fold increase in maternal mortality and morbidity has been seen with CS as against to a vaginal delivery.[31]

- PPH
- Infection or dehiscence at the wound site
- DVT leading to pulmonary embolism
- Ileus
- Atelectasis
- Urinary tract infection (UTI)
- Fever
- Post dural puncture headache
- Adhesions causing pain and complications in future pregnancies
- Abdominal wall hematoma
- Postpartum depression
- Incisional hernias
- Death.

In Baby

- Respiratory problems
- Lower APGAR
- Injury due to procedure.

Postoperative Management

- Monitoring of vitals, urine output, and amount of vaginal bleeding
- P/A examination to see for uterine contractility
- Volume resuscitation
- Early feeding which has shown to shorten hospital stay[32]
- Adequate analgesia
- Ambulation

- Initiation of breastfeeding
- SRC removal on day 2
- Discharge on postoperative day 2 to 4, in uncomplicated cases[33]
- Explain regarding recovery (six weeks for the body to heal completely) and suture removal after day 7
- Discuss regarding contraception as well as refraining from strenuous exercises and intercourse for 4–6 weeks postpartum.[34]

CLASSICAL CESAREAN SECTION

Definition

When a vertical incision is given over the anterior wall of the uterus in the upper active segment it is a classical CS.

Incidence

- Classical CS is an infrequently performed surgery with an incidence of 0.3% of all deliveries.
- There is an inverse relationship between gestational age at delivery and the likelihood of classical CS. An Australian study noted that at 24 weeks, 20% of all cesarean deliveries were of the classical type, while at 30 weeks, the rate was 5%, and at term, only 1%.[35,36]

Problem

This incision encompasses the active upper uterine segment (contractile portion of the uterus) thus causing a high risk of uterine rupture in future pregnancies (4–10%) and patients require a repeat classical CS in next pregnancy.[37]

Indications

- Placenta accreta syndromes
- Coexisting cervical cancer
- Lower uterine segment is not approachable:
  - Anterior placenta previa
  - Large fibroid in the lower uterine segment
  - Densely adhered bladder due to previous surgery
  - Preterm breech with ill formed LUS.
- Transverse lie (dorsoinferior position) especially with membrane rupture or impacted shoulder.
- Postmortem CS
- Morbid obesity
- Multifetal pregnancy.

Steps

1. Vertical incision is given over the abdomen and the abdomen is opened in layers.
2. Identify the bilateral round ligaments.
3. Taking care of the bladder which might be high up, a midline vertical incision is given extending from as low down to the upper uterine segment.
4. After entering the uterine cavity, extend the incision on both sides. If the placenta is in the way, displace it.
5. Deliver the baby as a breech, so that the delivery of the head can be guided with your hand.
6. Give oxytocics.
7. Clamp and cut the cord and hand over the baby to the pediatrician.
8. Deliver the placenta and membranes when the uterus contracts and if it fails to contact then do uterine massage and wait for oxytocics to act.
9. Then repair the uterus in 2 layers with ''1'' chromic catgut.
10. Mop blood and exudate from the peritoneal cavity, and close the abdomen in layers.

Postoperative Management

- Similar to LSCS
- Explanation regarding high risk of rupture in next pregnancy and need for elective classical CS in next pregnancy at 36–37 weeks.

Complications

- Greater degree of blood loss
- Longer operating time
- Difficult apposition
- Poor healing due to contraction and retraction of upper segment
- Rupture uterus in subsequent pregnancy during 3rd trimester or in labor
- High risk of placental implantation over scar in next pregnancy
- More chance of infection.[38]

CESAREAN HYSTERECTOMY

Definition

Removal of the uterus at the time of cesarean delivery.

Incidence

- It is becoming more common due to the rising primary CS rate.
- Knight et al.[39] showed that the incidence of cesarean hysterectomy is 1:30,000 if it is after a vaginal delivery, 1:1700 if it is after a cesarean delivery 1:220 if it is after two or more cesarean deliveries.

- Maternal morbidity associated with cesarean hysterectomy may be as high as 56%.[40]

Concerns

- It is a technically challenging procedure due to the anatomic and physiologic changes of pregnancy such as massive increase in blood flow to the uterus at term obscuring the operative field and making suturing pedicles more difficult.
- It is frequently performed in emergent, unplanned situations to save the mother's life.
- It permanently ends future fertility.

Pathogenesis

- Normally, the placenta attaches to the uterus via specialized endometrium known as decidua.
- Once the fetus delivers, the placenta separates and cessation of bleeding occurs due to contraction of the spiral arteries leading to decrease in the surface area of the exposed placental bed.
- In case due to any reason the placenta is not able to separate or the vessels are not able to contract even with medical management cesarean hysterectomy may be required as a last resort, i.e. as a life-saving procedure.

Risk Factors

- Maternal age over 35
- Parity ≥3
- History of cesarean delivery or any surgeries on the uterus.

Indications

The advent of broad-spectrum antibiotics and improved pharmacological therapy and procedures for controlling hemorrhage (e.g. embolization, B-Lynch suture), has resulted in a decline in the incidence of emergent cesarean hysterectomy.

1. Most common cause—abnormal placentation[41]

    Degrees:
    - Placenta accreta (adherence of the placenta to myometrium)
    - Increta (invasion through myometrium)
    - Percreta (invasion all the way through the myometrium into serosa, frequently into the bladder).

    Risk Factors:
    - Prior cesarean delivery
    - Placenta previa
    - Prior uterine surgery including myomectomy (fibroid removal) and curettage.

    Diagnosis
    - When suspected prior to delivery—based on ultrasonography or MRI or based on risk factors
    - Encountered unexpectedly at delivery.

2. Complications of CS such as Postpartum hemorrhage:[42]
    - Uterine atony
    - Hysterectomy is the last resort once all conservative management exausted.
3. Cancers such as cervical cancer, ovarian cancer and endometrial cancer. Cervical cancer is one of the most common cancers diagnosed in pregnancy.[41]
4. Uterine rupture.
5. Leiomyoma in pregnancy if symtomatic.
6. Infection (e.g. chorioamnionitis).
7. Extension of uterine incision at delivery.

Contraindication

Refusal of the procedure.

Approach Considerations

- Best abdominal entry technique: Midline vertical incision (due to best exposure) and in emergency, a low transverse incision may need to be converted to a midline vertical incision resulting in an inverted T-shaped incision which is:
    - More difficult to close
    - More painful
    - Less cosmetically acceptable
    - A longer recovery time.
- After entering the abdominal cavity, a typical cesarean delivery is performed.
- After the delivery of the baby, deliver the placenta which often leads to bleeding.
    - If the placenta delivers easily but heavy bleeding or uterine atony is present, medical management of PPH should begin followed by the various methods to treat the PPH which if fail, the decision of hysterectomy should be made.
    - If the placenta does not detach with gentle traction, accreta should be suspected and the anesthesiologist and family should be informed, and the hysterectomy should proceed. Forcibly trying to detach an abnormally adherent placenta can have serious consequences such as heavy blood loss and damage to nearby organs.
- After recognizing that the placenta is not detaching, it is left in situ and the uterine incision is quickly sutured

- and closed using a single running layer to decrease bleeding prior to starting the hysterectomy.
- The hysterectomy may be performed using the standard steps. However, if bleeding is severe, the steps may be hastened without suturing/tying off the pedicles (i.e. leaving clamps in place) until the uterine arteries have been clamped and bleeding significantly slows.
- Sharp dissection of the adhesions might be required in cases with history of previous surgeries.
- Serial clamping of structures done bilaterally:
  - Round ligament.
  - Cornual structures including the utero-ovarian ligament.
  - Uterine arteries.
  - The cardinal and uterosacral ligaments.
- If the surgeon decides to do a supracervical hysterectomy, the uterine fundus is "amputated," often with cautery or scissors, and the remaining part of the cervix (stump) may be sutured.
- If total hysterectomy is planned then after removing the uterus and cervix, vaginal cuff is closed.
- Finally, irrigation is done and hemostasis confirmed. Methylene blue test is advisable to confirm that no injury to the ureters or bladder has taken place.
- If there has been an inadvertent cystotomy, the area is dissected and the bladder is closed with two continuous layers of absorbable 4.0 polyglycolic sutures. It is necessary to give postoperative antibiotic coverage and Foley catheter drainage of the bladder for 7–10 days to allow repair.
- Then abdomen closed in layers.
- If placenta percreta with invasion into the bladder is a preoperative concern, a cystourethroscopy may be performed prior to the cesarean section, and if placenta is visualized invading into the bladder, then urologists should be called into the operating room for bladder reconstruction.

Postoperative Management

- Broad spectrum antibiotic coverage especially in case of urinary tract injury, history of chorioamnionitis and fever.
- Catheter care
- Blood and blood product transfusion
- Maintain adequate hydration
- Vital and urine output charting.
- Complete work-up and examination of the postoperative patient, including appropriate cultures, whenever significant fever exists.
- All women receive thromboprophylaxis for at least 7 days postoperatively, and use of graduated elastic compression stockings is advised.

Complications and Outcome[43]

- Fever due to multiple blood and blood product transfusions or due to infections
- Other blood transfusion reactions
- Infections in the abdominal wound or within the abdomen and pelvis, as well as in the urinary tract
- Vaginal cuff hematoma or pelvis hematoma and abscess formation
- Bleeding intraoperative or immediate postoperative due to vascular pedicles
- Urinary tract injury to the bladder or ureters including vesicovaginal fistulas.[41]
- Disseminated intravascular coagulation (DIC) can occur in case of excessive blood loss during the surgery thus requiring transfusion of multiple blood products; carrying the risk of spontaneous bleeding from multiple surfaces simultaneously
- DVT and pulmonary embolism[42]
- Ileus
- Hospital readmission
- Bowel injury
- Wound dehiscence
- Septic pelvic thrombophlebitis
- Pneumonia or atelectasis
- Subsequent laparotomy
- Death.

SURGERIES FOR UTERINE RUPTURE REPAIR

Introduction

- Uterine dehiscence or rupture is more common during labor but in previously scarred uterus it may occur during the third trimester.
- Management depends on prompt detection and diagnosis.

Classification

- Occult or incomplete rupture: Scar dehiscence present but the visceral peritoneum is still intact. They require strict monitoring to look for signs of scar dehiscence.
- Complete rupture (catastrophic) is a full thickness tear and requires urgent surgical intervention.

Causes:
- Traumatic:
  - Motor vehicle accident.
  - Incorrect use of oxytocics.
  - Operative vaginal delivery (e.g. breech extraction)
- Spontaneous:
  - Previous history of surgery of the uterus (CS, myomectomy, etc.)[44]
  - Multiparous females
  - History of cervical laceration.

Incidence

- Uterine rupture in an unscarred uterus occurs extremely rarely (6.1/10,000 deliveries).[45]
- Following a previous cesarean section the incidence increases to 22–74/10,000 deliveries if vaginal birth is attempted.[46]

Risk Factors

- Previous cesarean section (87%):
  - Classical, vertical and T-shaped incisions are at more risk than low transverse incision.
  - Short interconception period.[47]
  - Gestational age >40 weeks.
- Previous uterine surgery (e.g. myomectomy, D&C, MRP)
- Uterine anomalies, e.g. undeveloped uterine horn.
- Trauma, e.g. a vehicle accident.
- Instrumental delivery.
- Obstructed labor.
- Induction of labor.
- H/O Cervical laceration.
- Abnormal placentation.
- Macrosomia and fetal anomaly, e.g. hydrocephalus.
- Malpresentations and malposition.
- Multiple pregnancy.
- Choriocarcinoma/invasive mole.
- Maneuvers to relieve shoulder dystocia.

Presentation[48]

Vague Signs and Symptoms

- Fetal bradycardia on CTG[47]
- Severe abdominal pain
- Chest or shoulder tip pain
- Sudden shortness of breath
- Scar pain and tenderness
- Abnormal vaginal bleeding or hematuria
- Severe pallor
- Cessation of previously efficient uterine contractions
- Maternal tachycardia, hypotension or shock
- On P/A examination: Fetal parts felt in the abdominal cavity and absent FHS
- On P/V examination: Fetal parts have moved up.

Diagnosis

- Clinically
- Ultrasound to look for abnormal fetal position, hemoperitoneum or absent or thin uterine wall
- Intrauterine pressure catheters to see for loss of resistance.

Management[48]

- Resuscitation if the patient is unstable.
- Urgent laparotomy and delivery.
- Uterine rupture to be repaired if possible and hysterectomy to be considered as a lifesaving measure.
- If repair done with conservation of the pregnancy then postoperative tocolysis, progesterone support and dexa cover should be given followed by elective CS at 32 weeks. This technique is highly controversial.[49]
- Postoperative antibiotics and DVT prophylaxis.

Complications

- Postoperative infection
- Urinary tract injuries
- Amniotic fluid embolus
- Massive maternal hemorrhage
- Disseminated intravascular coagulation (DIC)
- Pituitary failure (Sheehan syndrome).

Prognosis[47]

- Perinatal death—6.2%
- Emergency hysterectomy needed for 14—33%
- Risk of repeat rupture if earlier one was repaired is 20%

Prevention

Due to unpredictability, we cannot prevent it but in patients who opt for a trial of scar continuous fetal heart rate monitoring should be done along with preparedness to deal with the complications.

REFERENCES

1. Pazol K, Creanga AA, Zane SB, Burley KD, et al. Abortion surveillance--United States, 2009. Centers for Disease Control and Prevention (CDC). MMWR Surveill Summ. 2012;61(SS-8):1–44.
2. Raymond EG, Shannon C, Weaver MA, et al. First-trimester medical abortion with mifepristone 200 mg and misoprostol: a systematic review. Contraception. 2013;87:26–37.
1. Combs CA, Laros RK. Prolonged third stage of labour: morbidity and risk factors. Obstet Gynecol. 1991;77:863-867.
2. Tandberg A, Albrechtsen S, Iverson DE. Manual removal of placenta. Acta Obstet Gynecol Scand. 1999;78:33-36.
3. Carroli G, Bergel E. Umbilical vein injection for management of retained placenta. Cochrane Database of Systematic Reviews, 2001, Issue 4. Art. No.: CD001337.
4. Chongsomchai C, Lumbiganon P, Laopaiboon M. Prophylactic antibiotics for manual removal of retained placenta in vaginal birth. Cochrane Database of Systematic Reviews, 2006, Issue 2. Art. No.: CD004904.
5. Last RJ. Anatomy Regional and Applied. London: Churchill Livingstone. 1984. p. 345.
6. Finn M, Bowyer L, Carr S, et al. Women's Health: A Core Curriculum. Australia: Elsevier; 2005.
7. Sultan AH. Obstetric perineal injury and anal incontinence. Clin Risk. 1999;5:193-6.
8. Koelbl H, Igawa T, Salvatore S, et al. Pathophysiology of urinary incontinence, faecal incontinence and pelvic organ prolapse. In: Abrams P, Cardozo L, Khoury S, Wein A (Eds). Incontinence. 5th ed. [place unknown]: ICUD-EAU; 2013. pp. 261-3596.
9. Baghestan E, Irgens LM, Børdahl PE, et al. Familial risk of obstetric anal sphincter injuries: registry-based cohort study. BJOG. 2013;120:831-37.
10. Smith LA, Price N, Simonite V, et al. Incidence of and risk factors for perineal trauma: a prospective observational study. BMC Pregnancy Childbirth. 2013;13:59
11. Kettle C, Tohill S. Perineal Care: Clinical Evidence; 2008.
12. Gurol-Urganci I, Cromwell DA, Edozien LC, et al. Third- and fourth-degree perineal tears among primiparous women in England between 2000 and 2012: time trends and risk factors. BJOG. 2013;120:1516-25.
13. Duggal N, Mercado C, Daniels K, et al. Antibiotic prophylaxis for prevention of post-partum perineal wound complications: a randomized controlled trial. Obstet Gynecol. 2008;111:1268-73.
14. Dutta DC. Textbook of Obstetrics, 7th edition; 2011.
15. Carroli G, Mignini L. Episiotomy for vaginal birth. Cochrane Database Syst Rev. 2009;21;(1):CD000081.
16. Hoffman BL, Schorge JO, Schaffer JI, et al. Williams Gynecology. 2nd edition; 2012.
17. Cunningham FG, Leveno KJ, Bloom SL, et al. Williams Obstetrics. 24th edition; 2014.
18. Saleem N, Ali HS, Irfan A, et al. Broad ligament hematoma following a vaginal delivery in primigravida. Pak J Med Sci. 2009;25:683-5.
19. Muthulakshmi B, Francis I, Magos A, et al. Broad ligament haematoma after a normal delivery. J Obstet Gynaecol. 2003;23(6):669-70.
20. Jain KA, Olcott EW. Magnetic resonance imaging of postpartum pelvic hematomas: early experience in diagnosis and treatment planning. *Magn Reson Imaging*. 1999;17(7): 973-7.
21. Gilstrap LC, Cunningham FG, VanDorsten JP. Operative Obstetrics. 2nd edition; 2002.
22. Cunningham FG, Leveno KJ, Bloom SL, et al. Williams Obstetrics. 24th edn. 2014.
23. Births - Method of Delivery. Centers for Disease Control and Prevention. July 6, 2016.
24. Mishra US, Ramanathan M. Delivery-related complications and determinants of caesarean section rates in India. Health Policy Plan. 2002;17:90-8.
25. [Guideline] Barclay L. Longer labor okay to avoid cesarean, new guidelines say. Medscape Medical News from WebMD. 2014 Feb 19.
26. Caughey AB, Cahill AG, Guise JM, et al. Safe prevention of the primary cesarean delivery. *Am J Obstet Gynecol*. 2014; 210(3):179-93.
27. Notzon FC, Cnattingius S, Bergsjo P, et al. Cesarean section delivery in the 1980s: international comparison by indication. Am J Obstet Gynecol. 1994;170(2):495-504.
28. Bujold E, Goyet M, Marcoux S, et al. The role of uterine closure in the risk of uterine rupture. Obstet Gynecol. 2010;116(1):43-50.
29. Landon MB. Vaginal birth after cesarean delivery. Clin Perinatol. 2008;35(3):491-504, ix-x.
30. Patolia DS, Hilliard RL, Toy EC, et al. Early feeding after cesarean: randomized trial. Obstet Gynecol. 2001;98(1):113-6.
31. Tan PC, Norazilah MJ, Omar SZ. Hospital discharge on the first compared with the second day after a planned cesarean delivery: a randomized controlled trial. Obstet Gynecol. 2012;120(6):1273-82.
32. Committee Opinion No. 670 Summary: Immediate Postpartum Long-Acting Reversible Contraception. Obstet Gynecol. 2016;128(2):422-3.
33. Bethune M, Permezel M. The relationship between gestational age and the incidence of classical caesarean section. Aust N Z J Obstet Gynaecol. 1997;37(2):153-5.
34. Chauhan SP, Magann EF, Wiggs CD, et al. Pregnancy after classic cesarean delivery. Obstet Gynecol. 2002;100(5 Pt 1):946-50.
35. Landon MB. Vaginal birth after cesarean delivery. Clin Perinatol. 2008;35(3):491-504, ix-x.
36. LS, O'Connell CM, Baskett TF. Maternal and perinatal morbidity associated with classic and inverted T cesarean incisions. Obstet Gynecol. 2002;100(4):633-7.
37. Knight, et al. Cesarean delivery and peripartum hysterectomy. Obstetrics and Gynaecology 2008;111:97-105.
38. Rossi, et al. Emergency Postpartum hysterectomy for uncontrolled postpartum bleeding. A systematic review. Obstetrics & Gynaecology. 2010;115:3.
39. Shellhaas CS, Gilbert S, Landon MB, et al. The frequency and complication rates of hysterectomy accompanying cesarean delivery. *Obstet Gynecol*. 2009;114(2 Pt 1):224-9.
40. Bateman BT, Mhyre JM, Callaghan WM, Peripartum hysterectomy in the United States: nationwide 14 year experience. *Am J Obstet Gynecol*. 2012;206(1):63.e1-8.

41. Shellhaas, et al. The frequency and complication rates of hysterectomy accompanying cesarean delivery. Obstetrics and Gynaecology. 2009;114;224-9.
42. Kieser KE, Baskett TF: A 10-year population-based study of uterine rupture. Obstet Gynecol. 2002;100(4):749-53.
43. Zwart JJ, Richters JM, Ory F, et al. Severe maternal morbidity during pregnancy, delivery and puerperium in the Netherlands: a nationwide population-based study of 371,000 pregnancies. BJOG. 2008;115(7):842-50.
44. Birth After Previous Caesarean Birth; Royal College of Obstetricians and Gynaecologists; 2007.
45. Guise JM, Eden K, Emeis C, et al. Vaginal birth after cesarean: new insights. Evid Rep Technol Assess (Full Rep). 2010;(191):1-397.
46. Edmonds DK (Ed). Dewhurst's Textbook of Obstetrics and Gynaecology, 8th edition. 2012. John Wiley & Sons; 2012.
47. Shirata I, Fujiwaki R, Takubo K. Successful continuation of pregnancy after repair of a midgestational uterine rupture with the use of a fibrin-coated collagen fleece (TachoComb) in a primigravid woman with no known risk factors. Am J Obstet Gynecol. 2007;197:e7-9.

28

CHAPTER

Gynecological Disorders in Pregnancy

Niharika Dhiman

FIBROID IN PREGNANCY

CASE SCENARIO

Primigravida with 8 months amenorrhea with acute pain abdomen.

A 26 years old, Mrs X, wife of Mr Y, resident of Sadar Bazaar, a homemaker, came to gyne casuality on 1/5/17 with complaints of:
- Eight month amenorrhea
- Acute pain in abdomen × 2 days

Her LMP was 14/9/16 making her period of gestation (POG) 32 weeks and 2 days on 1/5/2017.

History of Presenting Complaint

- Patient was a booked antenatal case and presented to the gyne emergency with complain of pain in lower abdomen for 2 days.
- The pain was acute in onset mainly localized in the right side of the abdomen.
- Severe in intensity, was associated with vomiting and low grade fever.
- There are no aggravating or relieving factors.
- Pain was not associated with any bloody mucoid discharge or bleeding per vaginum (P/V) or leaking per vaginum or any hardening of the abdomen.
- There is no associated history of burning micturition or pain during micturition, no bowel complaints.
- There is no history of decreased fetal movements.
- There is no history of any abdominal trauma.
- She was showing regularly in the antenatal period and was a diagnosed case of fibroid uterus during this pregnancy only.

Course in the Hospital

She was admitted to the labor room after her abdominal and internal examination.

She received intravenous fluids and few injections in her buttocks. She was also given some oral medications and monitored for abdominal pain and fetal heart. After 3–4 hours, she was relieved of her symptoms. An ultrasound was also done for her. Blood sample was taken in the labor room.

- Level II ultrasound was done at 5th month of pregnancy and she was told that there is a mass arising from the right side of the uterus most probably a fibroid. All other parameters were normal.
- Repeat scan, at 6th month, showed an increase in the size of the fibroid.
- Patient was counseled regarding certain warning symptoms (pain in abdomen, bleeding per vaginam, leaking per vaginum or fever) and was advised to report to the emergency in presence of any of the symptoms.
- There is no history of breathlessness, easy fatigability, swelling over the feet, abnormal weight gain, leaking or bleeding P/V, recurrent urinary infection or increased blood sugar.

Menstrual History (M/H)

- Menarche—attained at 13–14 years
- LMP—14/9/16, EDD—22/3/2017. Previous cycles were regular, 4–5 days of bleeding with 28–30 days cycle with normal flow. No history of dysmenorrhea, menorrhagia. No history of pills intake for contraception or missed periods prior to conception.

Contraceptive History

Barrier method.

Diagnosis on History
Primigravida with 32 weeks and 2 days POG with acute abdomen probably red degeneration of fibroid.

Examination
- Temperature—100 °F
- Pulse rate—100/minute, regular, rhythmic, good in volume, normal in character, with no radiofemoral or radioradial delay. All peripheral pulses are palpable.
- Blood pressure—110/80 mm of Hg in right arm in sitting position.
- Respiratory rate—16/minute
- Average built with normal gait, normal hairline, and average orodental hygiene
  - Height: 155 cm; Weight: 65 kg
  - No pallor/icterus/cyanosis/clubbing/edema
  - Thyroid: normal
  - No lymphadenopathy

Abdominal Examination
Inspection
Abdomen is uniformly distended all quadrants moving with respiration. Umbilicus is central and everted. Linea nigra and striae gravidarum present, no other scar marks are seen. All hernial sites are free.

Palpation
- Uterus is relaxed, fundal height—36 weeks; symphysis fundal height (SFH)—36 cm
- Abdominal girth—38 inches.

Obstetric Examination
Fundal Grip
A soft broad irregular structure felt at fundus, suggestive of breech. Another mass 8 × 10 cm felt arising from right side of the fundus, local temperature over the mass is raised. It is tender on touch, firm to soft in consistency with restricted mobility.

Lateral Grip
Smooth, resistant and curved structure felt on the right lateral side of the abdomen, suggestive of back. Multiple knobby parts felt on the left side, suggestive of limbs.

Pelvic Grip
A hard, globular smooth and ballotable structure felt on palpation, suggestive of head. Head is freely mobile, not engaged.

Auscultation
Fetal heart sound was heard at the right spinoumblical line 134 beats/min, regular.

Diagnosis after Examination
Primigravida with 32 weeks POG with single live fetus with cephalic presentation with fibroid uterus with red degeneration.

Q1. What is the incidence of fibroid during pregnancy?
- The incidence of fibroid during pregnancy varies from 0.09–3.9%.
- Incidence is much higher and varies from 12–25% in older women who are postponing childbearing or have taken infertility treatment.[1]

Q2. What is the differential diagnosis of a gravid uterus with fibroid?
- Early gestation: Twin gestation, ectopic pregnancy, ovarian mass, bicornuate uterus and retroverted uterus.
- Late gestation: Ovarian mass.

Q3. What are the differential diagnosis of acute pain in abdomen during pregnancy?

Early Pregnancy
- Abortion
- Ectopic pregnancy
- Torsion of ovarian cyst
- Cystitis
- Pyelonephritis

Late Pregnancy
- Preterm labor
- Abruptio placentae
- Chorioamnionitis
- Degeneration of fibroid
- Rupture uterus

Others
- Acute appendicitis
- Acute cholecystitis
- Acute pancreatitis
- Acute peritonitis

Q4. How will you diagnose a case of fibroid during pregnancy?

On the bases of history:
- Prepregnancy pelvic scan for documentation of presence, size and site of fibroid (already diagnosed).

- First trimester: History of (H/o) bleeding per vaginum (BPV), threatened abortion, pelvic sonography for documentation of fibroid.
- Second and third trimester: H/o preterm labor, BPV, LPV, acute pain abdomen, fever, vomiting, and malpresentations.
- Obstetric history: Previous H/o missed abortions, recurrent pregnancy loss (RPL), threatened abortion, malpresentations and antepartum hemorrhage.
- In the intrapartum period—H/o prolonged labor or obstructed labor, cesarean section for fibroid uterus.
- In the postpartum period—H/o retained placenta, postpartum hemorrhage and puerperal sepsis.

On Examination

It is relatively difficult to make a diagnosis of fibroid clinically as the pregnancy progresses because of the growing size of the uterus and the change in shape of the fibroid (intramural).
- Size of uterus more than the period of gestation.
- Asymmetrically enlarged gravid uterus (early gestation).
- Larger fibroids >5 cm can be identified as a mass per abdomen along with the gravid uterus. Tenderness over the mass with associated features of vomiting and fever is suggestive of red degeneration in the fibroid.
- Subserosal and pedunculated fibroids can present as adnexal mass.
- Cervical fibroid can be identified as polyp on per-speculum examination.

Radiological Findings

Ultrasonography: The first trimester anomaly scan can be the best time to look for any fibroids, if a fibroid is seen the followings points related to the fibroid should be noted:
- Number
- Position (anterior, posterior, corporeal or cervical)
- Type, size and relation of the fibroid to placenta and the uterine cavity (Fig. 1).

Fibroids appear as:
- Well-defined mass.
- Echogenicity similar to the myometrium (isoechoic).
- A circumferential vascularity on color Doppler.
- Degeneration may have a complex appearance, with areas of cystic change and absence of color flow on Doppler.[2]
- A sequential scan should also be done at the beginning of third trimester to note the increase in size of fibroid and for fetal biometry to rule out any fetal growth restriction[3] (Fig. 1).
- A sonographic evaluation should be done in late third trimester to assess the feasibility of vaginal delivery.

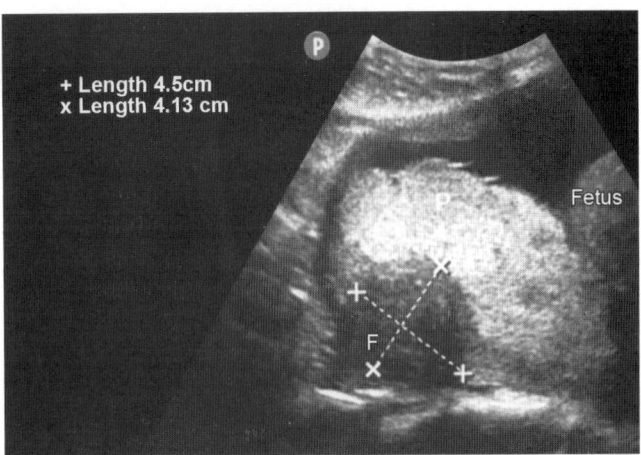

Fig. 1: Ultrasonography of a 27 years lady diagnosed with fibroid uterus who had presented with pain abdomen at 28 weeks of gestation. The fibroid is present in the retroplacental space

- Multiple fibroids may pose difficulty during a cesarean delivery therefore mapping of uterus (sonographically) by the surgeon is the best way to find the appropriate site for incision.

MRI: Non-degenerating fibroids appear as well-defined masses of low-signal intensity as compared to the myometrium on T2W images and isointense to the myometrium on T1W images.
- Fibroids undergoing degeneration have heterogeneous appearance, with minimal or irregular enhancement.
- The fibroid may have a peripheral rim of low signal on T2W images and high signal on T1W images due to the peripheral obstructed veins.
- Areas of hemorrhage within the fibroid produce varying signal, depending on the age of the blood products. Recent hemorrhage shows high signal on both T1W and T2W images; there will be no enhancement as the blood supply is obstructed.
- MRI mapping of fibroid is indicated in case multiple fibroids are diagnosed on ultrasonography or a single large fibroid is present in the lower part of the uterus, in such cases it may be helpful in deciding the mode of delivery[4] (Fig. 2).

Q5. What are the effects of pregnancy on fibroid?

1. **Size:** 60–80 % of the fibroids do not show any significant change in size or volume. The remaining 20–40% may increase in volume by 12% ± 6%.
   - This growth occurs mainly in the initial 10 weeks of the pregnancy.
   - There is very little growth in the second and third trimester.

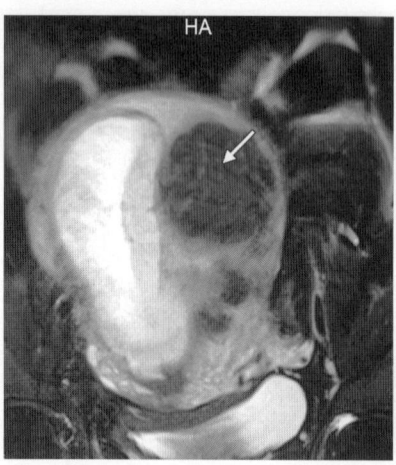
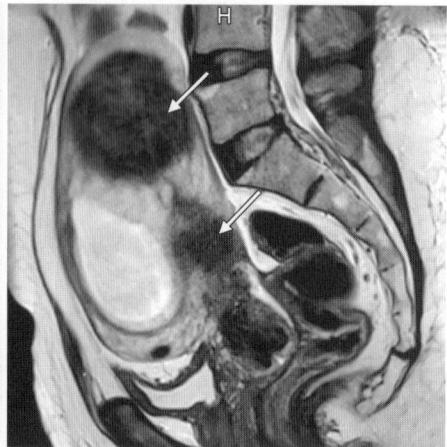

Fig. 2: MRI films of a 27 years old lady diagnosed with fibroid uterus who had presented with pain abdomen at 28 weeks of gestation. The fibroid is present in the retroplacental space depicted by arrows in the coronal and sagittal views

- Smaller and larger fibroids (≥6 cm) have different pattern of growth, smaller fibroids tend to grow faster as compared to larger fibroids which remain unchanged or may decrease in size because of degenerative changes.
- During puerperium 7.8% of the fibroids will decrease in size by 10%.[5]

2. **Shape:** During the course of pregnancy fibroids become softened and more flattened.
   - The shape may become discoid.
3. **Degenerative changes:** Red degeneration (5–15% of all fibroids in pregnancy) is the commonest change during pregnancy.
4. **Symptoms:** Pain in abdomen is the commonest symptom followed by fever.
5. Pedunculated fibroids may undergo torsion, posterior wall fibroid can cause uterine impaction.
6. Rarely fibroids may get infected during pregnancy and puerperium.[5]

Q6. What are the causes of red degeneration and associated pain during pregnancy?

Red degeneration has been seen with fibroids >5 cm in size and is commonly seen in the second and third trimester of pregnancy, pain of varying intensity is associated with 70% of the fibroids undergoing red degeneration. Three theories have been postulated which explain the cause of red degeneration and associated pain:
- Rapidly growing fibroid outgrows its blood supply leading to tissue anoxia, necrosis and infarction.
- Even in the absence of growth of fibroid the enlarging uterus causes kinking of the vessels supplying blood to the fibroid thus leading to ischemia and necrosis.
- The cellular damage caused by the ischemia releases prostaglandins (PG) which causes pain of varying intensity and is effectively relieved on taking PG synthetase inhibitors.[6]

Q7. How will you manage the above mentioned case of red degeneration?

All cases of red degeneration should be managed conservatively.
- Admit the patient
- Bed rest
- Maintain hydration
- Analgesia
  - PG synthetase inhibitors (Tablet ibuprofen 200-400 mg 4-6 hourly). PG synthetase inhibitors should be used with caution especially for >48 hours during the third trimester as it has been associated with premature closure of the fetal ductus arteriosus, pulmonary hypertension, necrotizing enterocolitis, intracranial hemorrhage and oligohydramnios.
  - Narcotic analgesia (tablet tramadol 50-100 mg orally every 4-6 hours)
  - Epidural analgesia.
  - Surgical management in the form of myomectomy can be considered in case of intractable pain because of degenerating fibroid.
- Antenatal steroids: Injection dexamethasone 6 mg intramuscular 12 hourly four doses.
- Ultrasonography with Doppler: Size, location and relation of fibroid with the placenta. Ascertain fetal well-being (biometry, rule out gross congenital abnormalities and malpresentations).

The pain because of red degeneration usually subsides in the next 2-3 days and patient can be discharged. She should be advised to follow up regularly in the antenatal clinic. Warning signs such as pain in abdomen, fever, BPV and LPV should be explained and a provisional plan for the mode of delivery should be made and discussed with the couple before discharging.

Q8. What are the effects of fibroid on pregnancy?

Nearly 10–30% of the women with fibroid during pregnancy develop complications.[6]

Proposed mechanisms by which fibroids cause adverse pregnancy outcome are:
- Decreased uterine distensibility
- Mechanical obstruction
- Increased uterine irritability
- Poor placentation[6]

Early Pregnancy[7,8]

1. **Abortion:** The risk of spontaneous abortion is higher in pregnancy associated with fibroid as compared to a normal gravid uterus (14 vs 7.6%). The risk increases further when associated with multiple fibroids as compared to single fibroid (23 vs 8%). Intramural and submucosal fibroids and fibroids located in the uterine corpus increase the risk of spontaneous abortion.
2. **Bleeding in early pregnancy:** The closer the placentation to the fibroid more is the chance of bleeding **late pregnancy.**[7,8]

Late Pregnancy

1. **Preterm labor**
2. **Abruptio placentae:** The risk increases to three fold multiple fibroids, retroplacental clots and fibroid volume > 200 cc are independent risk factors.
3. **Placenta previa:** The risk increases to two-fold.
4. **Fetal growth restriction and fetal anomalies:** Dolichocephaly, torticollis and limb reduction defects are associated with large submucosal fibroids.

Intrapartum Complications

Large fibroids, multiple fibroids, fibroids in the lower segments and submucosal fibroids are independent risk factors for malpresentations and cesarean section.

1. Malpresentations
2. Labor dystocia
3. Cesarean section
4. Postpartum hemorrhage
5. Retained placenta

Puerperium

Red degeneration, infection of fibroid, uterine inversion and sub-involution.

Q9. Indications of cesarean section in fibroid with pregnancy?

Cervical fibroid, broad ligament fibroid, malpresentations and any other obstetric indication.

Q10. Indications for antepartum myomectomy?

Persistent severe pain abdomen failing medical management, torsion of subserosal or pedunculated fibroid. Myomectomy should preferably be done during the first and second trimester.[9]

Q11. What are the methods for decreasing blood loss while performing cesarean section in a gravid uterus with fibroid?

When cesarean section is indicated in a gravid uterus with fibroid:
- It should be planned electively with adequate arrangement of blood and blood product.
- Preferably it should be performed by a senior obstetrician.
- Avoid giving incision over the fibroid or its capsule to deliver the baby.
- If the fibroid is located in the lower uterine segment a classical section may be preferred.
- Uterine artery ligation and bilateral uterine artery embolization can be performed after delivery of the baby.
- In case the above measures do not reduce the blood loss one may proceed ahead with cesarean hysterectomy.[10]

OVARIAN TUMOR IN PREGNANCY

CASE SCENARIO

G2P1L1 with nine months amenorrhea with ovarian tumor.
A 26 years old, Mrs F, wife of Mr M, resident of Karol Bagh, a homemaker, was a referred case to the antenatal clinic of our hospital with an USG report of ovarian mass.
Her LMP was 1/4/17 making her period of gestation (POG) as 19 weeks and 2 days on 14/8/2017.

History of Presenting Complaint

Patient was referred from a primary health center with an ultrasonography report which showed a mass arising from one of the ovaries and a pregnancy of 5 months. She complained of severe pain in the lower abdomen and difficulty in passing urine × 5 days. There is no history of burning micturition or blood in urine. There was no episode of bleeding or leaking per vaginam. There is no history of backache, radiation of the pain, any aggravating or relieving factors. No history of any abnormal bowel symptoms.

In her prior USGs, no evidence of any abnormality was there.

Course in the Hospital

She was admitted to the obstetric ward after performing abdominal examination and her bladder was catheterized and internal examination was done. Ultrasonography with color Doppler was done. Blood investigations were sent. She was prepared for laparotomy in view of symptomatic ovarian tumor.

Diagnosis on History

G2P1 L1 with 19 weeks and 2 days POG with ovarian tumor with retention of urine.

Abdominal Examination

Inspection

There is fullness in the lower abdomen. All quadrants moving with respiration—linea nigra and striae gravidarum present, no other scar marks are seen. Umbilicus is central and inverted—all hernial sites are free.

Palpation (done after catheterization of bladder)

Fundal height—20 weeks. A mass 8 × 8 cm felt separately from the uterus occupying the right iliac fossa.
- The mass is tender on touch, no guarding, no rigidity.
- Cystic in consistency with well-defined margins and smooth surface.
- Side to side mobility is restricted, lower limit of the mass could not be reached.
- There is no fluid thrill, no shifting dullness.
- No other organomegaly noted.

Auscultation

Normal bowel sounds heard.

Perineal Examination

External genitalia normal, no bleeding and no leaking observed.

Per Speculum Examination

Os closed, cervix long, no discharge, bleeding or leaking observed.

Per Vaginal Examination

- External os closed, cervix soft, long and posterior.
- Cervical motion tenderness present.
- A mass felt right anterior to the gravid uterus measuring 10 × 8 cm, cystic in consistency, with smooth surface and well-defined margins and tender on touch.
- Per rectal examination—gravid uterus felt no fullness or nodularity in POD and rectal mucosa is free.

Diagnosis After Examination

G2 P1 L1 with 19 weeks plus 2 days POG with ovarian tumor and acute urinary retention.

Q1. What is the incidence of ovarian tumors in pregnancy?

- The incidence of ovarian tumor varies from 1 in 10,000–25,000 pregnancies.
- About 1 in 600 pregnancies are complicated by adnexal mass which are discovered as incidental findings on routine obstetric ultrasonography.
- Ovarian malignancy is estimated to occur in approximately 2–3% of the masses identified during pregnancy.[11]

Q2. What is the risk of ovarian torsion in pregnancy and what are the features in above mentioned patient in favor of diagnosis of ovarian torsion?

- Risk of ovarian torsion increases 5 times in pregnancy though it is not that common in second trimester.
- Complain of lower abdomen pain, tenderness and cervical motion tenderness can be suggestive of ovarian torsion.

Q3. What is the differential diagnosis of ovarian mass in pregnancy?

Differential diagnosis of ovarian mass in pregnancy (in order of occurrence):
1. Functional ovarian cysts—follicular, corpus luteum, and theca-lutein cysts.
2. Benign cystic teratomas, serous cystadenomas, para-ovarian cysts, mucinous cystadenomas, endometriomas.
3. Malignant tumors—non-epithelial tumors are the commonest followed by low malignant potential tumor and epithelial ovarian tumor.[11]

Q4. What are the other investigations required in the above mentioned case scenario?

The main aim of investigation is to know the nature of the ovarian mass, whether benign or malignant, uncomplicated or complicated along with preanesthetic workup in case surgical management is planned.

Imaging[11-13]

- **Ultrasound examination** is safe and reliable modality, it should determine the origin of the mass, as well as its location, size, internal structure (existing vegetation or septa) and should classify it into benign or malignant according to the morphological index (unilocular, unilocular-solid, multilocular, multilocular-solid, or solid) (Fig. 3).

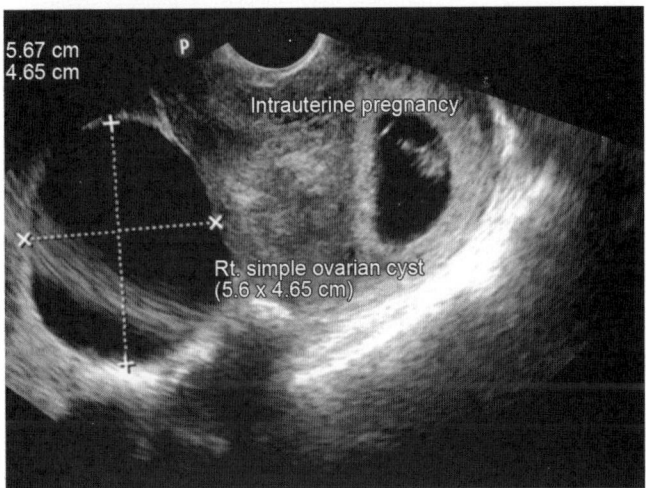

Fig. 3: A 23 years old lady presented to antenatal clinic at 2 months of gestation, on examination a right adnexal mass was found, an ultrasonography done shows a simple right ovarian cyst with 8 weeks intrauterine pregnancy

- **A color Doppler** imaging should also be performed to obtain a vascular map of the ovarian mass and to rule out ovarian torsion.
- **Pelvic MRI** with gadolinium injection should be avoided during the first trimester. This second line examination should only be indicated during pregnancy to remove any doubt or to provide additional information if the ultrasound examination is not sufficient for the assessment of ovarian cancer.
- Pelvic CT scanning is not indicated during pregnancy.
- Measurement of tumor markers like CA125, β-hCG and α fetoprotein may give false high results in pregnancy and are not recommended to formulate a diagnosis but can help in follow up after pregnancy.

Q5. In the above mentioned case ultrasonography shows a dermoid cyst (7 × 6 cm) arising from the right ovary, how will you manage this case?

Before the management of any ovarian mass in pregnancy the following questions need to be answered:

- What is the nature of the mass?
- What is the likelihood that it is malignant?
- Is there a possibility that the mass may regress?
- Will the mass undergo torsion, possible rupture, or will it cause obstruction during delivery (impaction)?

This case is a large dermoid cyst which is a benign tumor of the ovary diagnosed at 19 weeks of gestation. It is causing urinary retention and has high chances of undergoing torsion, possible rupture, and may likely cause obstruction of labor if left untreated. Hence the plan of management is ovarian cystectomy (laparotomy or laparoscopy).

Q6. What are the indications for surgical management of ovarian tumor?

- Persistent (>16 weeks) or larger ovarian mass (>5 cms).
- Tumors high risk for an acute abdomen, ovarian torsion, or rupture.
- Tumors causing obstructive symptoms.
- Suspected ovarian malignancy.
- During labor tumors impacted in the pelvis below the presenting part should undergo cesarean section followed by removal of the mass in same sitting.
- During labor large ovarian tumor above the presenting part should be removed surgically in the postpartum period.

Q7. What are the indications for conservative management of ovarian tumor in pregnancy?

Mass that is simple in nature by ultrasonography (USG), less than 5 cm in diameter, and diagnosed before 16 weeks.

Q8. What are the precautions to be taken during surgery for ovarian tumor in pregnancy?

- Adequate maternal monitoring before, during and after the surgery is mandatory to avoid hypoxia, hypotension and hypoglycemia.
- A left lateral tilt should be given to avoid caval compression.
- Prophylactic tocolysis has no role during surgery and should only be considered when a diagnosis of preterm has been established.
- Ovarian masses, especially suspicious ones, must be removed intact when possible. Spillage or rupture of

a malignant ovarian cyst is associated with decreased survival.
- Lower extremity sequential compression devices should be used during intraoperative and postoperative period.
- A midline or vertical incision should be given to enter the abdomen.
- During exploration the uterus should not be manipulated, i.e. *Hands Off the uterus approach.*[14]

Q9. What are the precautions during laparoscopy?

It is safe to perform laparoscopy between 16–20 weeks of pregnancy as most of the benign masses resolve by this time, the size of uterus is optimal for better visualization of the ovarian mass and the risk of preterm delivery is the least.
- Patient should be put in a Trendelenburg position slowly with a slight left lateral tilt, this helps in avoiding hypotension, hypoxemia and hypovolemic.
- The preferred method for primary trocar insertion should be the open laparoscopy and supraumbilical port placement to limit the possibility of uterine perforation by insertion of a Veress needle.
- Pneumoperitoneum by CO_2 is safe for the fetus.
- The maximum pressure of 10–13 mm Hg, an experienced surgeon and limited operation time (25–90 minutes) is considered.

A guideline from the Society of American Gastrointestinal and Endoscopic Surgeons, published in 2011, makes the following recommendation: "Laparoscopy is safe and effective treatment in gravid patients with symptomatic ovarian cystic masses. Observation is acceptable for all other cystic lesions provided USG is not concerning for malignancy and tumor markers are normal. Initial observation is warranted for more cystic lesions less than 6 cm in size."[15]

Q10. How will you manage a malignant ovarian tumor diagnosed during pregnancy?

The following issues should be considered before deciding on the definitive management of ovarian cancers in pregnancy (Table 1):
- High suspicion of malignant ovarian tumor
- Type and stage of ovarian malignancy
- Period of gestation
- Fetal effect of therapy
- Timing of delivery
- Route of delivery
- Completion of therapy after delivery.

Table 1: Management of ovarian cancer in pregnancy[16,17]

Type of cancer	Treatment
Low malignant potential tumor	Treated conservatively by U/L adnexectomy and peritoneal cytology and exploration with biopsies. This diagnosis should never lead to the end of the pregnancy.
Non-epithelial ovarian malignancies	Unilateral adnexectomy with peritoneal cytology and exploration with biopsies (only one ovary is involved) followed by adjuvant chemotherapy. Bilateral adnexectomy with peritoneal cytology and exploration with biopsies with progesterone support if operated before 12 weeks followed by adjuvant chemotherapy.
Epithelial ovarian tumor	**Stage I disease unilateral (IA)/bilateral (IB)**—adnexectomy + peritoneal cytology + complete abdominopelvic exploration. Adjuvant chemotherapy in this stage depends upon the histological type and extent of the tumor and is indicated as in non-pregnant women **Advanced stages (II-IV):** 1. <24 weeks—termination of pregnancy followed by staging laparotomy and adjuvant chemotherapy. 2. Operable disease **beyond 32 weeks** a cesarean section should be performed along with staging laparotomy/complete surgery for the ovarian malignancy. 3. 24–32 weeks the aim is to avoid prematurity and fetal toxicity without deferring the mother's treatment. Biopsy should be ordered in such cases and can be performed by ultrasonography/laparoscopy/minilaparotomy. For operable disease surgery (adnexectomy + exploration) should be performed followed by chemotherapy, whereas in inoperable cases neo-adjuvant therapy should be considered followed by surgery. The time gap between last chemotherapy session and delivery should be at least 3 weeks.

CERVICAL LESIONS (PREMALIGNANT AND MALIGNANT) IN PREGNANCY

CASE SCENARIO

Case 1: G2P1L1 with nine months amenorrhea came to ANC OPD with report of abnormal pap smear (LSIL) on routine screening.

Case 2: G4P3l3 with nine months amenorrhea with painless bleeding per vaginum on and off for 8 months.

On local examination an ulcerative lesion measuring 1 cm at 7 o'clock position with irregular margins is identified. On Per vaginum examination the lesion is hard in consistency and bleeds on touch. Assessment of parametrium could not be made easily because of the gravid uterus.

Q1. What is the incidence of cervical lesions in pregnancy?

The incidence of carcinoma cervix is 0.1 to 12 per 10,000 pregnancies and for premalignant lesions the incidence varies from 1.30 to 2.7 per 1000 pregnancies.[18]

Q2. What are the methods used for screening cervical cancer in pregnancy?

All pregnant women should undergo screening for cervical cancer during their antenatal examination if not screened previously.

- The preferred methods are: **Pap smear, VIA (visual inspection by acetic acid), LBC (liquid based cytology) and colposcopy.**
- The reliability of Pap smear during pregnancy is same as that in non-pregnant state.
- There are certain pregnancy related changes in the cervix which can mimic malignancy or a high grade lesion during examination (local/colposcopy) and cytology.
- During pregnancy under the influence of hormones the squamocolumnar junction is pushed onto the ectocervix and the columnar cells are thus exposed to the acidic pH of the vagina leading to metaplasia which may then mimic dysplastic changes. Increased vascularity, hypertrophy and hyperplasia of the endocervical glands could mimic cervical intraepithelial neoplasia (CIN).
- Other physiological cellular changes, such as degenerated decidual cells (Arias–Stella phenomena) and trophoblastic cells may mimic a high grade lesion. Thus, increasing the false-positive results if the cytopathologist is unaware of the pregnant state.

Endocervical curettage is contraindicated during pregnancy as it can have adverse obstetric outcome. However, brush cytology can be safely done during pregnancy.

Q3. What are the factors which need to be taken into consideration before management is started?

Gestational age, histological subtype, stage, nodal status, obstetrical complications and also patients' wishes concerning continuation *versus* termination of pregnancy.

Q4. How will you manage Case 1—abnormal Pap smear (premalignant disease)?

Premalignant lesions of cervix are managed conservatively during pregnancy unless a progression is suspected. A close follow-up with Pap smear and colposcopy is to be done every 12 weeks. In case of any progression a colposcopy guided biopsy is performed.

Q5. What is the course of premalignant disease during pregnancy?

Table 2: Course of premalignant lesions of cervix during pregnancy[19]

Type of lesion	Regression	Persistence	Progression
HSIL	50%	40.3%	9.7% (progression to microinvasive)
LSIL	48.8%	29.2%	22% (progression to HSIL)

Q6. What are the indications of conisation during pregnancy and risks associated with the procedure?

Indications

- Suspicion of invasive cancer which cannot be ruled out on colposcopic biopsy.
- Microinvasive carcinoma.

Risks

Spontaneous abortion (25%), hemorrhage (5–15%), abortion, preterm labor and infection.

Conisation when indicated should be done between 14–20 weeks of gestation. Cone biopsy can be done by using any of the following methods: LLETZ (large loop excision of the transformation zone), laser and cold knife conisation. A shallow cone is preferred over a deeper one to prevent adverse pregnancy outcome.

Q7. How will you proceed with the management case 2?

Case 2 is an early stage carcinoma cervix most probably **clinical stage IB1**. After histological confirmation by taking a biopsy a MRI should be ordered to determine the tumor size, stromal invasion, amount of healthy stroma, vaginal and parametrial invasion, and lymph node infiltration. An early stage disease (Stage IB1) at 9 months amenorrhea should be delivered by cesarean section along with modified radical hysterectomy and pelvic lymphadenectomy.

Q8. How will you manage late stage disease (Ib2, IIb, IIIb)?

At Early Gestation

- *Option A:* Radical hysterectomy with pelvic lymphadenectomy with fetus in situ.
- *Option B:* External beam radiotherapy with fetus in situ followed by termination of pregnancy and intracavitary brachytherapy.[20]

Q9. What is the mode of delivery in women with cervical lesion?

All premalignant lesions and very early stage disease (Stage IA with negative cone margins) can undergo vaginal delivery. For lesions > stage IA should be delivered by cesarean section for the fear of hemorrhage and dissemination of malignant cells during vaginal delivery.[20]

PROLAPSE WITH PREGNANCY

Q1. What are the effects of pregnancy on prolapse?

- The cervix becomes hypertrophied and edematous.
- The degree of uterocervical descent increase with the progression of pregnancy, rectocele and cystocele become more evident and stress urinary incontinence aggravates.
- Vaginal discharge becomes copious, decubitus ulcer may develop if the cervix remains outside.
- Incarceration of uterus may occur in severe degree of prolapse.

Q2. What are the effects of prolapse on pregnancy?

- Antepartum period: Abortion, uterine incarceration, premature rupture of membranes, chorioamnionitis.
- Intrapartum period: Cervical dystocia, prolonged labor rupture of uterus and operative intervention.
- Postpartum period: Subinvolution and puerperal sepsis.

Q3. How will you manage a case of third degree prolapse during pregnancy?

- The aim of management is to prevent edema and infection of the prolapsed part by keeping it inside the introitus. During early pregnancy this can be achieved by inserting a ring pessary or by inserting a tampon soaked in acriflavine and glycerin.
- During the third trimester if the cervix is lying outside the introitus tamponing should be done with foot end elevation of the bed. During labor vaginal packing with glycerin and acriflavine should continue, prophylactic antibiotics to continue, careful watch for descent of head and cervical dilation to be made. In case of delay in dilation and descent of head cesarean section has to done.

REFERENCES

1. Klatsky PC, Tran ND, Caughey AB, et al. Fibroids and reproductive outcomes: a systematic literature review from conception to delivery. Am J Obstet Gynecol. 2008;198:357-66.
2. Roy C, Bierry G, El Ghali S, et al. Acute torsion of uterine leiomyoma: CT features. Abdom Imaging. 2005;30:120-3.
3. Eze CU, Odumera EA, Ochie K, et al. Sonographic assessment of pregnancy co-existing with uterine leiomyoma in Owerri, Nigeria. Afr Health Sci. 2013;13(2):453-60.
4. Ueda H, Togashi K, Konishi I, et al. Unusual appearances of uterine leiomyomas: MR imaging findings and their histopathologic backgrounds. Radiographics. 1999;19:S131-45.
5. Lee HJ, Norwitz ER, Shaw J. Contemporary management of fibroids in pregnancy. Rev Obstet Gynecol. 2010;3(1):20-7.
6. Katz VL, Dotters DJ, Droegemueller W. Complications of uterine leiomyomas in pregnancy. Obstet Gynecol. 1989;73:593-6.
7. Parker WH. Etiology, symptomatology, and diagnosis of uterine myomas. Fertil Steril. 2007;87:725-36.
8. Benson CB, Chow JS, Chang-lee W, et al. Outcome of pregnancies in women with uterine leiomyomas identified by sonography in the first trimester. J Clin Ultrasound. 2001;29:261-4.
9. Lolis DE, Kalantaridon SN, Makrydimas G, et al. Successful myomectomy during pregnancy. Hum Reprod. 2003;18(8):1699-702.
10. Walker WJ, McDowell SJ. Pregnancy after uterine artery embolization for leiomyomata: a series of 56 completed pregnancies. Am J Obstet Gynecol. 2006;195:1266-71.
11. Amant F, Brepoels L, Halaska MJ, et al. Gynaecologic cancer complicating pregnancy: an overview. Best Pract Res Clin Obstet Gynaecol. 2010;24:61-79.
12. Amant F, Halaska MJ, Fumagalli M, et al. Gynecologic cancers in pregnancy: guidelines of a second international consensus meeting. Int J Gynecol Cancer. 2014;24:394-403.
13. Han SN, Verheecke M, Vandenbroucke T, et al. Management of gynaecological cancers during pregnancy. Curr Oncol Rep. 2014;16:415.
14. Nick AM, Schmeler K. Adnexal masses in pregnancy. Perinatology. 2010;2:13-21.
15. Pearl J, Price R, Richardson W, et al. Society of American Gastrointestinal Endoscopic Surgeons. Surg Endosc. 2011;25(11):3479-92.
16. Mancari R, Tomasi-Cont N, Sarno MA, et al. Treatment options for pregnant women with ovarian tumors. Int J Gynecol Cancer. 2014;24:967-72.
17. Di Saia PJ, Creasman WT. Clinical Gynaecologic Oncology; 8th edition; Elseviers; 2012.
18. H Al-Halal, et al. Incidence and Obstetrical Outcomes of Cervical Intraepithelial Neoplasia and Cervical Cancer in Pregnancy: A Population-Based Study on 8.8 Million Births. Arch Gynecol Obstet 2012;287(2):245-250.
19. Robova H, Rob L, Pluta M, et al. Squamous intraepithelial lesion-microinvasive carcinoma of the cervix during pregnancy. Eur J Gynaecol Oncol. 2005;26(6):611-4.
20. Hunter MI, Tewari K, Monk BJ. Cervical neoplasia in pregnancy. Part 2: current treatment of invasive disease. Am J Obstet Gynecol. 2008;199(1):10-8.

29 CHAPTER

Miscellaneous

Poonam Kashyap, Nuzhat Zaman

ULTRASOUND IN OBSTETRICS

CASE SCENARIO

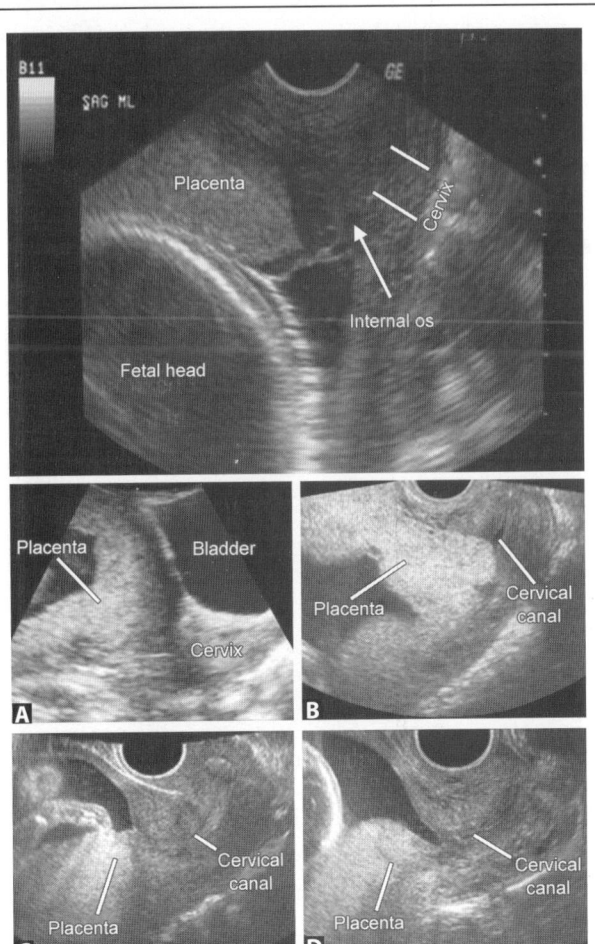

Fig. 1: Placenta previa

Q1. What is the likely diagnosis?

This ultrasonograms are showing placenta previa of different grade.[1,2]

Q2. What are the clinical implications of this condition?

The patient may present with vaginal bleeding after the 20th week of gestation.

- Usually the bleeding is painless, but it can be associated with uterine contractions and abdominal pain.
- Bleeding may range in severity from light to severe.

CASE SCENARIO

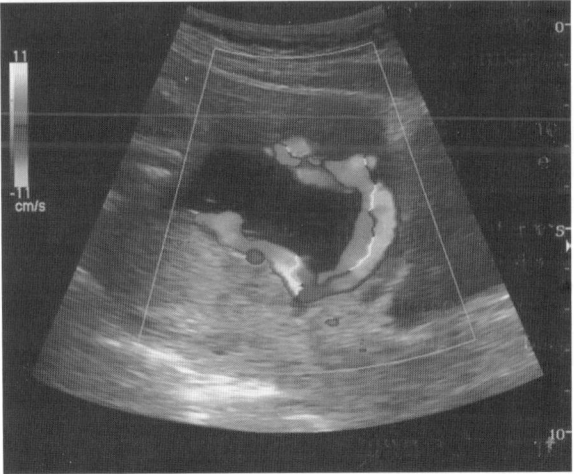

Fig. 2: Vasa previa (For color version, see plate 1)

Q3. What does this ultrasound image depict?

This image shows vasa previa with posterior placenta and umbilical cord abutting the cervical os. There is vilamentous insertion of cord.

Q4. What is the clinical presentation of the patient?

Unfortunately, in some cases there are no warning signs of vasa previa, which generally cannot be diagnosed until labor, when the fetus is already at risk, or until after a stillbirth. There may be sudden onset of painless vaginal bleeding, especially in their second and third trimesters. A Telltale Clue is the color of the blood. Bright red blood is well oxygenated, and this means it comes from the mother, not the baby. The baby's blood is a darker red color due to the naturally lower oxygen levels of a fetus.[3]

Q5. Which test can be performed to diagnose this condition?

Fetal hemoglobin can be diagnosed by alkali denaturation testin vaginal blood, as fetal hemoglobin is resistant to denaturation in presence of 1% NaOH.

CASE SCENARIO

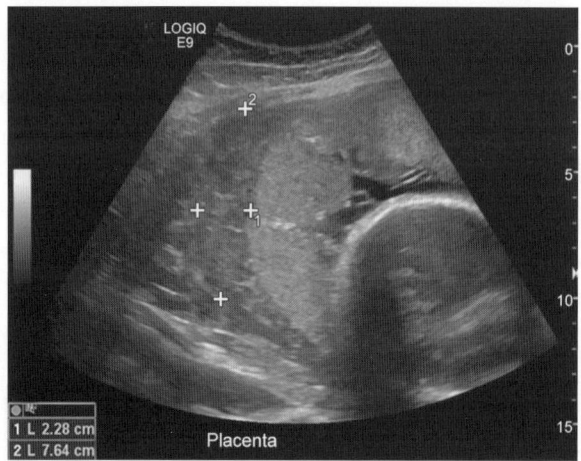

Fig. 3: Retroplacental hematoma

Q1. What are the findings in this ultrasonogram?

This image is showing a retroplacental hematoma and intraplacental anechoic areas:
- Separation and rounding of the placental edge
- Thickening of the placenta: often to over 5.5 cm
- Thickening of the retroplacental myometrium: usually should be 1–2 mm unless there is a focal myometrial contraction
- Disruption in retroplacental circulation.[4]

Q2. What are the causes of this condition?

Maternal trauma:
- Age 35 years or older
- Cigarette smoking
- Cocaine use
- Thrombophilia
- Previous placental abruption
- Chorioamnionitis
- Prolonged rupture of membranes
- Preeclampsia and maternal hypertension: often seen in as many as 50% of cases
- Short umbilical cord
- Increased parity.

CASE SCENARIO

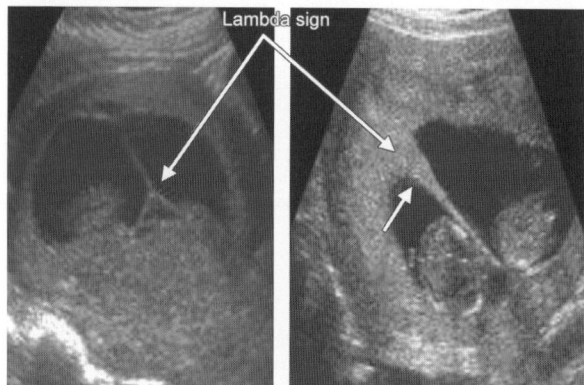

Fig. 4: Lambda sign in dichorionic in diamniotic pregnancy

Q1. What is this Lambda sign?

The twin peak sign [also known as the lambda (λ) sign] is a triangular appearance of the chorion insinuating between the layers of the inter twin membrane and strongly suggests a dichorionic twin pregnancy. It is best seen in the first trimester (between 10–14 weeks).[5]

CASE SCENARIO

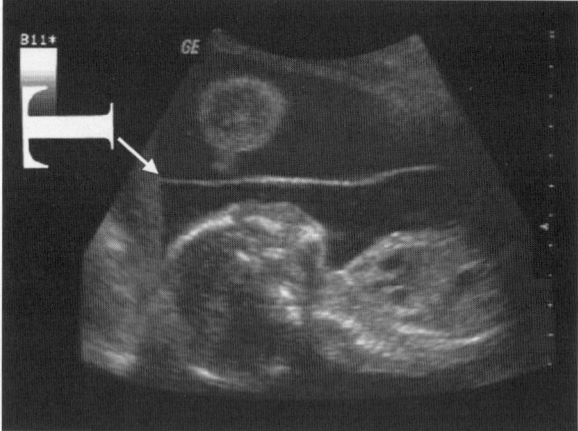

Fig. 5: "T-sign" in monochorionic diamniotic pregnancy

Q1. What is this T-sign and its significance?

The "T-sign" is really the absence of a twin-peak sign (or lambda sign) and is used in ultrasound assessment of a mulifetal pregnancy.

It refers to the lack of chorion extending between the layers of the intertwin membrane, denoting a monochorionic pregnancy. The intertwin membrane comes to an abrupt halt at the edge in a T configuration.[6]

CASE SCENARIO

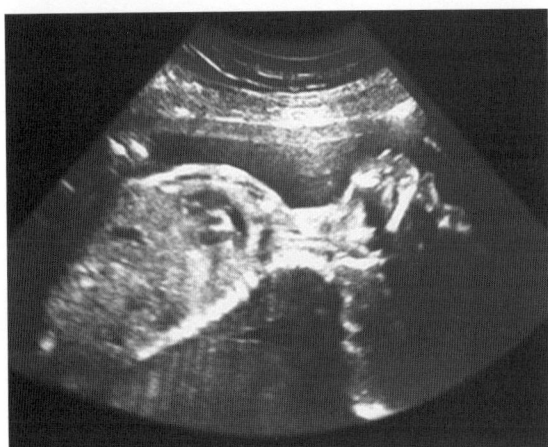

Fig. 6: Hyperextended fetal head

Q1. What is the clinical importance of hyperextended head of fetus?

If the fetal head is the presenting part, hyperextension leads to face presentation. If the fetus is in breech presentation, this fetus is called star gazing fetus. During labor, there may be injury to the cervical spine of the fetus especially in breech vaginal delivery.[5,6]

Q2. What are the conditions leading to hyperextension of fetal head?

There may be fetal anomalies, such as structural abnormalities, conjoint twins, fetal neck masses, iniencephaly, nuchal cord, polyhydramnios. Uterine anomalies and fibroid uterus can also lead to hyperextension of fetal head.[6]

DRUGS USED IN OBSTETRICS

CASE SCENARIO

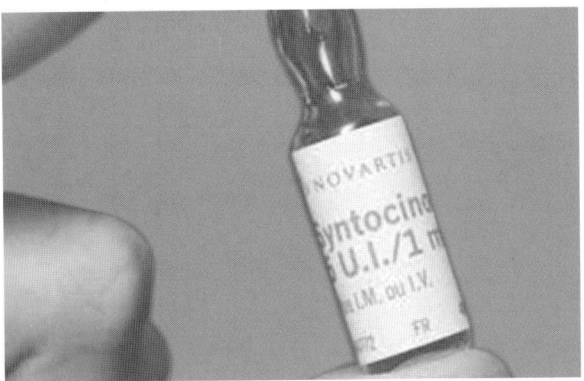

Fig. 7: Syntocinon drug

Q1. What are the uses of this drug?

The drug is used in following conditions:

Early Pregnancy
- To accelerate abortion
- For induction of abortion
- In molar pregnancy at the time of evacuatiom.

Late Pregnancy
- To induce labor
- For cervical ripening.

Labor
- Augmentation of labor
- Uterine inertia
- Active management of 3rd stage of labor.

Puerpurium
- Control of post partum hemorrhage.

Q2. What is active management of 3rd stage of labor?

Active management of the third stage of labor as a prophylactic intervention is composed of a package of three components or steps: (1) Administration of a uterotonic, preferably oxytocin, immediately after birth of the baby; (2) controlled cord traction (CCT) to deliver the placenta; and (3) massage of the uterine fundus after the placenta is delivered. Massage of fundus is not recommended if prophylactic oxytocin has been given.[7]

CASE SCENARIO

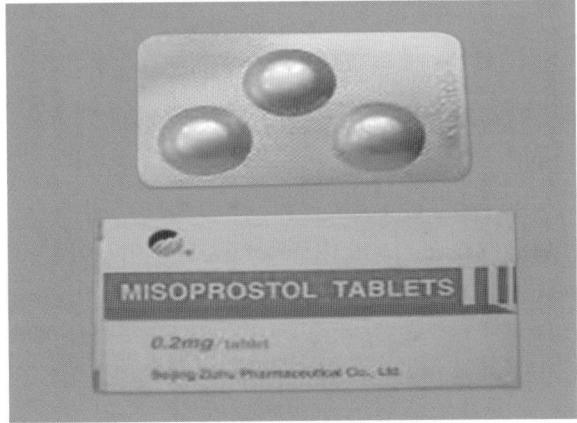

Fig. 8: Misoprostol tablets

Q1. What are the indications of use of this drug.

Indications
- Medical abortion: Misoprostol along with mifepristone used within 63 days.

- Used for induction of abortion in case of miscarriage and for completion of abortions up to 12 weeks of gestation.
- Effective as cervical ripening agent prior 1st trimester surgical abortion
- Used for induction in 2nd trimester for termination of pregnancy and induction of labor in case of intrauterine fetal death.
- Used for cervical ripening and induction of labor for a viable fetus, 25 microgram of vaginal misoprostol every 4 to 6 hours up to a maximum of six doses can be given.[8]
- Also used for prevention of PPH in dose of 800 microgram per rectally and for treatment of PPH, 1000 microgram rectally.

Q2. What are the contraindications of use?

It should not be used in patients with allergy to misoprostol, during pregnancy and lactation.

CASE SCENARIO

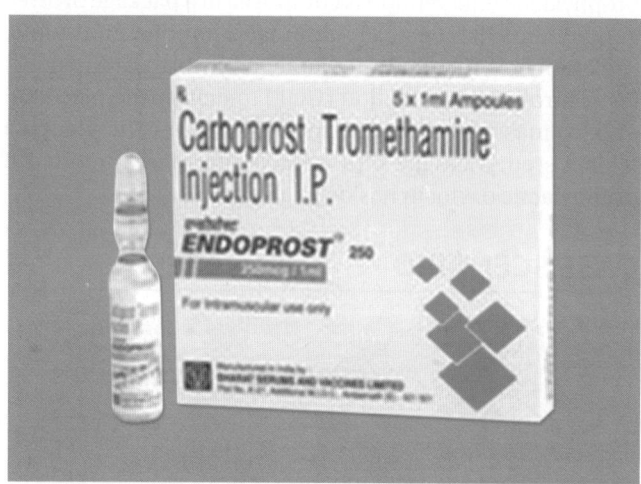

Fig. 9: Carboprost tromethamine injection

Q1. What are the indications of use?

Used for treatment of postpartum hemorrhage caused by uterine atony and not controlled by other medical methods.

Q2. What are the contraindications?

Hypersensitivity to prostaglandins and caution should be given in asthmatic patients.

Note: Drugs used in obstetrics are many but few more, i.e. ergometrin, magnesium sulfate, methyl dopa, labetalol, dexamethasone, betamethasone, nifedipine, atosiban, isoxsuprine and many others too can be kept for spotting and asked.

CARDIOTOCOGRAPHY

CASE SCENARIO

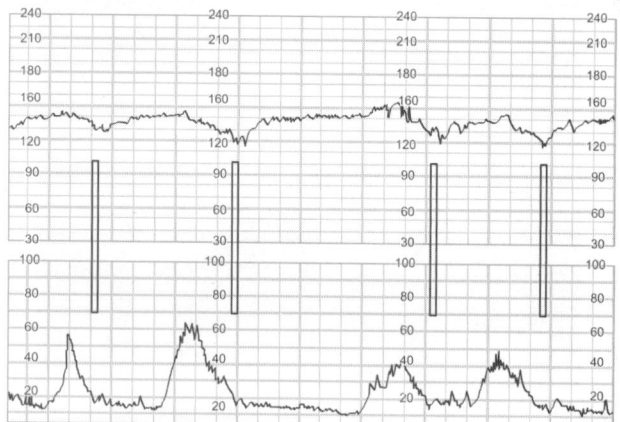

Fig. 10: Cardiotocography shows late decelerations persisting after the contraction has finished

Q1. What is the normal fetal heart rate?

Normal fetal heart rate is 110 to 160 bpm.

Q2. What is the interpretation of this CTG finding?

Late decelerations are a result of placental insufficiency, which can result in fetal distress. A 'gradual' deceleration has onset to nadir of 30 seconds or more, the low point of fetal heart rate occurs after the peak of the contraction, and returns to baseline after the contraction is complete.

Q3. How is it different from prolonged deceleration?

Prolonged deceleration is decrease in FHR from baseline greater than or equal to 15 bpm, lasting greater than or equal to 2 minutes, but less than 10 minutes. A deceleration greater than or equal to 10 minutes is a baseline change.[9]

CASE SCENARIO

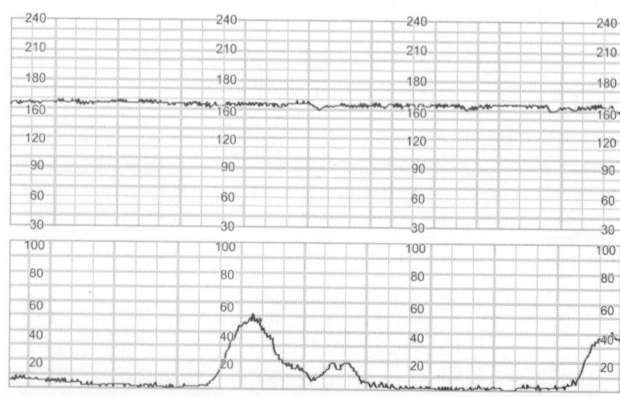

Fig. 11: Cardiotocography shows reduced varibility less than 10 bpm over a period of time

Q1. What is the normal beat to beat variability in CTG?

Normal beat to beat variability is 5 to 25 bpm.

Q2. What is the significance of reduced variability?

Presence of moderate baseline variability reflects delivery of oxygen to the fetal central nervous system and no hypoxia. Lack of moderate baseline FHR variability may be a result of the fetal sleep cycle, or a result of medications, extreme prematurity, congenital anomalies, or preexisting neurological injury.

PARTOGRAM

CASE SCENARIO

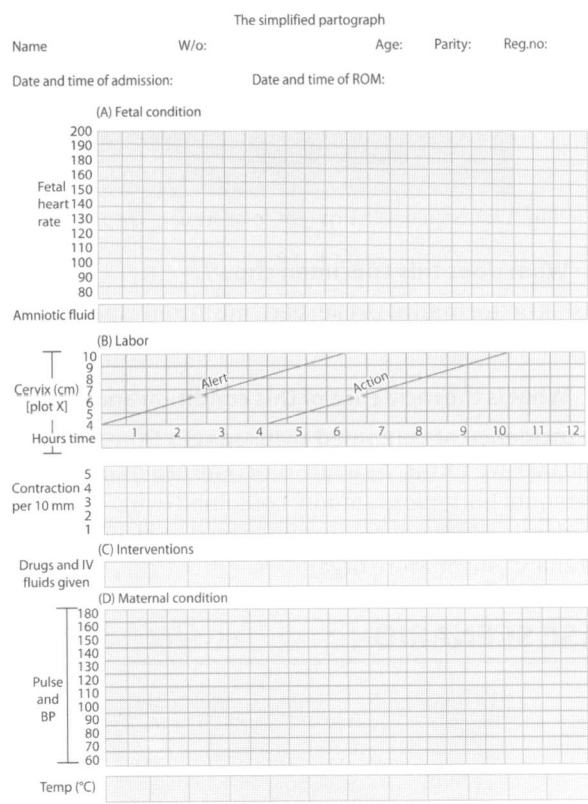

Fig. 12: Partogram

Q1. What is a partogram?

Partogram is graphical information about the progress of labor in which the salient information about fetal well being, maternal well being and the progress of labor are recorded into a chart.

Q2. What are alert and action line?

These two lines are designed to warn to take action quickly if labor is not progressing normally. The alert line starts at 4 cm of cervical dilatation and it travels diagonally upwards to the point of expected full dilatation (10 cm) at the rate of 1 cm per hour. The action line is parallel to the alert line, and 4 hours to the right of the alert line.[10]

INSTRUMENTS

CASE SCENARIO

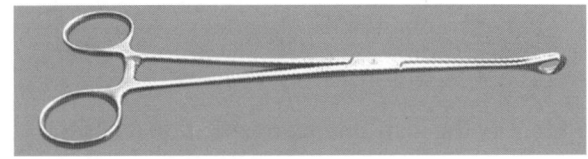

Fig. 13: Sponge holding forceps

Q1. Which is this instrument?

This is a sponge, holding forceps. It has ring shaped ends with transverse serrations on inner surface to prevent slipping.

Indications

- Used for holding sponge or a gauze piece for painting the area before operation, such as preparation of vagina, vulva and abdominal wall before surgery.
- To hold the pregnant cervix during insertion of Foley's Catheter in 2nd trimester for termination using ethacridine lactate.[11]
    - Removal of POC during abortions and MTP
    - To diagnose and repair of cervical tears
    - For postpartum Cu T insertion
    - For doing uterine packing in PPH
    - For removal of retained placental tissue
    - To hold the cut ends of lower segment during lower segment cesarean section (LSCS)
    - For pushing the bladder down with sponge on a holder in hysterectomy
    - Atraumatic clamp over ovarian vessels during myomectomy/metroplasty.

CASE SCENARIO

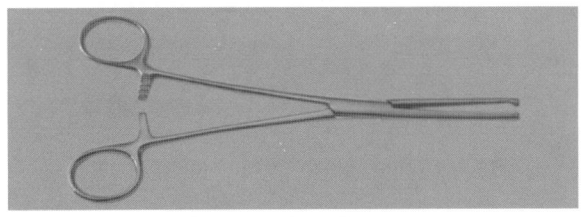

Fig. 14: Kocher's forceps

Q1. Identify the instrument and describe its uses.

This is Kocher's Forceps.
- It is used for rupturing the membrane artificially during vaginal delivery.[11]
- Used for holding uterine artery in hysterectomy.
- Used for uterine angles in hysterectomy.

CASE SCENARIO

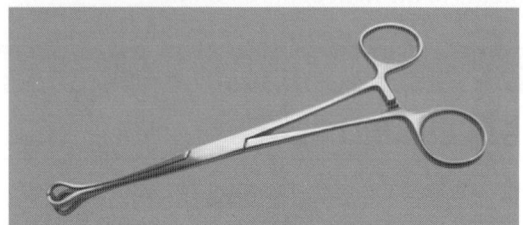

Fig. 15: Babcock's forceps

Q1. Identify the instrument and mention its uses.

This is a ratcheted, nonperforating atraumatic forceps used for holding delicate tissues. The jaws are circumferential and the tips are triangular and fenestrated with horizontal serrations.
- It is used for holding tubes for ligating tubes during sterilization
- It is frequently used with intestinal and laparotomy procedures

Note: All instruments used for LSCS, laparotomy, digital evacuation, instrumental delivery (forceps, vacuum) and episiotomy can be asked.

SPECIMENS

CASE SCENARIO

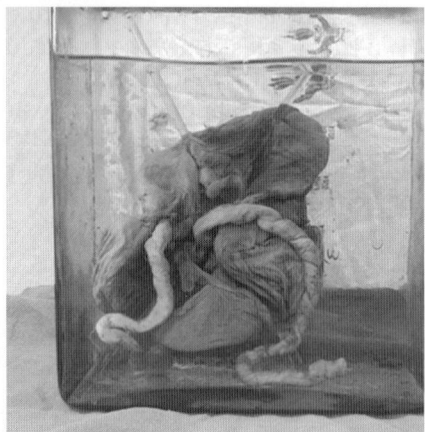

Fig. 16: Monochorionic, diamniotic placenta
(For color version, see plate 2)

Q1. What is the specimen?

This is a mounted specimen of monochorionic, diamniotic placenta.

Q2. What will be the findings on gross examination of placenta?

In monochorionic diamniotic placenta, there is no thick membrane between the twins. It looks like one sac with two embryos in the uterus. There is only one outer sac, the chorion. In monochorionic monoamniotic placenta there is only one chorion and one amnion, with both embryos inside the same amnion.[12]

CASE SCENARIO

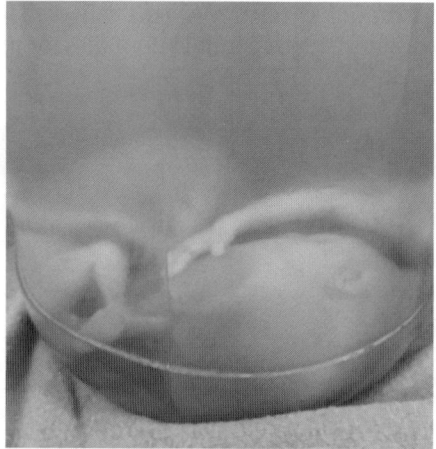

Fig. 17: Conjoined twins *(For color version, see plate 2)*

Q1. What does this specimen show?

This is a formalin preserved mounted specimen of Conjoined twins.

Q2. What is the incidence of this condition and its cause?

The incidence of conjoined twins ranges from 1:50,000 to 1:100,000 live births. As a rare outcome of a monoamniotic and monochorionic gestation, conjoined twins occur when two identical individuals are joined by part of their anatomy and share one or more organs.[13]

CASE SCENARIO

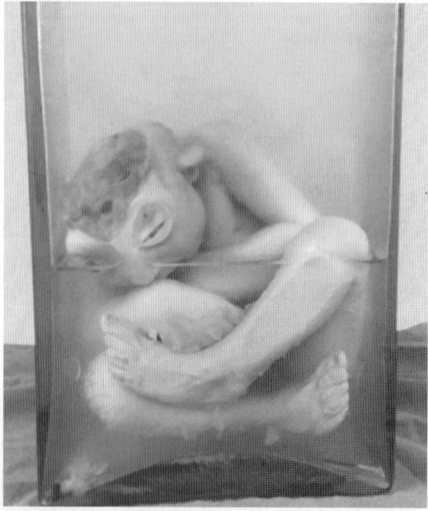

Fig. 18: Anencephaly *(For color version, see plate 2)*

Q1. What is the specimen?

This is a formalin preserved mounted specimen of fetus with anencephaly.

Q2. What is the useful imaging modalities in evaluating anencephaly? What is the utility of the procedure, including limitations and accuracy?

Anencephaly can theoretically be diagnosed as early as 8 weeks on ultrasound; however, it can be missed in the first trimester. There is 100% accuracy in the second trimester for this diagnosis by ultrasound and it has overall 97% sensitive and 100% specific in diagnosing an open neural tube defect.[14]

CASE SCENARIO

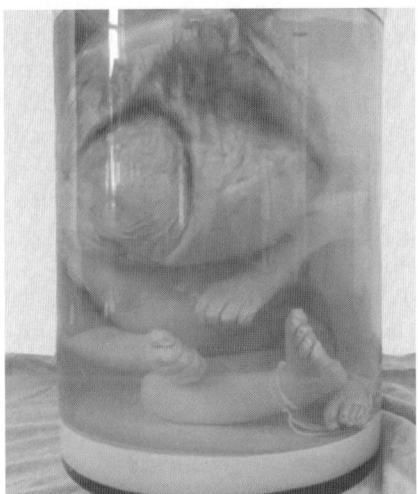

Fig. 19: Hydrocephalus *(For color version, see plate 2)*

Q1. What does this specimen show?

This is a formalin preserved mounted specimen of fetus with hydrocephalus.

Q2. What are the causes of congenital hydrocephalus?

Hydrocephalus is caused by a variety of medical problems including birth defects, in-utero infections and malformations within the brain. Aqueductal stenosis is the most common cause. Other causes are meningomyelocele, Chiari II malformation, tumors in posterior fossa, arachnoid cyst, Dandywalker syndrome.[15]

Note: These are few examples, specimens of meningocele, encephalocele, omphalocele, abortus, salpingectomy specimen (ectopic pregnancy), cesarean hysterectomy (ruptured uterus, atonic (flappy uterus, adherent placenta), cornual pregnancy and many more can be there.

REFERENCES

1. Miller DA, Chollet JA, Goodwin TM. Clinical risk factors for placenta previa-placenta accreta. Am J Obstet Gynecol. 1997;177:210-4.
2. Elsayes KM, Trout AT, Friedkin AM et al. Imaging of the placenta: a multimodality pictorial review. Radiographics. 29(5):1371-91.
3. Merz E, Bahlmann F. Ultrasound in obstetrics and gynecology. Thieme Medical Publishers. 2005. ISBN:1588901475.
4. Dashe JS, Mcintire DD, Ramus RM, et al. Persistence of placenta previa according to gestational age at ultrasound detection. Obstet Gynecol. 2002;99 (5 Pt 1):692-7.
5. Trop I. The twin peak sign. Radiology. 2001;220(1):68-9.
6. Benson C. Ultrasonography in obstetrics and gynocology, a practical approach, Thieme. 2007. ISBN:1588906124.
7. Lovold A, Stanton C, Armbruster D. How to avoid iatrogenic morbidity and mortality while increasing availability of oxytocin and misoprostol for PPH prevention? Int J Gynaecol Obstet. 2008;103(3):276-82.
8. Walraven G, Wanyonyi S, Stones W. Management of postpartum hemorrhage in low-income countries. Best Pract Res Clin Obstet Gynaecol. 2008;22(6): 1013-23.
9. Intrapartum care: NICE guideline. CG190 (February 2017).
10. Yisma E, Dessalegn B, Astatkie A, Fesseha N. Completion of the modified World Health Organization (WHO) partograph during labour in public health institutions of Addis Ababa, Ethiopia. Reproductive Health. 2013.
11. Text book of Obstetrics by Dr. DC Dutta, 6th Edition. ISBN 81-7381-142-3.
12. Nair M, Kumar G. Uncomplicated monochorionic diamniotic twin pregnancy. J Obstet Gynaecol. 2009;29(2):90-3.
13. Spencer R. Anatomic description of conjoined twins: a plea for standardized terminology. J Pediatr Surg. 1996;31(7):941-4.
14. Mehta TS, Levine D. Ultrasound and MR Imaging of Fetal Neural Tube Defects. Ultrasound Clin. 2007;2: 187-201.
15. Hannon T, et al: Epidemiology, natural history, progression, and postnatal outcome of severe fetal ventriculomegaly. Obstet Gynecol. 2012;120:1345-53.

30
CHAPTER

Common Mistakes in Case Presentation

Nilanchali Singh, Pushpa Mishra

'To Err is Human.' However, simple errors in case presentation may not be acceptable in Examinations. After, evaluating series of case presentations, we came across some common errors in history taking and examination by the medical students. Common sense is the most uncommon one, in the same way, the most basic thing in a case presentation is to know the basics. A lesson learnt in third semester to take history and do examination, is never outdated.

Common Errors in History Taking

- First mistake, quite commonly done, is not taking history in patient's language. Adding your own inferences in history is not a good idea.
  Example 1: Patient is giving history of intake of blood thinning drug in second trimester which she takes orally once a day. She stopped taking the medications in first trimester, as advised by her doctor and was kept on daily injections twice a day. (This history clearly shows, patient was on warfarin and heparin in 2nd and 1st trimester respectively). One may add 'likely to be warfarin' or 'likely to be heparin' after the description but refrain from directly mentioning the drugs if not mentioned by patient.
  Example 2: A patient comes with symptoms of leaking at 7 months of amenorrhea not preterm prelabor rupture of membranes (PPROM).
- Patient might be well-educated and may be able to tell you her diagnosis, investigations or even the treatment she is taking. If the patient has told these particulars, one should include them in their history.
- *Booked patient:* If she has three or more visits, with at least one in third trimester. Once admitted to the facility, she is considered to be booked there.
- *Registered patient:* If she has one visit or less than required for being called a booked one.
- *Un-booked patient:* If she has presented for the first time in the hospital.
- Always remember the sequence of events and mention it to accordingly too. Also, the headings of history should be in universally prescribed sequence. The history should portray the events clearly, rather than jumbling up from one event to another, without giving heed to its sequence.
- History should not be asked with leading questions. Leading questions should only follow the patients' complaints and its description.
- The GPLA formula, i.e. Gravida (G), para (P), abortion (A) and live babies (L) should be clearly understood and presented. It commonly has mistakes as follows:
  - Current pregnancy, even beyond period of viability is not added in 'Parity'. For example, a patient who is pregnant for the second time, with history of one vaginal delivery and live baby, who is 34 weeks pregnant has the formula, G2 P1L1.
  - If one does not give importance to A and P, management changes from recurrent pregnancy loss to repeated preterm births.
  - All twins/triplets have single parity (were parous one time!). If a patient comes with second pregnancy and had delivered triplets with all alive babies then she is G2P1A0L3.
  - L stands for child alive in present date and not 'Live Born.'
- Presenting complaints should be in chronological order with the symptom which is oldest to be presented first. Therefore, in obstetrics patients, history of amenorrhea is usually the first one to be mentioned.
- If the complaint of the patient is of a longer duration, and you have described it in detail, there is no need to again elaborate it in 'Trimester History'. You may simply mention 'The patient presented with such complaints and was managed as described earlier'.

- One should always take history of 'Course during hospital Stay'. It is a very significant history especially in patients with longer hospital stays. This may be mentioned after 'Trimester History' or prior too.
- Patients may not mention that they have taken or not, teratogenic drug but mention that some drugs were taken for their health condition, which may be teratogenic. For example, blood thinning drug in valve replacement patient, antiepileptic drug in epilepsy patients.
- Patients usually do not give history of preeclampsia, FGR, hypertension, diabetes, thyroid (unless a known case) but they give history of symptoms suggestive of certain diseases. These symptoms suggestive of particular conditions need to be mentioned.
- In menstrual history, details like history of prolonged cycle or shortened cycle need to be mentioned as they may affect the calculation of patient's gestational age. Similarly, history of heavy menstrual bleeding may indicate pre-existing anemia.
- A patient conceived in early lactational period may grossly be wrong dated and few do not have proper periods for a year or two.
- There are many errors and insufficiencies in obstetric history. Following points should be taken care of:
    - A simple line, booked/unbooked, immunized or not, IFA intake, home/hospital delivery and breastfed, immunized baby with normal mile stones avoid a lot of viva in the exam.
    - One often misses the antepartum period of previous pregnancy. It has a significance.
    - Any vaginal delivery is not normal vaginal delivery (NVD), i.e. intrauterine demise (IUD), preterm, fetal growth restriction (FGR), breech, etc. may be vaginal delivery but not normal vaginal delivery. Remember the definition!
    - Indication for lower segment cesarean section (LSCS) cannot be preeclampsia with nonprogress of labor (NPOL) with failed induction. Here preeclampsia is the indication for induction of labor and if patient does not have established labor pains then indication is failed induction and if patient went in active labor and then progress is halted, now indication is not NPOL but arrest of labor. There should be clarity of thought and should be depicted in history presentation.
    - Missed abortion and IUD is not synonymous, both have different definitions.
    - Similarly, there is a difference between IUD and stillbirth. All IUDs are still birth, however, all stillbirths are not IUDs.
    - History of stillbirths should be elaborated in terms of cause, investigation, management and counseling for next pregnancy.
    - Macerated and fresh stillbirths may have different etiologies and implications and therefore need a different periconceptional evaluation, counseling (folic acid in NTDs) or advice.
- Past/Medical/Family history:
    - Relevant history should be taken, i.e. a h/o incision and drainage of a small abscess in the arm, 2 years back is not relevant but 10 years back pelvic surgery is very much relevant and should be assessed carefully. However, any surgical or medical history needs to be mentioned, otherwise, as in prior case one may keep on wondering about the scar at arm!
    - Same way all the medical problems in the parents/family, e.g. death due to road traffic accident is not relevant but history of diabetes and hypertension is significant.
    - History of malignancies in relatives is important especially the ones with hereditary linkage, i.e. breast and ovarian malignancies.
- Some commonly used terms in history are often, not properly understood and described. One should be completely thorough with terms like, 24-hour recall method for dietary history, modified Kuppuswamy Scale, etc.
- Contraceptive history should not be forgotten. It should be mentioned either separately or along with obstetric history.

Points to Note while Examining a Patient

- While doing examination, patient should be explained about the full procedure and made comfortable.
- Bladder emptying and proper exposure is quite commonly missed examination steps but carry substantial reward.
- One should stand on the right side of the patient to examine.
- Patient should be in the right position for abdominal examination, i.e. lying supine without any pillow, with legs slightly flexed and abducted at hip joint, arms lying by the side.

- Warming hands before examination especially in winters and showing normal etiquettes always fetches more marks.
- General well-being, state of consciousness, orientation, comfort, hydration status of the patient, are all necessary to mention.
- Calculating the body mass index (BMI) is important. Prepregnancy weight should ideally be used to calculate it.
- Pulse rate, blood pressure, temperature and respiratory rate are important for every patient.
- Examination should be done from Top to Bottom, i.e. from Head to Toe. It should follow vital examination.
- Hairline, pallor, icterus, cyanosis, orodental hygiene, thyroid, pedal edema, any obvious lymphadenopathy needs evaluation and mention.
- Any deformity, if present, needs mention, e.g.
  - Postpolio residual paralysis (Patient may not complain but incidental finding do affect mode of delivery and labor outcome)
  - Spinal deformity (Has importance if patient has to be given spinal anesthesia for cesarean section and might be a cause for abnormal lie and presentation of the baby).
- Breast examination should never be missed. Both normal and abnormal changes in pregnancy need to be mentioned. Condition like inverted or cracked nipple need to be mentioned as they are very important part of patient and neonatal care.
- Systemic examination, i.e. cardiovascular, respiratory system, etc. should follow the general physical examination. One should especially focus upon the systems likely to be involved like cardiovascular system (CVS) in heart disease.
- While inspecting the abdomen, one often mentions that all hernial sites free. It is important to know the various hernial sites, and how to elicit it. The sites that need to be mentioned are umbilical, inguinal, femoral and incisional, in case, of prior surgeries.
- Symphysio-fundal height (SFH) is in centimeters and abdominal girth is mentioned in inches. There is a significance to it, as it corresponds with gestational age.
- During SFH measurement, following points should be taken care of:
  - Confirming empty bladder
  - Uterine deviation should be corrected
  - Straightening of the legs after marking the height and before taking measurement.
  - Properly locating the superior border of pubic symphysis
  - Keeping the centimeters side below, to avoid bias.
  - Starting measurement from variable to fixed point, i.e. Symphysis pubis.
- The various grips need to be mentioned only after commenting upon the fundal height, clinical assessment of liqour, uterine contour, and presence/absence of contractions.
- Though majority of times back of fetus is on one side and limbs are on other (lateral grips) and fetal heart is easily localized on the side of back, sometimes back is posterior and fetal heart is either located in the far flanks or midline just below the umbilicus. Do not get confused and do not modify the findings!
- Scar tenderness should be elicited at the uterine scar which lies just behind the symphysis pubis. A common mistake is to elicit scar tenderness at the abdominal scar!
- Speculum examination should be done, especially if it has not been done earlier to look for any abnormal findings.
- Vaginal examination should be done only in term patients for pelvic assessment and assessing the pre-induction cervical status (Bishop's score). If it has been done earlier, one should not repeat it, as more the number of vaginal examination, more the chances of puerperal and neonatal sepsis. You may omit this step during examination stating this reason.

How to Answer Management of the Case?

The common question asked after history and examination is, 'how will you manage the patient?'

- All patients come with certain symptoms or signs or abnormal investigations or referred due to certain reasons that should be given due importance while discussing management.
- A common mistake is omitting important part of diagnosis, e.g. 'previous cesarean', while mentioning the diagnosis. Once, diagnosis is made, we proceed for management.
- First thing that needs to be done is counseling of the patient and relatives. For example, in patient with abnormal sugar levels, one needs to explain the patient and relatives regarding treatment, risks to mother and fetus, stay in hospital (if required).
- Counseling and informed consent are two different things, i.e. telling a patient regarding her need of surgery for good size breech baby (>4 kg) along with its risks and consequences with vaginal delivery/LSCS

would be counseling while getting a consent signed that she is willing to undergo LSCS with all its risks and consequences, is informed consent.
- Next, we need to investigate the patient for either making or confirming a diagnosis or accessing its severity.
- After counseling and investigating the focus is on, how to optimize the patient (like diet, OHA, insulin according to period of gestation and sugar levels for patient with diabetes; anti-hypertensives for Hypertension patients).
- Then the monitoring part is equally important. Monitoring of both mother and fetus is important.
  - *Maternal:* Routine and specific to the condition (e.g. sugar monitoring in diabetes)
  - *Fetal:* Daily fetal movement record (DFMR), intermittent auscultation, nonstress test (NST), biophysical profile, biometry, Doppler (as indicated)
- Area specific management is also important. For example, thalassemia screening in north west India, Sickle cell in central India, etc.

Common Errors while Answering in Management

- Starting with drug treatment directly like, 'I will start the patient on insulin'
- Fetal monitoring directly with NST without clinical management, i.e. DFMR.
- Gestational diabetes mellitus (GDM) and a known case of diabetes mellitus are not same and their implications and management differ.
- Similarly, various hypertensive disorders have different management. The risks, investigations, treatment, monitoring and fetal outcome vary, if she has gestational hypertension, chronic hypertension or preeclampsia.
- Magnesium sulfate is not an antihypertensive, for sure.
- Talking about hi-fi investigations at first go. For example, in anemics, one should talk about Hemoglobin and hematocrit first, followed by peripheral smear (type of anemia) and RBC's indices, then comes the role of ferritin level, folate level and B12 levels.
- Management of labor should be answered for Ist stage (latent and active), IInd stage and IIIrd stage separately.

One should never answer higher investigation before mentioning basic diagnostic ones.

Follow-up

- Various medical problems, i.e. hypertension, GDM, etc. have their time bound follow-up as mentioned in standard text books.
- Routine postnatal patients should be followed up for contraceptive advice.

SUMMARY

One should be very careful while answering during examinations. Errors while answering basic questions may have a negative impact on the examiners. Avoiding simple mistakes can fetch you more marks.

And only then can you move forward with your extraordinary preparation to extraordinary viva.

Appendices

APPENDIX 1: MODIFIED KUPPUSWAMY SCALE (2017)

Education of head of family	Score
Profession or honours	7
Graduate or postgraduate	6
Intermediate or post high school diploma	5
High school certificate	4
Middle school certificate	3
Primary school certificate	2
Literate	1

Occupation of Head of Family

Profession	10
Semiprofession	6
Clerical, Shop-owner	5
Skilled worker	4
Semiskilled worker	3
Unskilled worker	2
Unemployed	1

Monthly Income of Family

In 2017 (January 2017 CPI)	
>41430	12
20715–41429	10
15536–20714	6
10357–15535	4
6214–10356	3
2092–6213	2
<2091	1

Socioeconomic class		Total score
I	Upper	26–29
II	Upper middle	16–25
III	Lower middle	11–15
IV	Upper lower	5–10
V	Lower	<5

APPENDIX 2: BMI (BODY MASS INDEX)

Classification	Asian Range	World wild range
Underweight	<17.50	<18.50
Normal weight	17.50–22.99	18.50–24.99
Over weight	23.00–27.99	25.00–29.99
Obese	>28.00	>30.00

30.0–34.9	class I obesity
35.0–39.9	class II obesity
≥ 40.0	class III obesity

APPENDIX 3: GRADING AND RANKING

Key to evidence statements and grading of recommendations, using the ranking of the Canadian Task Force on preventive health care quality of evidence assessment*

I: Evidence obtained from at least one properly randomized controlled trial.

II-1: Evidence from well-designed controled trials without randomization.

II-2: Evidence from well-designed cohort (prospective or retrospective) or case-control studies, preferably from more than one center or research group.

II-3: Evidence obtained from comparisons between times or places with or without the intervention. Dramatic results in uncontroled experiments (such as the results of treatment with penicillin in the 1940s) could also be included in this category.

III: Opinions of respected authorities, based on clinical experience, descriptive studies, or reports of expert committees.

Classification of Recommendations[†]
A. There is good evidence to recommend the clinical preventive action
B. There is fair evidence to recommend the clinical preventive action
C. The existing evidence is conflicting and does not allow to make a recommendation for or against use of the clinical preventive action; however, other factors may influence decision-making
D. There is fair evidence to recommend against the clinical preventive action
E. There is good evidence to recommend against the clinical preventive action
F. There is insufficient evidence (in quantity or quality) to make a recommendation; however, other factors may influence decision-making.

---

*The quality of evidence reported in these guidelines has been adapted from The Evaluation of Evidence criteria described in the Canadian Task Force on Preventive Health Care.
[†]Recommendations included in these guidelines have been adapted from the classification of Recommendations criteria described in The Canadian Task Force on preventive health care.